ELAINE R. RUBIN

EDITOR

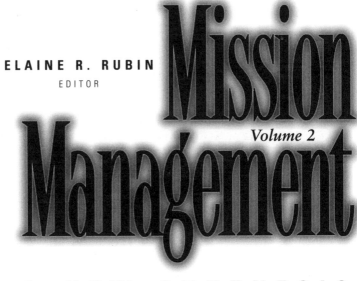

# Mission

*Volume 2*

# Management

## A NEW SYNTHESIS

D1114068

ASSOCIATION OF ACADEMIC HEALTH CENTERS

The Association of Academic Health Centers (AHC) is a national, nonprofit organization comprising more than 100 institutional members in the United States that are the health complexes of the major universities. Academic health centers consist of an allopathic or osteopathic school of medicine, at least one other health professions school or program, and one or more teaching hospitals. These institutions are the nation's primary resources for education in the health professions, biomedical and health services research, and many aspects of patient care.

The AHC seeks to influence public dialogue on significant health and science policy issues, to advance education for health professionals, to promote biomedical and health services research, and to enhance patient care. The AHC is dedicated to improving the health of the people through leadership and cooperative action with others.

The views expressed in this book are those of its authors and do not necessarily represent the views of the Board of Directors of the Association of Academic Health Centers or the membership at large.

### Library of Congress Cataloging-in-Publication Data

Mission management: a new synthesis / Elaine R. Rubin, editor.

    p.       cm.

    Includes bibliographical references (p. ).

    ISBN 1-879694-12-3 (v. 2)

    1. Academic medical centers- -United States.       I. Rubin, Elaine R.

RA981. A2M56 1998

362.1' 0973—dc21                      98-19149

                                            CIP

Available from:
Association of Academic Health Centers
1400 Sixteenth Street, N.W. Suite 720
Washington, D. C. 20036
202/265-9600; Fax 202/265-7514
Price: $30.00 (plus $5.00 shipping/handling)

Design and production by Fletcher Design, Washington, DC

# CONTENTS

SECTION 3
## Lessons from Corporate America and the International Scene

## FOREWORD

T HE SIGNIFICANT ROLE THAT ACADEMIC HEALTH centers play in both the nation's health care system and the world of higher education is well known, and the resulting synergistic relationship—in which the clinical setting helps educate students and the academic setting yields students who help provide services—has been acknowledged, accepted, and ultimately supported by the public for decades.

Today, however, accepted attitudes, values, and modes of behavior are being questioned and reassessed. One result is that many experts, both within and outside the academic health center, fear that the academic health center's tripartite mission of education, research, and service is becoming unbalanced and perhaps on the verge of collapse, with the amount of attention paid to clinical services beginning to overshadow the two traditional academic missions.

Tremendous thought is going into strategies that academic health centers can employ to maintain the patient-care component of their mission. Moreover, current concerns about the bottom line raise questions about ways to balance the corporate, or entrepreneurial mindset with academic traditions and values.

The growth of managed care and the expansion of other organized delivery systems, demands for price rollbacks in clinical services, and state and Federal budget cuts in education and health care services, are the major threats to the ability of academic health centers to pay for education and research. Academic health centers are now hard-pressed to maintain this traditional patchwork of financial support, which also includes institutional funds such as endowments, state funds, and public and private grants. Compounding the financial challenges are new societal demands for accountability that are affecting all institutions of higher education.

Academic health centers have responded to the revolutionary, new environment by reevaluating and redefining how they are organized and operated. But although the new health care scene poses enormous challenges for academic health centers, it is also providing them with special opportunities for responding to changing societal needs. This repositioning process includes changing management and governance structures, defining leadership roles and decision-making processes, developing new faculty incentive systems, and establishing new educational and research partnerships.

However, little is known about the effects of these changes on the education and research facets of the academic health center mission. To fill this gap, the Association of Academic Health Centers undertook a study to examine the impact of an emerging new clinical environment on the education and research components of the academic health center mission. Part of this effort involved commissioning essays from experts on a broad range of interrelated issues, from higher education to organizational behavior. These commissioned pieces, along with several related papers presented at recent annual meetings of the association, provided the study with essential background material.

Volume 1 of this report contains the study findings. The background papers comprise this book, volume 2; they define institutional priorities, analyze educational and research problems, identify conflicts, provide insights into misunderstood or unresolved problems, and present new perspectives on academic and organizational structures within the academic health center environment. We anticipate that the papers will contribute to the dialogue on new directions for the academic health center and suggest new areas for exploration and emulation.

Together, the two books make an important contribution to the literature on academic health centers. They not only highlight critical issues and emerging initiatives that demand attention but also offer new perspectives on approaches that educators, administrators, and policy-makers in today's higher education and health care worlds are taking to prepare for the next century.

A multitude of people deserve thanks for conceptualizing and developing volume 2. First, we thank the authors for contributing their expertise through these published essays. Dr. Elaine Rubin, assistant vice president for program at the Association of Academic Health Centers, deserves special mention for her fine editing of their work and structuring of the book and her overall dedication to both author and readers. Finally, we would like to thank the Robert Wood Johnson Foundation and the University HealthSystem Consortium for their generous support of the study that made this book possible.

Roger J. Bulger, MD
President, Association of Academic Health Centers

Marian Osterweis, PhD
Executive Vice President, Association of Academic Health Centers

## PREFACE

THIS BOOK EXAMINES THE BACKGROUND AND raison d'être for many of the changes occurring within academic health centers today as well as the many programs, policies, and practices currently under debate. In so doing, it highlights the internal and external forces that may well be unbalancing the academic health center's tripartite mission—education, research, and service—and outlines recent institutional initiatives aimed at creating a new synergy between these mission components.

Section one develops a framework for understanding the world of higher education, the changing shape of university-academic health center relationships, and a rationale for the transformations currently underway. Robert Atwell addresses the public's ambivalent attitudes toward the vast higher education enterprise and outlines key issues that cloud its future. Eli Noam confronts transformation in the university from the standpoint of technology's implications for the future, questioning whether the economic foundation of the current university system can be sustained in the face of the new ways in which information flows.

The three essays concluding this section address organizational culture and leadership, critical issues of concern within the university today. Carol Aschenbrener widens our thinking on the institutional environment, discussing socioeconomic, political, and global issues that must be considered as universities and academic health centers redefine their missions. Gregory Eastwood provides insight into the personal attributes required of leaders, the changing nature of leadership, and the route to leadership in academic health centers. Finally, Jane

Henney examines the many dimensions of leadership as they relate to developing new governance structures for an academic health center.

In section two, authors examine the specific mission components and the forces shaping change. Five chapters highlight educational issues; three focus on research; and two chapters analyze the service component.

John Naughton and Paul Batalden and his colleagues take a look at the history of innovations in education, thus setting the stage for understanding critical concepts and issues under exploration. Naughton describes the evolution of health professions education from a cottage industry to the sophisticated complex enterprise manifested in the academic health center, and asks if the academic health center concept is still valid in a health care setting dominated by competition and cost-containment. Paul Batalden, John Evans, and Jeanne Ryer discuss innovation and quality in both education and health care delivery.

DeWitt Baldwin argues the case for the relatively new concept of interdisciplinary education in the health professions and suggests how academic health centers can continue to nurture this important concept. My paper describes the meanings and functions ascribed to tenure over the centuries, the relevance of tenure today, and the societal, professional, and institutional issues requiring consideration in any attempt to alter or abandon the system.

Judith Swazey and Melissa Anderson analyze the role of mentoring, emphasizing that recruitment and retention of future health professionals and graduate students may well depend on the type of people who mentor them, whether formally or informally. The authors argue that instilling values in new health professionals and their socialization to their professions are integral to mentoring. Meredith Gonyea presents a powerful methodology for shaping responsible strategies at all levels of policy making in her chapter on resource requirements, costs, and sources of support for health professions education programs.

The next three chapters in this section address the endangered research mission. David Blumenthal discusses some of the strategies academic health centers are adopting to protect this mission. Ralph Snyderman examines efforts to restructure academic health center research as a business operation, suggesting ways that needless deficits in both research and education can be minimized. Karl Hittelman and Mary Beth O'Connor provide details and insight into a restructuring model designed and implemented at the University of California, San Francisco.

The final two chapters of the section deal with the health care marketplace. Robert Baker summarizes key studies from the University HealthSystem Consortium on the changing market for clinical services, reviewing the consortium's market classification tool and analyzing the implications of market forces for the academic health center mission. Alan Hillman looks closely at one specific market, Philadelphia, tracing the evolution of market stages and their impact on the city's academic health center networks. Both authors suggest future strategies related to organization, marketing, and contracting for academic health centers.

Section three highlights issues and trends in other sectors of American society and also the global community that affects academic health centers. Charles Snow brings the experiences of corporate America to bear in his analysis, reminding the reader that, as the academic health center mission changes, so must the organization's structure and management systems; he suggests that the organization of the future will likely be a cellular, or self-managing, organization.

John Owen describes the many facets of the globalization of health care, from health services to technological developments and how globalization impacts academic health centers, and highlights some new facets of the traditional mission areas for academic health centers to consider as they orient their organizations toward the future.

As this book goes to press, I want to thank some very special people whose work behind the scenes were invaluable. Cynthia Spriggs deserves special mention for her administrative support throughout the project. Shirley Sirota Rosenberg of SSR, Incorporated, deserves a generous acknowledgment for her editorial know-how; her appreciation for the English language is a rare commodity in today's world, and her expertise, advice, and counsel contributed greatly to the value of the final product. And, of course, many thanks to Richard Fletcher of Fletcher Design whose graphic skills helped structure and fine-tune the authors' intent.

—ERR

# CONTRIBUTORS

**Melissa S. Anderson, PhD,** is assistant professor, Department of Educational Policy and Administration, University of Minnesota.

**Carol A. Aschenbrener, MD,** is senior vice president of Kaludis Consulting Group.

**Robert H. Atwell** is president emeritus of the American Council on Education.

**Robert J. Baker** is president and chief executive officer of the University HealthSystem Consortium.

**DeWitt C. Baldwin, Jr., MD,** is scholar-in-residence and senior associate at the Institute for Ethics of the American Medical Association.

**Paul B. Batalden, MD,** is director of health care improvement leadership development at Dartmouth Medical School.

**David Blumenthal, MD, MPP,** is executive director of The Commonwealth Fund Task Force on Academic Health Centers, and Chief, Health Policy Research and Development Unit, Massachusetts General Hospital, Partners HealthCare System, Boston, and associate professor of medicine and health care policy at Harvard Medical School.

**Gregory L. Eastwood, MD,** is the president of the State University of New York Health Science Center at Syracuse.

**John P. Evans, PhD,** is a professor at the Kenan-Flagler Business School, University of North Carolina-Chapel Hill.

**Meredith A. Gonyea, PhD,** is president of The Center for Studies in Health Policy, Inc., in Washington, D.C.

**Jane E. Henney, MD,** is vice president for health sciences at The University of New Mexico Health Sciences Center.

**Alan L. Hillman, MD, MBA,** is director, Center for Health Policy, Leonard Davis Institute of Health Policy, and associate dean, School of Medicine, University of Pennsylvania.

**Karl J. Hittelman, PhD,** is associate vice chancellor for academic affairs, University of California, San Francisco.

**John Naughton, MD,** is professor of medicine, physiology, social and preventive medicine, and rehabilitation medicine in the School of Medicine and Biomedical Sciences at the State University of New York at Buffalo.

**Eli Noam, PhD,** is professor of finance and economics and director of the Institute for Tele-Information at Columbia University.

**Mary Beth O'Connor, MBA,** is a partner in the Higher Education Consulting Practice, Coopers & Lybrand, LLP.

**John Wyn Owen, CB,** is secretary of The Nuffield Trust, London.

**Elaine R. Rubin, PhD,** is assistant vice president for program at the Association of Academic Health Centers.

**Jeanne C. Ryer, MS,** is a principal with Ryer Associates.

**Charles C. Snow, PhD,** is Mellon Bank Professor of Business Administration, The Smeal College of Business Administration, The Pennsylvania State University.

**Ralph Snyderman, MD,** is chancellor for health affairs and dean of the School of Medicine, Duke University Medical Center, and CEO, Duke University Health System.

**Judith P. Swazey, PhD,** is president of The Acadia Institute, Bar Harbor, Maine.

# A NEW UNIVERSITY
# FOR A
# NEW MILLENNIUM

UNIVERSITIES IN THE
21ST CENTURY

TECHNOLOGY'S
TRANSFORMATION OF
THE UNIVERSITY

LEADERSHIP, CULTURE, AND
CHANGE: CRITICAL ELEMENTS
FOR TRANSFORMATION

LEADERSHIP AMID CHANGE:
THE CHALLENGE TO ACADEMIC
HEALTH CENTERS

CONFRONTING THE REALITIES
OF CREATING AN INSTITUTIONAL
CULTURE

# UNIVERSITIES IN THE 21ST CENTURY

*Robert H. Atwell*

MUCH OF AMERICAN HIGHER EDUCATION today is beset with perplexing views. On the one hand, we hear that our higher education enterprise (to call the entire enterprise a "system" is far too simple) is the envy of the world. On the other hand, we get strong, negative messages about high prices for tuition, low standards for graduation, excessive political correctness (usually meaning a left-leaning faculty left over from the 1960s), excessive research and insufficient teaching, slovenliness hiding behind tenure, and the little attention paid to the job market awaiting students after graduation. The list goes on.

Yet college graduates in America typically still display college and university decals on their auto windows, root for the athletic teams of their alma maters, and generally take the position that although problems abound, "my school was and is great and gave me a good education."

These ambivalent attitudes are understandable. By most measures, the higher education enterprise has served this nation with distinction. It has provided more educational opportunity for a larger share of the population than any other nation. It has blended public and private support in a manner that has strengthened the institutions, in general, and created healthy competition and

---

*Robert Atwell is president emeritus of the American Council on Education.*

cooperation between public and private institutions, in particular. Its research enterprise has simultaneously served as an engine of economic growth, a key to improving the health of our citizens, and a bulwark for our national defense. It has also earned our nation a preeminent position in scholarly research productivity in most fields, whether measured by Nobel laureates or citations in scholarly journals.

Recently, of course, the achievement test scores of secondary school graduates in some other nations have surpassed those in America. Nevertheless, except for the greater proportion of undergraduate students abroad who go on to complete their degree programs, the United States is still far ahead internationally in most measures of higher education performance.

## WHY WORRY?

Given this extraordinary record, why should we worry?

In general, we should worry so that, like the most successful corporations in this country, we do not lapse into the IBM syndrome, that is, waxing complacency after being number one for a long time. More specifically, we should worry because some of the issues we confront today are clouding the future of American higher education.

1. In the long run, American colleges and universities will be no better than the products of America's public schools that enter them. However, except for a few shining exceptions, the products of our public elementary and secondary schools are woefully deficient by international standards, in part, because the schools are being asked to compensate for the deterioration of the family. In a similar manner, colleges and universities are being asked to compensate for the poor products of public education; we call the process "remediation," and its demands have arguably reduced academic standards and placed burdens on colleges and universities for which they are ill-prepared.

2. The public funds on which both public and private colleges and universities have depended for growth and improvement for many years are under severe stress as a result of taxpayer revolts, on the one hand, and competing demands from such other societal systems as prisons, Medicare, welfare, the environment, transportation, and the public schools, on the other. Several of the funds for these competitors come either from entitlements or are mandatory.

Higher education, however, is discretionary in Federal and state budgets.

3. As public funding of higher education either diminishes or fails to keep pace with rising demand, costs are being shifted from taxpayers to students and families. A rising debt burden is, therefore, falling on students and families who have to pay for tuition price increases well in excess of inflation. The public anger and worry about this situation is fueled by the media, which focuses on a few high-priced selective private colleges and universities when it discusses the cost of higher education. In addition, price and financial aid decisions are made by different offices within universities.

4. Even as resources are stable to diminishing, many institutions find themselves caught between increased numbers of students knocking on their doors and the difficulty of achieving greater productivity in such a people-intensive enterprise.

5. Technology is devouring budgets as institutions struggle to keep up with the state-of-the-art lest they find themselves working with outdated technology. In many cases, faculty members themselves are resistant to technological change even as they come face to face with students who are more computer-literate than they.

6. Students today are older, increasingly part-time, less well-prepared, and from more diverse racial and ethnic backgrounds than their predecessors. With budgets falling and resistance to affirmative action building, institutions worry about how they can continue to be accessible to these students.

7. The governance of colleges and universities is not well equipped to deal with new realities, which require quick decisions as higher education moves into new markets. Members of governing boards are either bound to nostalgia or serving the perceived agenda of an electorate or political appointing authority that put them in office. Thus, they are increasingly less inclined to see themselves as guardians of, and advocates for, the institution.

8. Shared governance between faculty and administration is characterized by indecision, the veto powers of small segments of the community, and the reluctance of the faculty, particularly in institutions focused more on teaching than on research, to make difficult but necessary decisions that may, in turn, adversely affect their colleagues.

Another area for change involves governance and accountability, which encompasses the purview of external governance and accountability systems including governing boards, multicampus systems, state oversight arrangements and accreditation. It also includes "shared governance," or the arrangements for decision making at the campus level that includes administration, faculty, staff, and students. These systems, if not broken, are in serious disrepair.

The revenue of colleges and universities exceeds $200 billion, or about 3 percent of gross domestic product. The proportion of our GDP that goes to higher education is the highest in the world. These numbers, however, are a bit misleading since higher education elsewhere is almost entirely financed by government, making it mostly free to the students. If we compare only government funding, which accounts for only about half of U.S. higher education monies, with the situation abroad we would find other countries spending more of their GDP on higher education.

---

THERE ARE ABOUT 3,600 NONPROFIT COLLEGES AND UNIVERSITIES IN THE United States, and about the same number of for-profit institutions; the latter is a rapidly growing but still small sector. Together, their students total about 14 million. This huge number, representing close to 5 percent of the population, reflects our extraordinarily high participation rates in higher education. No other nation comes close to a situation in which about 50 percent of its high school graduates immediately go on to postsecondary education and 60 percent eventually do so in their lifetimes.

Although half of our higher education institutions are private, fourth-fifths of higher education students are in public institutions. About half of our undergraduates are in the nation's 1,200 community colleges; most of these colleges did not exist forty years ago. In addition, only about 12 percent of our undergraduates fit the outdated notion that a college student is someone who is between the ages of 18 and 22, a full-time resident student, and slated to graduate in four years from the institution in which she or he started. Instead, about half the students are what we used to call the "nontraditional" student. Today, they are clearly part of a growing proportion of students on campus. The average age of community college students today is 29, and the parking lots at the school are filled at night.

---

## DECLINING REVENUES

In the United States, less than half of higher education revenue comes from Federal, state, and local governments, and this share is declining. As public funding declines, the students, and their families, share of revenue increases. Gifts and investment income are important at the margins for many colleges and universities, but only at a few institutions do these sources come close to constituting even a fifth of total income. Furthermore, the $100 billion or so in endowments of all colleges and universities is concentrated heavily in only about twenty institutions, most of them private.

## INCREASED DEMANDS

Thus, the rising numbers of students demanding enrollment, the diminishing resources, and the increasing expectations for the latest technologies will combine to become the overriding issue today.

After some years of decline in the number of high school graduates, we are now experiencing some modest increases overall and some sharp increases in the Sunbelt states of Arizona, California, Florida, and Texas. In California, the expectation is that there will be almost 500,000 more students knocking on the doors of colleges and universities within the next few years than there were in the early 1990s. This situation has given rise to the phrase "Tidal Wave II." (The first tidal wave comprised the baby boomers.) However, there are simply no plans in place for dealing with the implications of these numbers and, in the absence of such plans, California faces the prospect of having to deny access to hundreds of thousands of applicants. This state of affairs would signal the end of the much-envied, but already seriously frayed, Master Plan whereby any California high school graduate is assured admission to one of the three public higher education segments (University of California, California State University, and the California community college system). Although the numbers are less dramatic in other states, most of the other high-growth states will also face rising expectations in terms of higher education, with few or no public policy proposals on hand to deal with them.

This failure of public policy at the state level reflects a prevailing antitax sentiment in both state and Federal legislatures. Furthermore, this attitude comes at a time of rising demands from entitlements such as Medicaid and welfare, and

COLLEGES AND UNIVERSITIES EMPLOY ABOUT 2.5 MILLION PEOPLE, AND ONLY about one-third are members of the faculty. An ever-larger proportion of the faculty are part-time or adjuncts; thus they are not on the tenure track and not able to participate in governance (or fringe benefits) to the extent available to those with tenure or on the tenure track. Two-thirds of staff are not even faculty members; they range from highly paid surgeons and football coaches to maintenance workers, graduate assistants, and a host of people who keep the trains running. Most are also disenfranchised in terms of participating in shared governance and are usually lumped in a category that actually describes them in terms of what they are not, namely "nonacademic staff." Their importance far exceeds their status on campus.

from such semi-entitlements as prisons. Together, they consume more state dollars than higher education. There is also competition for public funding from a broken elementary-secondary school system, our also-broken children's services, and an environment of ever-diminishing discretionary state funding.

We are a seriously undertaxed nation both in comparison with other countries and in terms of our need for improved public services. But any politician who takes this position is doomed to ridicule and defeat. In this regard, it is interesting to note that the states that are the worst off in terms of budget difficulties are those that do not levy all of the "big three" taxes, namely, property, income, and sales.

Historically, the property tax has been the principal source of funds for elementary and secondary education and, in some states, also for community colleges. This local tax is probably the least popular tax. Because of the reluctance to raise this local tax, states are now assuming an increasing share of elementary and secondary school and community college financing. Nevertheless, the responsibility and power over schools continue to reside in the 16,000 local school districts and community college districts.

The decline in state support is so dramatic that there is increasing talk of privatizing in a number of flagship institutions in some states such as Virginia, where state support over a five-year period recently dropped from 32.7 percent of operating revenues to 20.7 percent. To escape state regulation, these institutions would give up all or most of their state funding. Some of this is just talk, but it is getting more serious in a few states.

At the Federal level, entitlements, defense, and interest on the public debt consume about four-fifths of tax revenues, leaving little for discretionary domestic programs. The recent agreement on the 1998 Federal budget, which is designed to balance the budget by the year 2002, leaves the accumulated national debt of about $7 trillion untouched but will throw the many claimants for Federal discretionary spending into fierce competition. The Federal government accounts for only about one-fifth of higher education's revenue through student financial aid and research. Thus, the seemingly generous increases in funding for higher education proposed by President Clinton will not substantially improve higher education's revenue picture. Because of the Federal spending crunch in discretionary domestic spending, the Administration is increasingly turning to tax policy, in the form of tax credits and tax deductions, as a way to assist students and their families. It is understandable that this approach is being met in some quarters of higher education with considerable skepticism; here the argument is that tax credits and tax deductions will largely benefit those who are attending college already and do little to promote access and affordability for lower-income students.

One of the factors driving up the price of tuition is the cost of technology. The cost not only includes the expense of installing new systems (running fiber optic cables throughout the campus, acquiring hardware and software, linking incompatible databases, equipping at least some classrooms with state-of-the-art interactive video and computer technology) but also the continuous servicing of equipment and training of required staff.

There is no shortage of software vendors for most administrative applications, but there is the insistent need to keep updating the technology even as there is a shortage of persons experienced in the management of a high-volume, high-tech educational environment. Until recently, the administrative and academic sides of the higher education house were separate. For example, professionals in academic computing belonged to the national association Educom. Those concerned with administrative applications associated themselves with the national association CAUSE. The senior professionals in the computer field are now discussing merging the two organizations—a situation reflecting the fast-changing world of higher education. We now have a person on many campuses known generically as "chief information officer," or CIO. Some institutions cannot afford the increasingly high salaries commanded by these very important people, and smaller institutions are increasingly considering outsourcing all or most of the information technology activities.

Colleges and universities must face the fact that information technology and distance education are here to stay and will require a continuously high level of investment in dollars, support staff, and released time for faculty training. Some people argue that institutions should anticipate spending 2 percent of their operating budgets on information technology. For institutions that are behind the times in this respect, the investment may be larger.

## INCREASED COMPETITION

The ability to provide distance education through technology represents a great strength of the best of the commercial providers of education. These commercial providers are continually increasing their market share in applied technology fields, and offer stiff competition to many sectors of higher education, particularly community colleges. Community colleges, however, have a comparative advantage in their relatively low prices. Like commercial providers, they go to where the business is, trying to meet consumers' education and training needs in convenient locations (sometimes at the work site) and at convenient times. But few community colleges can afford the high-tech environment that many commercial providers offer; commercial providers also tend to offer smaller classes and are as diligent as some community colleges in placing their graduates.

## POSSIBLE SOLUTIONS

Given the difficulties posed by the decrease in public funding and increase in demand, colleges and universities face three choices: increase student fees, increase gifts and investment income, or cut costs. All three options are being tried with varying levels of success.

The solution of choice for universities in the early 1990s (and earlier in the case of private institutions) was to increase student fees. To promote the socioeconomic and racial diversity of their student bodies, all private and increasingly many public institutions also accompanied this increase in the sticker price with deep discounts for students with demonstrated need. It is not unusual to find a private institution where half or more of the increase in student fees is channeled back into need-based aid, a phenomenon sometimes referred to as "Robin Hooding." We even find a similar phenomenon in the public sector with the University of California, for example, plowing more than one-third of the increased fees back into need-based aid.

But we have now reached the point where the price of some of the higher-priced private colleges and universities is driving students in the middle-income category beyond the reach of need-based aid. As a result, we now have many student bodies at private schools that consist of the poor and the rich. In 1975, the mean annual household income in the United States was 30 percent more than the price of four years at a private institution and three times more than the price of a four-year public institution. By 1994, the price of attending a private institution for four years was twice the annual median household income. By 1998, the price of four years at a public institution will exceed the annual median household income, thereby erasing the 1-to-3 price-to-household income ratio of the recent past. In the case of public institutions, the almost theological belief that low tuitions are the best way to ensure access and to realize the societal benefits of higher education has become an artifact.

Most public policy analysts would still argue for targeting taxpayer subsidies to needy students (and thereby push public sector prices even higher). However, the political pressures generated by several years of very large fee increases seem to be slowing increases to something closer to inflation. For different reasons, the same situation is happening at the private institutions. In the past, selective private institutions competed for students on the basis of quality (in the form of new and modernized facilities and more favorable student-faculty ratios). But today's families are more likely to opt for lower priced private or public institutions rather than for the more costly, prestigious institutions.

Gifts and investment income amount to less than 10 percent of the revenue of all institutions, but represent a significantly higher proportion in the most affluent and well-endowed institutions. These institutions, which also charge the highest prices, always argue (correctly) that even their high tuition fees sometimes cover only half of the cost of education. Gifts and investment income cover the other half. (The differences in cost of education per student between affluent and less-affluent private colleges is astonishing). The reality, however, is that in only perhaps 200 institutions, most but not all private, do gifts and investment income contribute more than 15 percent of total revenue for operations, not counting the capital improvement projects that are attractive to donors and which both public and private institutions are increasingly aggressive in pursuing.

Given the modest though essential role played by philanthropy and the increased competition for philanthropic dollars from other worthy causes, I believe that even a rising tide of college tuition dollars will not be able to raise all the boats.

This situation brings us to cost reductions as the remaining option for dealing with financial stringency. Theoretically, the first step to take is reduce the size of the faculty. But conventional wisdom holds that because higher education is such a people-intensive business, with at least one-fourth of expenditures going into salaries and benefits, downsizing faculty makes increased productivity more difficult to achieve. This situation may explain why downsizing has been slow to take hold in academe.

I think the resistance to downsizing on campus also reflects a more humane approach to human resource issues than prevalent in the world of commerce. Perhaps more important is the possibility that as long as colleges and universities could raise student fees at a rate commensurate with cost increases, there was little need to downsize. Institutions would prefer to compete on the basis of quality rather than price. The ability to maintain quality, however, seems to be changing quite rapidly along with the slowdown in the rate of price increases. Most colleges and universities are looking for new sources of income by forming partnerships with businesses to reduce the costs of operation. The next ten years will see increasing reliance on cost reductions and less reliance on price increases as a way to deal with financial stringency.

## PROBLEMS OF ACADEMIC
## HEALTH CENTERS

Academic health centers, in particular, could face major financial difficulties in the short term. If Medicare reimbursement policies for the higher patient-care costs at academic health centers should drop or welfare reform results in states changing their policies on reimbursing institutions for the care of the indigent, academic health centers could experience fiscal trauma shortly. The Federal budget "deal" struck between the President and Congressional majority for the 1998 budget, and perhaps in the future budgets, includes cuts in Medicare that will fall most heavily on the providers. Recognizing that the academic health centers cannot absorb severe cuts in Medicare reimbursements—and should not be asked to do so because of their vital role in training health care professionals—some members of Congress are proposing establishing a medical education trust fund to be funded at the Federal level from a combination of general fund revenues, surcharges on insurance premiums, and transfers from managed care providers.

Teaching hospitals now provide almost half of the uncompensated medical care in the nation. If Medicare reimbursement of patient care at these hospitals drops, or if, with the shift of much welfare responsibility to the states, states change their policies of reimbursement for indigent patients, teaching hospitals may have to turn patients away or else face large financial problems.

## SERVING THE DIVERSE STUDENT BODY

The increasing presence of a diverse student population at most senior institutions calls for changes in many aspects of campus life from class times and locations to arrangements for registration and payment. It also calls for a more aggressive marketing effort targeted less to high schools and more to people at work sites and shopping centers, and viewing television.

Institutions of higher education also have to take into account a population group on campus that does not possess the reading, writing, and computational skills necessary for college-level work. Colleges and universities with more or less open admissions policies (this includes most institutions) are forced to undertake substantial remediation. Most of this remedial work is not credited—nor should it be—toward an associate or a baccalaureate degree. Nonetheless, it places heavy demands on higher education institutions trying to compensate for the sorry state of many of our public schools.

Increasingly, legislatures and governing boards are questioning the remediation function of colleges. This unfortunate turning away from educational responsibility is yet another manifestation of how low-income students are being deprived of good educations.

Another manifestation of this lack of access to a good education is the fact that the rising price of tuition is coupled with the shift in need-based aid from grants to loans. I believe it is wrong to ask an academically high-risk student to undertake a substantial loan burden before he or she has become academically established. Many low-income students are wisely deciding not to take such a financial risk, but the result is that they are deprived of an education and society is deprived of their potential.

Challenges to affirmative action from judicial, legislative, and higher education governing bodies represent additional barriers to the education of low-income students. In the name of fairness and equality, many anti-affirmative action policies, laws, and regulations actually have the effect of denying education and training to our low-income, minority populations so that they can become taxpaying rather than tax-absorbing citizens. Anti-affirmative action measures will also effectively cut back on a diverse student body that, as many cogently and passionately argue, enriches the educational experience for all.

## GRADUATE EDUCATION

In fields where academe is the principal option for newly minted PhDs, we are both overproducing PhDs and, at the same time, producing the wrong products. There are virtually no incentives for cutting production (quite the reverse is true) and little incentive for changing the product. Doctoral education is largely in the hands of the major national research universities where scholarly production is the sine qua non for advancement. Clearly, we need a few such institutions; they are national treasures and should be nurtured and protected. But it does not follow that most of the PhDs turned out by major national research universities should also primarily be scholars rather than teachers.

Of course, one can draw too fine a line between teaching and research. And the argument that it is difficult if not impossible to be a good teacher unless one is involved in scholarly activities is persuasive. Nevertheless, the question here is one of equating scholarship with teaching activities, more than just the number of publications in refereed journals. Learning how to teach also requires learning how to achieve a balance between the depth of specialization that scholarship requires and the breadth of pedagogical knowledge that good teaching requires.

Doctoral education in our country, however, typically involves far more depth than breadth. It is not unusual for students to spend a quarter of their graduate careers taking courses and the rest of their time on dissertation research. The time needed to obtain a degree, already too long, is rising as a result of increasing specialization, further compromising preparation for teaching. There seems to be little recognition that most of the academic positions that PhDs can aspire to will be in institutions where teaching is the primary function. These institutions may be less interested in the intensity or depth of specialization and more interested in the range of courses that the job candidate can teach. Few new PhDs can expect to teach courses that come even close to their dissertation, and many will find themselves having to teach courses for which they have had little preparation.

The consequences of overproduction and overspecialization do not only include unemployment or underemployment of PhDs. Those who do find jobs will be frustrated over high teaching loads and insufficiently prepared students. In such a situation, teachers often take out their frustration on the employing institution by trying, usually inappropriately, to push the university toward the research university model. This is only a single model of excellence when what we need are multiple models of equally worthy, but quite different, institutions.

Indeed, we have the models; what must change is the very notion of a pecking order. We brag about the diversity of American higher education, but our behavior does not match our rhetoric.

## GOVERNANCE

Most colleges and universities pay at least lip service to according primacy to the faculty and the curriculum. (In some instances, "consultation" might be a more appropriate word than "primacy.") In general, the role of the faculty is stronger at research universities and selective private colleges than at community colleges and some regional state universities. It is interesting to note that the historically black colleges and universities (HBCUs) are generally deemed to accord a stronger role to administrators than to faculty.

I have argued elsewhere that faculty governance works well in stable fiscal environments with good institutional citizenship; it works poorly in times of fiscal stress or in the absence of institutional loyalty. And in institutions where research comes first and teaching comes second, the faculty see themselves less as citizens of an institution and more as members of a worldwide discipline. Although this state of affairs is less of a problem in mainstream institutions, faculty members everywhere tend to view adverse fiscal circumstances as someone else's problem to solve—usually the president—or something to be denied.

Shared governance almost always disenfranchises the majority of the institution's staff, namely, the part-time or adjunct faculty and nonacademic staff. Students, in turn, are also usually accorded a minimal role in institutional governance, which is generally limited to making decisions about the use of student activity fees.

But the worst feature of shared governance is the veto power of a vocal minority. In both formal and informal ways, the system usually permits more obstruction than is consistent with the need to make decisions. And the delays in decision making are increasingly intolerable. Addressing the tyranny of a small minority demands that all parties set forth clear lines of responsibility and authority within a shared governance framework, establishing and holding to timelines for particular decisions, and making tireless efforts to improve the communication and trust that are indispensable to improving internal governance.

Chief executives are often caught between the dysfunctional decision-making apparatus of shared governance and an equally flawed situation at the governing board or multicampus system level.

Most four-year public institutions and many community colleges are parts of multicampus systems. There were usually sufficient reasons for the current trend in this direction, but it has resulted in the increased bureaucratization of decision making and compromised the individuality of campuses. By way of dissecting this dimension of governance in disrepair, I offer the following observations:

- The governing boards of public higher education systems are either elected or appointed. In both instances, they increasingly see themselves not as guardians of the institution, but as representatives of the special interests that led to their appointment or election. Faculty members elected to community college boards, for example, frequently represent the agendas of special interest groups. Others appointed by governors often see themselves as carrying out the governor's agenda. Thus, their potential advocacy for the institution as a whole is overcome by micromanagement. Many members of the board are understandably reluctant to speak out despite the reports by an overwhelming number of public-sector college and university presidents of a deterioration in the quality of board appointments and subsequently of board behavior.

- Many state legislators and governors, although not usually hostile to higher education, justify their inability to provide reasonable financial support by finding fault with tenure, faculty teaching loads, administrative compensation or other issues that, in the absence of severe fiscal constraints would not be of great concern. Thus, higher education bashing becomes a way to justify painful fiscal realities. Sometimes, this bashing is accompanied by intrusion or micromanagement.

- Governors and legislators have accurately discerned that too many public institutions aspire to be level 1 research universities, the traditional model of excellence. State policymakers understandably and properly resist, creating conflict between the campus and the multicampus governing board, the state legislature, governor, or coordinating agency for the state.

- Private college and university presidents are usually in a more favorable situation vis-à-vis governing boards than their colleagues in the public sector. Often presidents have the opportunity to build the boards of the institutions over which they preside. These governing boards usually are self-perpetuating, i.e., they elect each other. This inherently less-than-democratic process tends to produce boards that are devoted to the institution and often consist of a high proportion of alumni with the financial means to support the institution.

The downside of this situation is that presidents are often at the mercy of the major donors on the board who also tend to be quite conservative politically and educationally. And it is sometimes the case, particularly in the smaller institutions, that powerful faculty members have direct relationships with sympathetic board members. Sometimes these relations can undermine the efforts of presidents who are trying, often with board encouragement, to reposition the institution in the face of budgetary stringency.

## ACCOUNTABILITY

In most nations, colleges and universities are accountable to a ministry of education that also supplies most of their funding. In Germany, for example, faculty and staff members of universities are employees of the *Lander*, which are analogous to our states. Clark Kerr, the noted educator, has cogently argued that the lay governing board may well be America's greatest contribution to the governance of higher education. Historically, our institutions have resisted intrusion from above the level of the governing board—and sometimes they have even resisted the authority of the governing board. Witness the recent battles between the University of California Board of Regents and the faculty and administrators of the campuses.

During the period when dependence on Federal and state funds was growing, institutions faced a growing body of regulations and oversight. Some arose out of the need for accountability in the use of public funds. In other cases, states wanted a national plan for higher education as opposed to having a plethora of individual institutions making their individual cases to the political authorities. All too often, these institutions had aspirations that were unrealistic in terms of budgetary resources or more reflective of what the faculty wanted rather than what the state needed. And in some instances, the colleges and universities were simply one means for achieving other public objectives, such as achieving access for the disabled or protecting the environment from toxic wastes.

Although not always quarreling with these objectives, colleges and universities usually resisted oversight or regulatory initiatives. As an alternative, they often put forth the concept of "self regulation," for which voluntary accreditation remains the salient example.

For many years, accreditation has served as both higher education's defense against governmental intrusion and its principal means of assuring at least minimal performance standards.*

Although it is my belief that accreditation has done a better job of uphold-

---

*Institutional accreditation means that the entire institution is accredited by a regional or national accrediting body that is itself recognized as an accrediting body by the U.S. De-ing quality on campus than some of its critics believe, two major criticisms of accreditation have some validity. One holds that "the bar has been set too low." The second is that accreditation focuses too much on inputs (faculty qualifications and salaries, library holdings, financial resources, etc.) than on outputs (determined by assessing such factors as value added to students, their successes after graduation, or other measures).

Recently, the system of regional accreditation has come under fire for incorporating such issues as affirmative action and diversity into its standards. Even many people committed to these principles argue that they are not fit subjects for accreditation.

Programmatic accreditation has been plagued with some of the same issues facing institutional accreditation (e.g., excessive concern with inputs), but some different spins have been put on this situation. Presidents argue that specialized accreditation becomes special pleading, that is, the outside evaluators plead the case for their insider colleagues and thereby contribute to the balkanization of the campus.

Some educators argue that strengthening accreditation is essential if higher education is to make a better case for self-regulation and thereby resist further governmental intrusion. The recent formation of a Council for Higher Education Accreditation (CHEA) at the national level, following an unprecedented "plebiscite" of college and university chief executives, provides some evidence of a desire to strengthen self-regulation not only as a way to forestall governmental intrusion but because it is the right thing to do.

## RECOMMENDATIONS

True, today's strong economy has improved the fiscal position of most states. Nevertheless, it would be folly to believe that the current tendency of states to either cut taxes or channel more funds into what they perceive as higher priority social needs will be arrested. Colleges and universities should not look forward to going back to business as usual. Yet I sense that some higher education leaders believe that the recent upturn in state finances will spare them from

---

partment of Education. Programmatic accreditation means that specialized programs within an institution such as law, business, allied health, and other programs are accredited by specialists in these fields.

hard decisions.

What will it take to change from an old to a new way of doing business? Less production of PhDs would be a good idea, but major research universities usually contend that it is the "lesser" mainstream institutions, and not they, who should get out of the doctorate business. However, sometimes it is the mainstream institutions that are producing PhDs better suited for today's job market. Nonetheless, there is a persistent mythology that real universities have Division One football teams and PhD programs. We need fewer of both.

In addition, any reform of doctoral education should include more breadth and less depth to the PhD curriculum; more emphasis on pedagogy, including but not limited to supervised teaching by PhD students (i.e., not simply turning a teaching assistant loose on undergraduates); and more truth in advertising about job prospects for those accepted to doctoral programs.

I believe that the role of the state political structure is to determine the mission of the institution, that is, what student outcomes should be measured. But it should not interfere in the process by which the outcomes are to be achieved. Robert Zemsky,* Director of the Institute for Research on Higher Education at the University of Pennsylvania, calls this sharing of responsibility "the bargain." The upshot is that performance is measured by results rather than process, with the institution determining its own method of assessing student learning outcomes and the system heads, governing boards, and accrediting bodies passing judgment on the efficacy of this process but not imposing their own process. When institutions fail to address the outcomes question adequately, we can expect to see externally imposed quantitative measures, such as cookie-cutter standardized tests, that do not respect the different missions and student clientele of diverse institutions.

Governing boards of public systems or campuses should view their primary responsibility as supporting the system or the campus as a whole. The primary means of carrying out this responsibility is by appointing, and evaluating the work of, a chief executive officer.

Particularly in the smaller systems, roles for the system heads and campus

---

*Zemsky, R., and W.F. Massey. 1995. Toward an understanding of our current predicaments. *Change* 27 November/December.

heads are inadequately differentiated, it is almost axiomatic that system and campus heads will get in each other's way. Three kinds of "bargains," therefore, need to be made in the governance of multicampus public systems. One reasonable bargain would be to have the system head concentrate on the state political structure and on systemwide fiscal and academic issues, while allowing the campus heads considerable autonomy. A second bargain would be one between the system head and the governing board. In this situation, the governing board would set the overall parameters for the campus-system relationship and then hold the system head accountable for results based on stated goals and objectives. A third bargain, between the system head and governing board, would be that an oversight body will establish goals and objectives, giving those responsible for the system freedom to achieve the negotiated goals and objectives. Micromanagement or favoritism for a particular institution or subset within an institution should be eschewed.

Governing boards of both public and private institutions have serious fiduciary duties requiring that they receive sufficient information, presented in understandable terms, to carry out these responsibilities. Trustees are not universally sophisticated about fiscal matters, and administrators are not always forthcoming when the news is bad.

Tackling all the issues raised in this paper is a tall order. The good news is that they are all being addressed in one way or another in many places. The fact that change happens slowly in higher education is perhaps a virtue, and we should take comfort from Clark Kerr's reminder that most of the institutions that have survived over 500 or so years are colleges and universities. Change is necessary but so is stability.

# TECHNOLOGY'S TRANSFORMATION OF THE UNIVERSITY

*Eli Noam, PhD*

THE RECENT TREMENDOUS ADVANCES IN THE USE OF computer networks as tools of inquiry, including the growth of free communication links among scientific researchers and practitioners around the world, have resulted in a less stifling organizational hierarchy, a loss of governmental controls, and an ethic of sharing information instead of commercializing it. Technology, it seems, has created a new set of tools to facilitate research. The most exciting and important changes in society will not come simply from the use of machines such as computers but from the unlocking of information such as the DNA code by utilizing technology.

Communications technology has also linked the information resources of the globe. But as one connects in new ways, one also abandons old connections. Thus, although new communications technologies are likely to strengthen research in general (and medical research in particular), they will also weaken the traditional methods of education. Instead of prospering with the new tools, many universities will have their traditional functions superseded, their financial bases eroded, and their roles in intellectual inquiry reduced. This transformation will not be limited to universities because many major institutions of society will

*Dr. Noam is professor of finance and economics and director of the Institute for Tele-Information at Columbia University. This paper republished from* The Digital Decade, *Washington: Association of Academic Health Centers, 1997.*

also be affected. For example, studies on the banking industry demonstrate that many commercial banks are in deep trouble because of the Information Revolution: What is worse, many are unaware of the problems they face.

Higher education has three primary functions: conducting research and evaluating its validity, preserving information, and passing that information on. Accomplishing each of these functions is based on a set of technologies and economics. Changing the technology means that the economics, the primacy of these functions, and the institutions must also change.

## THE UNIVERSITY AS A SOURCE
## OF INFORMATION

Information institutions date back 5,000–8,000 years, a time when priests emerged as specialized preservers and producers of information. They also served as the primary information storage receptacles of their societies. Eventually, recording methods emerged, writers were trained, and schools appeared. Writing led to information storage institutions. Under one Assyrian king, the Royal Library stocked over 10,000 works. In these libraries, documents were arranged in separate rooms by subject matter. Wise men congregated in the new libraries to use the information and to add to it. Knowledge and inquiries were organized along lines strikingly similar to today's university departments.

This model of centrally stored information with a wide range of subjects grouped under one institutional roof was logical when information was scarce, reproduction expensive and restricted, and specialization low.

Perhaps the best illustration of this model is the most formidable information institution of antiquity, the Great Library of Alexandria. At its peak, this library amassed nearly 700,000 volumes, many of them medical treatises. Less recognized is the role of this library as a graduate university. From its inception, it recruited some of the foremost scholars of the region, such as the geometrician Euclid. These scholars were surrounded by disciples and apprentices who adored them, cleaned up after them, and supplemented their salaries, which were never high enough. They were joined by other scholars who came to the information storage, produced still more information in collaborative efforts, and hence attracted more students and disciples.

## INFORMATION TECHNOLOGY: THREAT OR SALVATION

This system of higher education remained remarkably stable for over 2,500 years but is now in the process of breaking down. The reason is not primarily technological, since technology merely enables change. Rather, the fundamental reason is that today's abundant production and rapid distribution of information is undermining traditional methods of information flow and thus the university structure itself. That structure is poised to collapse in slow motion should alternatives to its functions be found.

A major reason for this possible collapse is the systematic imbalance in the information environment. Since World War II, the production of information in the U.S. economy has increased at a rate of about 6 percent, and the growth rate itself is rising rapidly. Distribution of information is growing even faster by an estimated 10 percent or more. However, reaching a similar growth rate for the processing of information by individuals and organizations has proved difficult. This situation has serious implications for a wide range of institutions. (Indeed, virtually all aspects of society are affected by this imbalance and by the ensuing attempt to adjust the individual and processing rates of information to the demands that growth in the other stages have put on them.)

An example of the recent information explosion is the rapid proliferation of available scientific texts. It took *Chemical Abstracts* thirty-one years, from 1907 to 1937, to print its first one million abstracts. The second million abstracts were printed a mere eighteen years later. The most recent million took only one and three-quarter years. Thus, more articles on chemistry have been published in the last two years than in humankind's entire history before 1900.

Organizational response to this increased volume of information has been to try to improve processing capabilities by hiring more people, particularly more highly educated people, reorganizing internally, and investing in technology. However, the main strategy has been to break the information down by subject matter for use by specialists. Nowhere is this better illustrated than in the medical profession, where there are now dozens of specialty fields and probably hundreds of subspecialties. (There is nothing new about specialization; the Bible tells us that Adam's sons specialized, one in agriculture and the other in hunting.)

As specialization has grown, so has the means to create an invisible college of specialists. Just as air transport established the jet-setting professoriate, so are communications technologies creating new electronic communities that respond to the basic need for collaboration. Ironically, the university pays for the network that helps its resident professors shift their focus outside the university and join virtual communities in cyberspace. Along the way, the advantages of physical proximity of the researchers and professors to their respective universities, as well as to each other, decline even more rapidly.

For most universities, the volume of information doubles every five to ten years. Thus, for the university to keep up with all the work, research and specialization would also have to double every five to ten years. This situation is neither economically nor organizationally sustainable. Universities can no longer cover a wide range of specialties. They might still have a wide range of departments but can only offer a limited set of subspecialties. For that reason, the specialist finds fewer similarly specialized colleagues on campus for the purpose of collaborative work. Because interaction increasingly occurs with physically distant specialists, the university no longer functions as an institutional setting for collaboration.

The function of the university as a physical repository of information is also in jeopardy. It has been said that a university is only as good as its library, but here, too, economics and technology are changing everything. To return to the previous example: In 1940, Chemical Abstracts cost $12 per year, in 1977 it cost $3,500, and in 1995 it cost $17,400.

Comprehensive library collections have become unaffordable at the same time that electronic alternatives have become powerful in storage ability, broad in content, and efficient in retrieval. Therefore, universities are gradually shifting from investment in the physical presence of information to the creation or the provision of electronic access. This logical economic and organizational response undermines the fundamental role of the university as the primary location for specialized information. Soon the combination of laptop computer and telephone line will serve just as well as, and often better than, being there, and access to information will be available anywhere at any time.

The teaching function of university departments and professional schools also faces new problems. Given the rapid growth of technology, it is hard to imagine that the current low-tech lecture system will survive. Student-teacher interaction is already under stress from the widening gulf between the basic introductory teaching level and the specialization of researchers. This interaction also comes with a big price tag, approximately $50 per lecture hour per student at private universities, not counting the public and philanthropic support that most universities receive or the opportunity costs of student's time. Such high prices for face-to-face education are prompting alternative providers of electronically transmitted education to enter the market. Today's students who seek prestigious jobs or enter restrictive professions usually have no choice but to attend a university.

## ALTERNATIVE EDUCATION THREATENS UNIVERSITIES

However, universities are only as strong as their control over accreditation and over the public's acceptance of alternative credentials. So if alternative instructional technologies and credential systems can be devised, there will be an outmigration from the classic campus-based medical, professional, and general education. Medical education may be affected less than other areas because so much of this education is skills-oriented in the last years of study. Nonetheless, information transmission in medicine, as well as in virtually all other professional and undergraduate education, could be handled in other ways.

Alternative education possibilities might include videos, such as restored lectures by outstanding scholars, electronic access to interactive reading materials and study exercises, electronic interaction with faculty and teaching assistants, hypertextbooks, video and computer conferencing, and language translation programs. Although the advantages of electronic forms of instruction are often exaggerated by merchants, the superiority of face-to-face instruction is sometimes also romanticized in today's educational environment where students often attend mass lectures in groups of 250 and rarely speak with their lecturers.

Electronic communication also has an economic advantage because it can be provided at a dramatically lower cost than face-to-face instruction. The cost of obtaining a university education is increasing substantially. Last year, the cost rose by 6 percent at public universities and by 5 percent at private universities.

With the price of education so high and demand so great, it was inevitable that alternative providers would enter the market. A curriculum, once created, could be offered electronically not simply to hundreds of students but to tens of thousands of people around the world at substantially reduced costs. It could be provided, for example, by universities seeking additional revenues in a period of declining cohorts. Universities around the country are entering the distance education business and moving beyond the borders of their traditional service areas. The market for this expanded service includes students with full-time jobs, family obligations, limited mobility, or an impossibly long commute, as well as those in need of specialized courses.

An excellent example is the agricultural satellite network, AGSAT, which lets two dozen colleges of agriculture exchange their course offerings and thereby reduce the duplication of courses from campus to campus. The victims of the reduction in duplication, of course, resist these efforts at cost reduction and the faculty, which tends to define the mission and structure of many institutions, is as resistant to change as any other profession. Some university communities, however, have rejected attempts to add untraditional services. In Maine, when the president of the university system tried to establish an electronic distance college, he became subject to faculty resistance and eventually had to resign.

It does not seem likely that the ultimate providers of electronic education will be universities becoming "televersities." Universities will merely break the ice and legitimize the practice; it will be commercial firms that will capitalize on this opportunity. Textbook publishers, for example, will establish sophisticated electronic courses using the most effective and prestigious lecturers. Already available on video is the Greatest Lecturers series by America's Superstar Teachers, distributed by a company affiliated with the cable TV giant Jones InterCable, which advertises itself as your own private university. The same company also offers courses on its mind-extension university channel.

Moreover, if the university's hold over the accreditation system weakens, our society may witness something like a McGraw-Hill University, which will hand out degrees, certificates, or course credits just as today some companies offer in-house degree programs. If these programs become valued by society for the quality of students admitted, the knowledge gained, and the requirements that must be met, such programs will be able to compete with courses offered at traditional universities and professional schools without the substantial overhead of physical institutions. They may be able to put together an effective and often-updated teaching package that makes traditional teaching seem boring in comparison.*

## UNIVERSITIES: OBSOLESCENCE OR INNOVATION?

If the university's tuition base falters, its foundation will erode. In these days of budget constriction, most universities will not be able to offset tuition losses with more public funding. Universities and professional schools are worried about their viability. For example, teaching hospitals must compete with hospitals that do not have an educational or research component, and the government has reduced assistance for graduate medical education and research. Private donations will need to increase considerably but, if anything, such donations are likely to decline in the future along with the reductions in university centrality in research and teaching.

Of course, there are other good reasons to attend universities. Universities are also about attending football games and mixers. The associated social networking is similarly important. A significant aspect of university experience, social networking could be replicated in other ways as was the case in the thousands of years preceding mass college attendance. It might also be done in much more attractive locations and climates.

Whether universities will encounter problems with obsolescence will vary according to institutions and departments. On the teaching side, the greatest negative effect of new technologies will be at two extremes. On the one hand, mass education courses will be a tempting target for commercial outfits. At the other extreme, invisible virtual colleges of specialists may start to formalize themselves, not simply to communicate but also to offer some apprenticeship programs and certifications electronically. Those courses that attract few specialists will also migrate away from the traditional university environment.

However, types of instruction that fall between these two extremes will probably survive–in particular, those parts of education that are contact- and skill-intensive and therefore continue to demand face-to face instruction.

---

* This situation mirrors the way *Sesame Street* has raised the expectation level of preschool children: When they come to school, they expect a very lively, structured, edited type of educational experience that few real-life teachers meet.

On the research side of the university, disciplines that do not experience the rampant growth of specialization will be least affected by outmigration. Nonetheless, these disciplines will also be squeezed financially because they will lose subsidies from the parts of the university which are well supported by grants. Most affected will be highly specialized research areas where keeping up with the latest research is critical. Medicine is one such field. Research requiring physical teams and shared equipment will likely continue to be located on one campus, but the university's research unit will connect primarily to government. In effect, the university would exist somewhat like an office park, albeit an office park of semiautonomous units. The university administration is likely to become even more decentralized, being partly run from a distance by telecommuting staff or contractors.

The question is not whether universities will remain important to society, to knowledge, and to health care, but whether the economic foundation of the current system can be sustained in the face of the changed flow of information. Research and teaching will become increasingly important, while that larger institutional setting, the university, will come under pressure.

## A NEW EMPHASIS
## FOR UNIVERSITIES?

Universities and professional schools will have to place new emphasis on the advantages that personal interaction and physical environment offer to education. True teaching and learning are about more than information. Education is based on mentoring, on internalization or identification or role modeling, on guidance, group activities, and peer interaction. Universities are a traditional site where students participate in a rite of passage into adulthood. They are also about attending football games and mixers. The associated social networking is important. The strength of the future physical university lies less in pure information transfer and more in the college as a community, less in wholesale lecturing and more in individual tutorials. In research, the physical university's strength lies in establishing on-campus archipelagoes of specialized islands of excellence that benefit from physical proximity.

Furthermore, universities are becoming more important than ever in their role as validators of information. As the production of information grows exponentially, society requires credible screeners and validators of information. It has entrusted some of that function to the universities, medical and professional schools, and researchers. Society trusts those institutions more than it trusts commercial firms but, of course, the university must be careful to avoid undermining this trust by a creeping commercialization or self-censorship.

New technologies constitute a long-term threat to the central role of universities and their professional schools as research and teaching institutions. To remain viable, these institutions must undertake changes in focus and a more active management of priorities. In the future, universities will need to stress their functional strengths, such as tutorial aspects, while perhaps de-emphasizing information storage functions, to avoid being reduced to a collection of remaining physical functions like the research labs and the football team.

# LEADERSHIP, CULTURE, AND CHANGE: CRITICAL ELEMENTS FOR TRANSFORMATION

*Carol A. Aschenbrener, MD*

> *Organization is a process, not a structure...the process of organizing involves creating relationships around a shared sense of purpose, exchanging and creating information, learning constantly, paying attention to the results of our efforts, co-adapting, co-evolving, developing wisdom as we learn, staying clear about purpose, being alert to changes from all directions.*
>
> —Margaret Wheatley

A MUTUAL RELATIONSHIP EXISTS BETWEEN ANY large organization and its environmental context. For example, in many industries, market pressures to cut costs are stimulated by the emergence of new, strong global competitors; the availability of lower-cost, skilled labor abroad; and insatiable stockholder insistence on high-profit margins. Similar market pressures put academic health centers at a disadvantage because of their high costs of delivering health care. Market pressures also threaten the cross-subsidization of research that has prevailed for over two decades. Academic health centers, in turn, influence the focus and mode of health care delivery because of the factors they emphasize in their selection of students and trainees, the values they model in the learning sit-

---

*Dr. Aschenbrener is senior vice president of Kaludis Consulting Group.*

uation, and the stance they take on public health issues.

In the past, academic institutions succeeded financially despite inattention to their environmental context. Today, however, isolation and disconnection from context pose great danger to the survival of the academic health center, and those centers that ignore the societal context, the requirements of the people they serve, and the learning and developmental needs of their workforce do so at their own peril.

Many, perhaps all, academic health centers feel overwhelmed by the demand for change in health care delivery and the attendant sense of urgency. Changes need not have been so urgent; the signs of pressure for greater value and accountability have been apparent for at least twenty years. Many people ignored the context or put off change until it was inevitable and immediately necessary. Others believed that they would be rescued from the need to change because of their special or unique status. Some still believe this to be true.

In these times of turbulent global change, universities and academic health centers must understand the world as it is and as it is becoming if they are to have a chance for survival. But the ability to thrive will require much more. Universities and academic health centers must redefine their place in the world relative to the sociopolitical and economic global context and the needs of the constituencies they seek to serve. They must continually learn and improve in order to provide the best possible service and take advantage of market opportunities. And they must resolve critical issues of cost, access, and flexibility. Nothing less than institutional transformation will suffice. This paper discusses some of the ways in which academic health centers can affect successful change. Most of the points made also apply to their parent universities.

## CHANGES IN SOCIETY HERALD
## INSTITUTIONAL TRANSFORMATION

*Organizations will be needed even more than before. Precisely because there will be so much ambiguity, so much flexibility, so many variations, far more clarity will be needed in respect to mission, values, and strategy; in balancing long-range and short-range goals; in defining results. Above all, absolute clarity will be needed as to who makes ultimate decisions and who is in command in a crisis.*

—Peter Drucker

Context, by definition, is always dynamic. Choice of strategy, allocation of resources, selection of people, and rewards for certain behaviors all shape the future. Major actions such as selecting an industry partner for research or the decision to include only clinical faculty in an incentive-based compensation plan clearly set in motion streams of interconnected consequences. Even low-profile actions such as a decision to put signage in Spanish as well as English or to reconfigure student scholarship funds or to develop a marketing plan for Medicaid enrollment exert influence far beyond the action's intended target. Signals ignored, decisions deferred, changes postponed all create the future. Inaction is also action, and no action is without consequence. The aggregate consequences of choices, actions, and action deferred determine the future.

Five major socioeconomic developments help to define American society over the last thirty years: the emergence of a global economy, the diffusion of information and telecommunications technology, the maturation of the "baby boom" generation, the continued rise of individualism, and the deterioration of principles of economic justice.

The first development, a global economy, is the product of strong new competitors, primarily from the Pacific Rim; new global markets developing in the aftermath of the end of the Cold War; and a technology that allows customized manufacturing and nearly instantaneous communication. In this setting, the United States no longer reigns supreme. Across all sectors, wages have fallen, adjusted for inflation, since 1972 with the first slight rises evident only in the first six months of 1997. American business feels intense competitive pressure as new competitors flood markets with high quality products at lower prices. In an effort to become more cost competitive, business has put intense pressure on the health care industry to contain its costs, and has encouraged government to do likewise in hopes of reducing taxation.

Peter Drucker (1993) suggests that we are nearly fifteen years into the second development, a societal transformation that he calls a knowledge or information society, and he predicts that corporate turbulence and economic dislocation will accelerate. About 40 percent of U.S. households now have personal computers, and 92 percent of college students use personal computers. Technology is diffusing at an unprecedented rate. It took two dozen years for the fax machine to acquire ten million users but the World Wide Web reached that point in just ten months. With volumes of specialized information accessible on the Internet, people are questioning the cultural authority of their physicians and lawyers and bankers almost daily. In the face of these changes, how can the teacher-centered, lecture-focused model of higher education go unchallenged?

Changing population demographics is the third development. World population is expected to double by 2050, with 85 percent of the increase in developing countries. The mean age of the global population is declining, with 50 percent of the world's current population less than twenty years of age. Conversely, Western industrialized nations are "going gray," with a rising median age and a declining ratio of active workers to retired persons. In the United States, the maturation of the baby boomers will exert an increasing impact on organizations and markets. Across all industries and organizations, members of the baby boom generation are entering the executive suite. They replace members of the "silent generation" who grew up in a period of strong military and political leaders, a time when respect for authority was expected, the organization man was rewarded for conformity, and children were to be seen but not heard. The baby boom generation presents a striking contrast. Born between 1946 and 1964, they are the largest generation in U.S. history, almost 78 million strong. Beginning January 1, 1996, and continuing for the next eighteen years, a boomer will turn fifty every eighteen seconds, and his or her preferences and choices will affect every aspect of American life.

Boomers grew up in a period of unprecedented economic growth during which the United States had virtually no strong economic competitors. They grew up thinking they were special, that they could break the rules and still expect success. They have always questioned their teachers, blurred gender roles, and tried to push the system closer to their idea of perfection. During the

Vietnam War, the civil rights confrontations, and Watergate, they saw clearly the vulnerability of authority and they have been reluctant to accept any formal authority since (Smith and Clurman 1997).

Attitudes toward authority are related to reactions toward management in the workplace: those who have strong respect for authority are likely to accept or at least tolerate bosses who control, while those with little respect for authority will rebel or leave under the same circumstances (Conger 1997). As the boomers take over the reins in all sectors of society, we can expect to see a different approach to leadership and management. Their preference for a less authoritarian workplace will find support from members of Generation X, current ages 20–32, who have an aversion to authority and a decided preference for a balanced life. Boomers seek a different life. In a recent *Yankelovich Report*, 84 percent of the boomers said they felt the need to reduce stress, and 81 percent expressed a desire to "simplify life" (Smith and Clurman 1997). Baby boomers have less interest in the traditional perks of high position and express a desire to lead more as symbolic peers.

The fourth development, the increased emphasis on individualism (at the cost of collective responsibility), especially affects academic health centers. The rise in the standard of living since the 1950s has been accompanied by increasing emphasis on individual rights, with decreased recognition of responsibilities. As a nation, we seem to have forgotten the seventh-grade civics lesson that every right has a corresponding obligation. Some consequences of this development include fragmentation of the family, crumbling of the public school system, and growing public mistrust of government, business, and the professions.

The fifth development, again one that has special implications for academic health centers, is the deterioration, some would say "collapse," of principles of economic justice. Over the last twenty years, the distribution of both income and wealth have shifted to advantage the affluent. Income for the richest 5 percent rose 54 percent, and the top 20 percent enjoyed a 35-percent increase; the bottom 20 percent advanced only 1.5 percent (Hacker 1997).

Such a shift stimulates worries about the disappearance of the middle class and expansion of an "underclass" with little prospect of escaping from poverty. For example, according to *USA Today* (August 12, 1997), the cost of sending a child to a public university (tuition, room, and board) has risen from 9 percent of U.S. median family income fifteen years ago to 15 percent of median family income today. Older adults have fared better and children worse during this period. Since the enactment of Medicare in 1965, the distribution of Federal health dollars has shifted from a 50-50 balance between adults and children to a 90-10 distribution favoring seniors.

In 1965, the elderly were the largest group living in poverty; today, children hold that distinction, with 20 percent living below the poverty line. With the shift in distribution of wealth, the top 25 percent of our population might be expected to have even greater political leverage, supporting policies that maintain their advantage. Recent bipartisan action to reduce welfare benefits and reluctance to extend health care coverage to poor children are examples of policies with potential to increase growing economic imbalance.

These five societal developments pose major challenges for academic health centers and universities. The public is demanding services tailored to individual needs, value, and accountability in everything. Price competition in managed care puts academic health centers in danger of losing their ability to subsidize the academic mission. Public support for higher education is flat or declining in all states, and parents and students are alarmed at rising tuition. Demographic changes mean new and changing requirements and preferences by students, patients, other customers, and the workforce. Business is beginning to demand certification of competency, and all sectors of society insist on service and results.

The most significant internal change in academic health centers in this period has been the immense growth of the clinical enterprise, fueled mainly by a widening stream of Medicare and Medicaid dollars. The clinical faculty has been growing out of proportion to the needs of education and research for the last three decades. With the enactment of Medicare and Medicaid, university physicians and hospitals suddenly received payment for many people who had previously paid little or nothing for their care. For a major segment of the patient population, academic health centers went from being providers of care to the poor to vendors of clinical services for government payers. Clinical practice rapidly became the dominant activity and major source of income in most medical schools and, consequently, in the academic health center. In 1970–71, research revenues for U.S. medical schools were twice the medical service income. By 1980–81, medical service income had outpaced research funds and, by 1992–93, it was 2.5 times research revenues (Journal of American Medical Association 1977; 1987; 1997).

The faculty grew out of proportion to academic needs. Aided by capitation reimbursement, the aggregate medical student population grew by about 10,000 from 1976–96. But the faculty increased by 50,000, flipping the ratio of students to faculty from 1.4 to 0.7. Departments of internal medicine, surgery, and pediatrics nearly tripled, and basic science faculty increased by 50 percent. The only department that did not grow significantly was Preventive Medicine; the nationwide increase of only 65 faculty members over twenty years stands in contrast to the rhetoric about prevention and health promotion (Journal of American Medical Association 1977; 1987; 1997). With the recent efforts to restrict growth in Medicare and Medicaid expenditures, medical schools now have a growing imbalance between revenues and number of faculty.

## THE OLD WAY OF DOING BUSINESS

*The art of progress is to preserve order amid change*
*and to preserve change amid order.*

—Alfred North Whitehead

Walking the halls of an academic health center thirty years ago, one heard the following litany of complaints from patients: (1) "My doctor doesn't listen to me." (2) "My doctor doesn't answer my questions and sometimes seems angry at me for asking." (3) "I have to wait too long to get an appointment and then too long in the doctor's office." (4) "There are so many people participating in my care, but they don't seem to speak to each other. Sometimes it seems they dislike each other and use me as the go-between. Who's looking at the total picture?"

Comments overheard from students were similar across schools, and included the following: (1) "Why must I memorize so many facts when they seem irrelevant?" (2) "Faculty seldom talk with me about dying or sexual attraction to patients or anger at patients. Am I the only one who struggles with these feelings?" (3) "The referring physician is often portrayed as stupid or incompetent. Is that how they will talk about me when I am in practice?"

These concerns met with minimal response. Over the ensuing thirty years, complaints rang louder and louder about quality of service, workload for students and residents, cost of care, relevance to local communities, and lack of accountability for use of resources. Corporate America and government weighed in with their muscle and public attitudes grew increasingly critical of both higher education and health care in general. Mistrust of physicians and universities grew, and the public now clearly demands value and accountability and customization. Commenting on public sentiment about higher education, Zemsky and Massey (1995) concluded, "What has changed is not just the public's mood but its willingness to support institutions that allocate goods rather than serve customers and that value producers more than products."

The call for change can no longer be ignored. It is a call not for incremental change, but for transformation—for redefinition of purpose, renewed focus on mission and outcomes, and new structure to maximize quality, defined as "fitness for purpose at lowest cost to society." In a recent article in *Change*, Sir John Daniel (1997), vice chancellor of the Open University in the United Kingdom, asserted that universities are in crisis worldwide, with the common elements of crisis being cost, access, and flexibility. He notes that industries whose costs have risen faster over long periods than inflation almost inevitably wind up in serious trouble, either going out of existence or enduring grave upheaval to survive.

Higher education and health care fall in this category. Daniel suggests that return from crisis lies in reducing costs and increasing institutional differentiation, both of which entail reconsideration of the teacher-centered model of education that dominates in the United States. Warnings of impending doom for academic health centers also identify cost reduction and flexibility as being required elements for survival:

> Academic health centers have made enormous national contributions since their development following World War II . . . But these institutions cannot afford to rest on their laurels, for they are part of an industry that is undergoing sweeping change. Complacency could be deadly in such an environment. To remain as vital in the future as they have been in the past, academic health centers will find it necessary to change some of their traditional practices. They must become more efficient, find new ways to teach their students and relate more effectively to the outside world (Vanselow 1986).

Major change cannot occur without restructuring, for the authoritarian hierarchy typical of universities and health care institutions is inherently inflexible and internally focused.

The structure of universities and of most major organizations in our society is based on a mechanistic model, an authoritarian hierarchy with rigid organizational charts, strict role segregation, and internal competition. This model has its roots in medieval armies and the Catholic Church. The objective of this model was to get the task done and to manage workers in large organizations. Managers were considered to be the brains, the "heads," who interpreted the world to others and gave orders. Workers at all levels were considered "hands" who could not or should not make independent decisions.

Western health care adopted a similar model as evidenced by a hierarchy of professions, strict separation of scope of practice, specialized language, and an overriding belief that patients should obey physician orders rather than seek to understand treatment implications or health issues for themselves. Universities adopted mechanistic industrial values of standardization, memorization of facts (teacher interprets the world and gives orders about what to retain), and a strict system of credit based on time spent in instruction rather than competency achieved.

## CHANGES NEEDED NOW

The authoritarian hierarchy still evidenced today is anchored in principles of control and compliance. Information is hoarded by the managers who insist on one worldview and an unquestioning acceptance of orders. Hiring and advancement practices promote homogeneity of behavior and worldview, and the ability to fit in with the dominant pattern is strongly emphasized. Deviants are marginalized, and risk-taking is discouraged. "Don't rock the boat" and "If it ain't broke, don't fix it" are typical beliefs. Contracts with employees are often vague and general, without clearly defined expectations or a link to rewards, and they are rarely renegotiated.

This system provided predictability, order, and stability and worked well during the early decades of the Industrial Revolution. The authoritarian hierarchy is not bad, but it does not fit the contemporary context. It promotes a narrow view, preserves the status quo, impedes rapid change, and fails to stimulate optimum performance or innovation.

Hierarchy is needed for the order and stability that human beings require, but the authoritarian system doesn't serve people well in a world that is at once more complex, more polarized, and more cognizant of interdependence. It frustrates the needs of people in developed countries, who increasingly seek personal respect, meaning, and opportunity for growth in their work.

## Leadership: Critical to Effecting Change

*A leader is someone who understands where people are going and stands in front of them.*

—Gandhi

When the amount of change needed in response to environmental factors or market opportunities is low, little leadership is required. In stable times, such as during the twenty years of unchallenged economic growth after World War II, most organizations relied mainly on good management to keep operations running on time and within budget. As long as resources are flush and competitors few, there is little need to question budget allocation, establish priorities, or promote rapid innovation.

Management as we know it is a twentieth-century phenomenon designed to bring order and consistency to large complex organizations. The domain of management encompasses three processes: planning and budgeting, organizing and staffing, and controlling and problem solving. The focus is on identification of variances and consistency of results. Management may or may not be customer-focused depending on the culture of the organization (Kotter 1990).

The larger and more complex an organization, the greater the need for sound management. But although academic health centers are among the most complex organizations in our society, until recently many centers got by without well-developed management processes because resources were abundant and there were few serious competitors for their major revenue-generating activities. This situation was particularly true of medical schools. For example, it is not uncommon for a medical school to invest several million dollars of clinical practice revenues in research activities with no measure of the return on that investment and no assessment of public funds leveraged or improvements made in clinical care or integration into technology. Today there is growing realization that deans and department chairs in all the health colleges need management expertise in order to allocate resources to mission priorities, reduce costs, and maintain appropriate but not excess staff for the mission.

In the early 1970s, American business realized that it needed more leadership at all levels in the organization just to survive in the changing world. Leadership was increasingly seen as a necessary skill for all managers as well as executives because it is leadership, not management, that produces movement and change (Kotter 1990). As the magnitude of required change increases, so does the need for leadership. Today most large organizations seek significant leadership and effective management. In the executive team (those in the organization with organization-wide responsibility), it is advantageous to have people who are strong in both. The top team for academic health centers would include the CEO (vice president or chancellor equivalent) and staff who report to him or her directly: deans, directors of the clinical enterprise, and heads of some institution-wide centers. To respond effectively to the environmental context, academic health centers need strong managers who can ensure consistent results and leaders at all levels who can create and sustain change throughout the organization. "Leadership by itself never keeps an operation on time and on budget year after year. And management by itself never creates significant useful change" (Kotter 1990).

For centuries, the nature and development of leadership have been the subject of debate and speculation. One definition holds that leadership produces "actions that focus resources to create desirable opportunities" (Nair 1994). This definition imparts a value dimension to leadership: what resources shall be used to create which opportunities for whose advantage. There is broad agreement, however, that the essence of effective leadership involves the relationship between the leader and those who agree to be led. Competency, credibility, trustworthiness, and communication are repeatedly cited as key characteristics of good leaders (Kouzes and Posner 1992). An interview-study with one hundred well-known leaders from all sectors, including higher education, identified six key leadership needs in the twenty-first century: (1) leadership is needed throughout the organization, not just at the top; (2) leaders must facilitate excellence in others; (3) management and leadership are distinct from each other, and both are essential; (4) the humanistic dimension is increasingly important—leaders must care about employees as well as the bottom line; (5) a holistic approach will be required that can apply diverse skills to address interconnected systems; and (6) leaders must be able to master change, predicting and directing it rather than just reacting to it (McFarland et al. 1993).

## New Roles for Deans and Department Chairs

Although there may be differences in opinion about specific role-definitions for vice presidents or chancellors of academic health centers and deans of health colleges, there is broad consensus on two points: (1) the roles require skill at both management and leadership, and (2) the jobs carry high risk. When conditions require cost-effective use of resources and alignment across units, line management skills become critical. An MBA is not required, but the CEO and deans of the academic health center do need sufficient financial acumen to understand fund flows and capital financing and the payment dynamics of the health care delivery system. Both personnel management skills and interpersonal skills are important; the top team needs to understand the requirements of law and fairness in managing people and must be able to convey respect and develop rapport with employees and customers across broad societal dimensions.

Managing conflict has long been a major responsibility for academic health center executives. Given the complexity of today's environment and the rampant uncertainty and fear it stimulates, conflict management, including prevention by early attention and collaboration, may take 50 percent of the top team's time. Excellent listening, the ability to encourage expression of divergent views, and the skills of negotiation and mediation are increasingly important competencies for deans and CEOs. Finally, both complexity and change require an understanding of systems (interrelationships that create behavior) and process in order to achieve outcomes different from those of the past.

With respect to leadership, the challenge to vice presidents, deans, and department chairs at academic health centers is one of balance. As society moves through the upheaval of going from an industrial era to the information, or interactive, age, organizational leaders are challenged to balance seemingly contradictory characteristics. Across all sectors, the principle of individual freedom must be balanced with accountability for outcomes and prudent use of resources. At both organizational and personal levels, balance between reflection and action is essential, with people taking time to develop a systems perspective yet moving with the speed that the environment demands. Open communication is fundamental to continuous learning in the organization and must be balanced with a disciplined discretion that keeps confidential matters confidential. As leaders of academic health centers work to cultivate a strategic focus on priorities across the institution, they must also create an appropriate balance through support systems and incentives that foster innovation and initiative by individuals and teams. The strength of competitive market forces and rapid technological innovation require a new balance between directed decision making and shared leadership in the academic health center. With appropriate boundaries, as many decisions as possible should be pushed to the front line for speed and service, with some strategic decisions requiring fast executive action rather than the leisurely process of democratic deliberation.

Empowerment must be balanced with alignment. This approach means giving every faculty and staff member the latitude to act creatively to achieve outcomes, while rewarding people for pulling in the same direction. The model of leadership itself needs a reframing that provides a balance among order, collaboration, and autonomy appropriate to the times. Finally, a new balance is needed between specialization and wholeness, with a renewed emphasis on common ground across departments and health professions and a holistic approach to education and health care that considers the needs of body, mind, spirit, and community.

Because of the uncertainty, fear, and challenge that accompany any significant change, those who lead the change are always at risk. Unfortunately, as vice presidents and deans are asked to lead more sweeping change, university governance seems more impatient for quick success and less forgiving of missteps. For example, a recent study by the American Association of Medical Colleges (AAMC) identified the average tenure for medical deans appointed between 1980 and 1992 as being only 3.6 years. Increased politicization of public governing boards, faculty preference for the status quo, and faulty selection processes are often cited as causes for the high turnover. Alan Guskin, chancellor of Antioch University, cites turnover of university presidents as an additional concern, noting that 75 percent of new presidents come from outside the institution and most are new to the role (Guskin 1996).

Frequent turnover of executives is costly to the institution, disrupts the flow of change, and reinforces the expectations of those who oppose change that they can outlast any change agent. Turnover is especially costly for universities that undertake major restructuring; the process typically takes four to seven years for full implementation. As Marjorie Wilson (1984) noted, "One could conjecture that faculties not desiring change would seek out like members of the group for executive positions to avoid the introduction of radical approaches or insensitivity to 'the way we think' or 'the way we do things here'."

The role of the health college dean is changing, especially at colleges of medicine. In the past, the major functions of the dean were to (1) ensure that the educational programs met accreditation standards; (2) distribute resources, usually without having to disclose how much was given to whom; (3) aid department chairs in recruiting faculty; (4) keep people happy; (5) promote the college; and (6) reward outstanding achievement.

Today's deans must be concerned with (1) designing educational programs to address societal and workforce needs, (2) cutting costs, (3) right-sizing the faculty, (4) establishing direction and getting people to collaborate, (5) promoting integration with other academic health center units and outside partners, and (6) fostering alignment. In the medical school, several distinct models are evolving. In some academic health centers, the medical dean has academic responsibility and some role in managing the clinical enterprise, with the CEO of the academic health center or university president serving as integrator of all components of the academic health center.

In addition to the traditional academic role, some medical deans also have a significant fiduciary responsibility for an integrated health system; this responsibility may be shared with the CEO of the academic health center. Elsewhere, the dean has little or no responsibility for the clinical enterprise but may exert centralized oversight of academic functions. Whatever the model, the dean's role now clearly requires both management and leadership skills.

Kotter (1990) defines three major leadership processes: establishing direction, aligning people in that direction, and motivating and inspiring people to persist despite challenges and setbacks. A fourth process of understanding the environment seems fundamental to the other three. To understand the environment, the dean must be able to take a wide-angle view, synthesizing many data to project what might lie ahead, and then following trends that seem important.

Flexible thinking and the ability to change mental models are key skills for this work. Establishing direction entails the ability to develop a sense of shared purpose across the organization, implement strategic priorities, and identify possible consequences and opportunities related to action. The deans must be change agents, with a deep understanding of people and the dynamics of change. To align people in the desired direction, the dean must be a team builder as well as team player and must implement the structure to reinforce desired behavior. The structure would include performance management and compensation systems linked to productivity and institutional outcomes. In many cases, aligning people also requires that the dean play a major role outside the academic health center, building bridges with practicing health professionals, community partners, and potential donors.

Motivation and inspiration are essential to sustain change. Genuineness, tireless and effective communication, and an understanding of organizational culture are critical ingredients. People who have an agenda beyond just self-interest are more likely to be able to motivate others. To ensure appropriate succession, the dean also must take responsibility for developing others who can both manage and lead. This means identifying people throughout the organization who appear to have the interest and ability to lead or manage, or do both, and creating opportunities for them to gain the necessary skills and experience. Priority for development should be given to people who appear to have characteristics needed for the future, those who learn from their experiences and make continued learning a personal priority. The importance to the organization of developing people is highlighted when the dean includes it as an issue of accountability in performance expectations for all department chairs and other line managers. And, of course, deans need the financial acumen and discipline to cut costs without sacrificing quality or values. Unfortunately, faculty expectations of the dean may lag behind the realities of environmental demands, with many still looking to the dean to be a benevolent provider and ultimate arbiter of internal conflict who otherwise stays out of the way. The role of dean is not for the fainthearted or those who want to slow down. As Wilson (1984) concluded in her study of medical deans in the early 1980s, "A top administrative post in academic medicine is no place for one who wishes to avoid conflict or who requires immediate and tangible rewards and approval."

Roles for department chairs are clearly shifting, but the direction of change in roles seems less clear. The prevailing model of hiring or appointing chairs with the mandate to build departments catalyzed significant advance in research productivity for many health colleges and netted large increases in clinical revenues for many medical schools. However, this model also fostered internal competition for resources and often resulted in an aggregate of fiefdoms loosely united by fiberoptic cable and promotion and tenure policies. The fiefdom model runs counter to the recognized need for strategic focus, shared resources, and collaboration.

Many department chairs say they no longer know what is expected of them. It is likely that roles will differ across institutions, depending on the structure and local factors. Several themes are common in the efforts to redefine the role of department chairs. First, chairs will be expected to share collective responsibility for the welfare and success of their college and for the academic health center. This task calls for being well-informed about the environmental context, participating actively in strategic planning and implementation of plans, and modeling the core values of the academic health center.

Many department chairs may be asked to assume more accountability for managing the cost of education and research. In some medical schools, clinical department chairs will be expected to take more line management responsibility for the clinical practice; in other schools, chairs will retain accountability for the quality of clinical practice but management responsibility will shift to the head of the practice plan, the director of the clinical enterprise, or the dean.

Expectations for an entrepreneurial focus will increase, with chairs encouraged to explore new relationships with industry, health care partners, or government and community agencies. Regardless of how many structural units exist or whether they are called "departments" or "centers" or "institutes," the most important role of the department chair or the equivalent will continue to be the development of people. Specifically, the department chair will be entrusted with the critical roles of (1) selecting people who have the competencies needed to serve the institutional mission, (2) setting clear expectations for performance and assessing productivity in relation to those expectations, and (3) ensuring that faculty and staff in their care have the coaching, mentoring, and opportunities for learning necessary to continue their professional and personal growth across the career span. The chairs must also share with deans the accountability for succession planning.

## The Work of Leaders Is To Master Change

*Failure is only the opportunity to begin again more intelligently.*

—Henry Ford

If the work of leaders, as distinct from managers, is to produce movement, then leaders must be masters of change. This role means they must be able to foresee the need for change, develop a shared vision of change that is linked to the interests of their constituents, and guide people through the process of transition. William Bridges (1991) draws a distinction between change and transition. Change is situational and external, such as a new hiring policy, a new system to determine compensation, a new office configuration, or a new boss. Transition is the psychological process that people must go through to come to terms with the new situation. In Bridges's model, the process of transition entails three stages: an ending and a new beginning separated by a neutral or transition zone that is characterized by uncertainty and a sense of not belonging, of not fitting with either the old or the new.

The transition process occurs regardless of how the change is perceived. For example, even with the move to a fantastic new research building, faculty and staff still leave behind settings or ways of working that were familiar and comforting. Understanding this model of change and the behaviors that are likely to occur in each stage provides a template for planning interventions to manage the ending and the neutral zone, not just the beginning. This could include, for example, taking the time for a dialogue with faculty and staff about what they will miss and what they think they will lose in the changeover to a new information system provider. It would become an opportunity to share concerns, celebrate past success, and defuse the common polarization of old-bad and new-good that may arise in any change. Successful transition to the new situation, whatever it may be, depends on letting go of an old identity or reality. Finding ways to deal with people's feelings of fear, anger, sadness, and anxiety about endings and losses is difficult but necessary work that must be done by those leading change, and not be delegated to others. Postponing this work leaves concerns unresolved and may heighten expectations of rescue from the dreaded change.

Many academic health centers and universities are in the process of major restructuring in an attempt to enhance flexibility, speed of decision making, quality of service, and cost-effectiveness. This last is often given as the most urgent reason for change, yet it is the least likely to capture the hearts and minds of the people who are asked to change. Discussions of change strategies commonly speak to the need to create a "burning platform" or precipitate a crisis in order to catalyze movement. This approach is a movement of avoidance with the impetus to change often identified as the desire to escape loss—loss of money, jobs, status, patients, students, ranking, or competitive position—or all of these. Change that is perceived as movement toward a state or condition is more likely to capture the imagination, especially if it is linked to values esteemed by employees. It would be difficult to sustain creative energy and momentum through the long, difficult work of institutional restructuring without commitment across the organization to the creation of a desired future.

Ideally, the rationale for change includes a clear statement of realistic threats and opportunities in the environment and a compelling statement of what the future could be for the organization, that is, a combination of pushing people away from the old reality and pulling them toward the new. In restructuring, important roles for the executive team include developing a compelling vision of the restructured organization, focusing key players on the work over long periods of time, communicating urgency and facilitating continued momentum, and convincing the uncommitted that change is, indeed, likely to happen (Guskin 1996).

Human activity is ultimately driven by the desire to survive. In contemporary culture, survival commonly encompasses far more than meeting basic needs. For some, prestige, status, a role in decision making, guaranteed employment, or assurance of specific income levels may be perceived as survival issues. Thus, it is typical for a proposal for change to be met quickly with the question, "What's in it for me?" This is not to suggest universal selfishness as a prime motivator; instead, facing up to this reaction acknowledges the powerful human desires for connection, belonging, and meaning as being among those components of self-interest that go beyond basic survival needs. Until people feel some comfort with what they perceive as personal gains and losses from the change and until they have some conviction that the leaders are credible and trustworthy, significant movement is unlikely. Leaders who deeply understand the concerns of their constituents, invite open dialogue, and paint a clear vision of the altered state are more likely to meet success as change agents.

There are a number of patterns of reaction in change that are often labeled as resistance: foot-dragging, negativity, increased errors on the job, constant questioning about the need for change, increased absenteeism, low morale, gossip, and sabotage. In his book, *Leading Change*, James O'Toole (1995) suggests a number of reasons why people may resist change: "Resistance to change occurs when a would-be leader challenges the comfort of the group, the members' satisfaction with the established level of their power, prestige, privileges, position, and satisfaction with who they are, what they believe, what they cherish . . . in almost all instances, the majority of haves (people who have the power) resist the call to reform, not so much because they fear change, but because they bristle at having the will of others imposed on them."

Alternatively, behaviors labeled as "resistance" may represent grieving or fear rather than the intention to obstruct change. Gilmore et al. (1997) cite research suggesting that much of what is labeled as resistance of middle management is actually a predictable reaction to inadequate preparation or absence of support from top management when difficulties arise. Considering seemingly oppositional behaviors as evidence of lack of clarity, commitment, or connection suggests that the remedy lies with leadership's listening, clarifying the vision, responding to concerns, and making connections between the new reality and people affected by it. Conversely, labeling behavior as "resistant" suggests a cause for blame, shuts off dialogue, and promotes polarization between those who are committed and those who are not.

It is common to see circles of accusation and blame in any situation of change. Deans blame the faculty for being too conservative, the faculty question the dean's commitment to the academic mission, and both blame the department chair, but for different failings. Discomfort with major change such as restructuring may be great even at the highest levels of university administration. "Administrators believe in or accept the validity of the present system; they have become leaders by being able to manage successfully the present systems that will have to be overturned; and they have learned to be successful at creating change that occurs incrementally" (Guskin 1996).

In their assessment of why change initiatives fail, Robbins and Finley (1996) list seven "unchangeable rules for change."

1.  People do what they perceive is in their best interest, thinking as rationally as circumstances allow them to think.
2.  People are not inherently antichange. Most will, in fact, embrace initiatives provided the change has positive meaning for them.
3.  People thrive under creative challenge, but wilt under negative stress.
4.  People are different. No single "elegant solution" will address the entire breadth of these differences.
5.  People believe what they see. Actions do speak louder than words, and a history of previous deception multiplies present suspicion.
6.  The way to make effective long-term change is to first visualize what you want to accomplish, then inhabit the vision until it comes true.
7.  Change is an act of the imagination. Until the imagination is engaged, no important change can occur.

To increase the likelihood of sustainable change, leaders need to set clear direction, link the direction to the interests of those involved in change, listen deeply and often, and acknowledge feelings. They must also model the desired behaviors, reward others for those behaviors, and be open and honest about their own reactions and concerns. No change is made without loss, ending, uncertainty, or a potential unwanted outcome.

As O'Toole (1995) concludes, "What is required to guide effective change is . . . a new philosophy of leadership that is always and at all times focused on enlisting the hearts and minds of followers through inclusion and participation. Such a philosophy must be rooted in the most fundamental of moral principles: respect for people . . . Leaders must adopt the unnatural behavior of always leading by the pull of inspiring values."

## The Success of Change Depends on the Culture

*Individuals are what they believe, and groups are their cultures; hence to require a group to change its shared beliefs is to threaten its very existence.*

—James O'Toole

In any organization, culture determines what behavior is acceptable, what and who gets rewarded, and how information flows. Any significant organizational change stimulates reflection on some deeply held assumptions and, thus, is perceived as a challenge to the existing culture. For example, the incredible expansion of the Internet allows people to readily access specialized information that previously was held closely by the learned professions; this situation challenges the cultural authority of higher education and all the professions.

Webster's dictionary defines culture as "the total pattern of human behavior and its products embodied in thought, speech, action, and artifacts and dependent upon man's capacity for learning and transmitting knowledge to succeeding generations through use of tools, language, and systems of abstract thought." Edgar Schein (1992), one of the founders of the field of organizational psychology, describes organizational culture as "a pattern of shared basic assumptions that the group learned as it solved its problems of external adaptation and internal integration, a pattern that has worked well enough to be considered valid and, therefore, is to be taught to new members as the correct way to perceive, think and feel in relation to these problems."

Various definitions of societal and organizational culture incorporate four common themes: (1) culture is learned and is taught to new members of the group; (2) culture includes values, assumptions, beliefs, and customs; (3) the culture of any group grows out of successful problem solving; and (4) it is very difficult to change culture because so much of it is invisible and unconscious. Informally, culture may be thought of as who we are, what we value, and how we do things.

In the context of culture, "values and beliefs" encompass what deserves attention, what gets rewarded, what things mean, and which reactions are acceptable in a given situation and which are not. There is often a disconnect between the values espoused and those that actually guide daily interaction, that is, between the de jure and de facto cultures. For example, a dean may state emphatically that he wants to consult with all department chairs about making a specific decision, yet it is commonly known that the decision is actually made outside the group with only a few close associates.

Cultural assumptions are the deeply shared core that gives a group stability. This core includes assumptions that individuals bring to the work situation from national, regional, ethnic, religious, and other cultures. A common assumption in white America is if you work hard, you will be rewarded, even though this assumption no longer fits the social reality of concentration of wealth, stagnation of income, and growth of an underclass. Similarly, deeply encultured beliefs about the "proper" place of women influence beliefs about the role of the nursing profession and the range of acceptable behaviors between nurses and physicians.

Organizational cultures usually include assumptions about the inherent trustworthiness of people and how they are expected to behave. The belief that people respond best to the stick may be linked to a deep assumption that people are lazy and untrustworthy and won't perform without threat of punishment. A common assumption in academe seems to be "only experts speak," that is, the opinions of people who have advanced degrees are held in higher regard than the opinions of others, even when the issue at hand is outside their area of expertise.

Once established, basic assumptions are deeply held, often at an unconscious level. They are difficult to articulate, and people are often unaware of how these assumptions influence their own behavior. In academe, for instance, experimental data collected under controlled conditions are considered "objective" while other measurements are regarded as being "soft" and, therefore, of lower value. University faculty, for example, often discount perceptions as being "soft," which makes it difficult for them to accept the concept of customer service. The underlying assumption—that only science is objective, and that objectivity is always better—persists despite the work of Einstein and other physicists demonstrating how the position of the observer always affects the data collected.

In trying to understand and influence culture, it is essential to remember that we can never get beyond our own perspective and our own set of values, beliefs, and assumptions. We can enlarge that perspective, challenge it, learn its limitations, but we are always limited by our perspective. No one can see absolute reality. Culture is usually not consciously or deliberately constructed. Rather, it grows gradually from the assumptions that people make about others and about what works in the world. Organizational cultures are shaped most strongly by the actions and values of an organization's founders and early leaders. Early successes shape culture.

Over time, as actions within the culture become associated with success, people in the organization develop beliefs that current patterns of behavior are superior to any alternative ones and are guaranteed to bring success, regardless of circumstances. This attitude is evidenced by such comments as "We've always done it this way" and "It worked before, why change now?"

When things start going poorly in a strong culture, the tendency is to blame outside influences rather than look at beliefs and behaviors inside the organization. Because so many of the assumptions of a culture are deeply embedded, it is difficult for people to see why the old ways are no longer adequate when a major contextual change occurs. It is common for members of the dominant group in an organization, those who most resemble the founders in terms of their demographics, to be relatively blind to equally valid worldviews of other groups.

Universities and Western science, for instance, both have their foundations in the medieval Catholic church, an organization of white men privileged by virtue of being the most educated class of their time, and the values and assumptions of both institutions reflect a white-male perspective. Equating long hours with commitment to the work, valuing independence over collaboration, and using competition and winning as the dominant frame are common assumptions that can be linked to the values of these founders. Such values are not truth; they are only opinion.

One of the difficulties in organizational culture is that people often do not distinguish their own opinions and perceptions from fact. For example, assumptions about gender in the cultures of science and academe are so deeply buried that prior to the civil rights era, biomedical researchers rarely questioned the logic of conducting physiologic research on men and extrapolating results to women as if they were "little" men. It becomes critical to unearth and challenge cultural values and assumptions when attempting change that varies from the traditional model or entails close relationship with an outside entity.

One theoretical approach to culture, the nexus approach, is based on the premise that the organization is a microcosm of surrounding societal cultures and that the uniqueness, if any, of an organization's culture lies in the particular mix and interaction of occupational, ethnic, and other cultures (Martin 1992). The culture of an organization is embedded in and influenced by the macro culture of society. For example, U.S. national culture places high value on the individual, often to the detriment of the common good. This cultural position is reflected in the emphasis on individual achievement and the lack of recognition for teamwork in higher education. When systems to reward teamwork are proposed, they are often countered with objections that those proposing the new system don't value individual innovation. This approach presupposes a zero-sum game in which the elevation of one group can occur only at the expense of another group's status. The implication of the nexus approach is that one must understand the cultures outside the organization in order to understand the multiple, overlapping cultures within it.

Over time, the subcultures within an organization influence its larger culture. As members of groups different from the dominant group enter the organization, they are expected to assimilate and to learn and value the existing culture, usually without questioning it. This situation ensures maintenance of the status quo. When the number of new group members reaches a certain point (some say 15 percent), the subculture represented can no longer be ignored and there is opportunity to shape new elements of the larger culture.

This seems to be the case both in the cultures of groups and of nations. In U.S. society, for instance, the percentage of immigrants in the population is no larger than it was after World War II. However, a high percentage of immigrants are from Mexico, and they are settling in two states, creating the opportunity for political and cultural influence throughout the country, not just assimilation. Similarly, the number of women in academe is now sufficiently large that rigid up-or-out tenure guidelines are being revised and institutions are implementing more flexible leave policies, benefiting both sexes.

Schein (1992) identifies ten elements of organizational culture. Attention to these elements, which follow, can reveal much about an organization.

1. Artifacts—Visible manifestations that describe how people regularly interact. They may reveal little about underlying assumptions. (Artifacts include language, customs, traditions, rituals.)

2. Group norms—Implicit standards and values in the work group. Is a nurse permitted to disagree with the physician when others are present? Does the supervisor address those supervised by first name but expect to be addressed by title?

3. Publicly articulated values—Descriptions of the de jure culture. They may deviate widely from the de facto culture. For example, some academic health centers give a high profile to primary care in all institutional public relations materials, but high-achieving students may be discouraged by faculty from

entering primary care specialities.

4. Formal organizational philosophy—Philosophy reflected in broad policies and ideological principles. Faculty may be on the honor system for sick days, for example, while all other employees may be required to present professional corroboration for missing more than two days of work.

5. The rules of the game—Implicit guidelines for getting ahead. For example, in many professional organizations, it is considered impolitic to run for major office without first putting in time in the trenches; the assumption here is that one must not rise too quickly.

6. Climate—How the organization "feels." Climate is influenced by the physical facility and personal interactions. Do people have personal mementos or institutional slogans in their work space? Is the work space open or divided into enclosed offices? What is the general tone of the place?

7. Embedded skills—Special competencies. Most important are those passed on to new members without being written down.

8. Shared cognitive framework—Paradigms, mental models, and habits of thinking. "We are excellent" and "We are superior" represent different mental models. The cognitive framework of the academic health center culture typically reflects the physician worldview, with perspectives of other professions sometimes only a counterpoint or afterthought.

9. Shared meanings—Understandings created by group members. For example, comments to students about a referring physician may reflect an assumption that faculty physicians are more competent than those in practice.

10. Integrating symbols—Ideas, feelings, and images that groups develop to characterize themselves. The traditional white attire for health professionals is one example.

Every organization has a culture; some have many subcultures as well. Shared values are the core of any culture. In itself, a culture is not good or bad, helpful or detrimental. Culture provides a sense of continuity and stability, especially in times of turbulence when organizational values can be a source of both guidance and comfort. Every culture has strengths and limitations for particular circumstances. As circumstances change, the fit between culture and doing what needs to be done waxes and wanes.

In the traditional academic culture, most decisions are submitted to lengthy faculty deliberation with the goal of reaching consensus. This situation is typified in the notion of "a thousand points of veto" and the saw, "The vote was 95 for and 5 against so the motion failed."

Traditional faculty governance fits with values of individualism and academic freedom. It promotes collegiality and may work satisfactorily in times of societal stability, when institutions have the luxury of slow incremental change. In a fast-paced, highly competitive world, however, some decisions require the speed and expertise of informed executive action or the immediacy of frontline response to customer needs. A culture that balances shared governance, executive action, and dispersion of decision making to the front line is better suited to the times.

The literature of mergers, partnerships, reengineering, and other major corporate change is replete with examples of the relationship between culture and change. In times of turbulence and uncertainty, those who have held the most power and influence in an organization can be expected to reinforce the prevailing culture and, thus, the status quo. Conversely, one cannot expect to sustain any major alteration in direction, focus, or nature of outcomes without cultural changes. Workers, including professionals, will not persist in doing what they perceive is not valued. Thus, no amount of rhetoric or exhortation or program change will yield sustainable, learner-centered innovation in health professions education unless there is a system of reward and recognition that accords high value to this activity.

Inattention to issues of culture is perhaps the most frequently cited reason for failure of proposed or completed mergers and partnerships. In their description of the lessons learned in the successful Barnes-Jewish-Christian hospital merger, Lerner and colleagues (1997) note that some of their most vexing, persistent issues relate to the difficulty of bringing disparate cultures together.

There is no specific organizational culture that is superior or preferred. Rather, what is needed is congruence between outcomes that the organization seeks and its system of institutional values, beliefs, assumptions, and rewards. Across industries and firms, organizations identify the need to shift to a culture that is vision-driven, entrepreneurial, team-based, "boundaryless," and receptive to change (Gilmore et al. 1997). Organizations recognize the need for cultures that are more flexible and egalitarian, with less hierarchical reporting and decision making, and a greater sense of employee ownership.

Traditional academic culture is not change-ready. Decisions take a long time and require lengthy consultation with faculty. Conversely, frontline workers are rarely consulted, so a rich source of information about customer preferences is often missed. Administrative systems typically are slow and not models of cost-effectiveness. The reward system is narrow, consisting mainly of permanent rewards of promotion or salary increases that are tied to traditional academic measures and seniority.

The academic culture esteems faculty for their credentials rather than for present performance relative to expectations and institutional goals. Efforts to measure productivity are often seen as challenges to scholarly independence. Assumptions about uniqueness are manifest in isolation from the realities of the external world (ivory tower syndrome), an aversion to determining the cost of academic activities, and a dismissal of learnings from other professions or industries as irrelevant.

Two common assumptions of the academic culture are particularly problematic when speed, flexibility, collaboration, and best use of resources are priorities. The first is that a faculty position is akin to a hunting license to bag any and all resources, without consideration of institutional goals or impact on others. The other is that the domain of a department chair or manager is private turf, not to be intruded on, and that the members apportioned to that domain should work solely within its boundaries. Such assumptions must be challenged in order to achieve such goals as learner-centered education, optimal internal collaboration, customer focus, and seamless group practice.

Successful restructuring of academic health centers as flexible, innovative, responsive, entrepreneurial organizations will require culture shift. This does not mean the replacement of the existing culture but a reshaping that includes retention of essential, cherished values such as commitment to excellence and ethical conduct and the addition or increased prominence of other elements such as accountability, teamwork, and strategic focus.

Culture shift does not just happen. It requires comprehensive, planned interventions over long periods of time—interventions that bring congruence to institutional goals, reward systems, hiring practices, patterns of communication, and policies. The formation of initial institutional cultures is neither conscious nor deliberate, but the shift to a desired culture must be so. Patience and consistency are required in large measure.

The process of culture shift is uniquely local. There is no product to buy, no shortcut, no model to import. Each culture shift must integrate historic institutional strengths and the multiple cultures of the workforce with desired new elements. In shaping culture, academic health centers can, however, learn from each other and from organizations in other sectors. The work may be different in the corporate world, but human nature is the same and behavior is predictable.

Four steps seem to be critical in an attempt to reshape culture. First, the leaders must define clearly the characteristics of the desired culture, as well as behaviors that manifest the desired values and those that are no longer acceptable. Second, the entire senior management team must be committed and must "walk the talk," modeling institutional values in their daily interactions. The critical work of shaping culture and values cannot be delegated to middle management. People throughout the organization must be enrolled in the culture change and some, perhaps many, will rise to assume some leadership in the venture. But commitment and vigorous, continued participation cannot be optional for the senior team.

Third, all managers and leaders must be held accountable for their behavior. Accountability must be greater for those in high positions, and tolerance must be low for those who do not live the desired culture. A culture of openness will never occur if the dean or department chair is not taken to task for killing the messenger.

Finally, to sustain culture shift, the desired values and behaviors must be reflected in hiring practices, performance appraisal, advancement, and reward systems. Rewards and culture can and should reinforce each other. Introducing a new reward system without linking it to culture or trying to shape culture without implementing new rewards are recipes for failure.

Attempts to change culture are fraught with risk. Gilmore et al. (1997) suggest that there are four unanticipated side effects of any cultural agenda, and they argue that these effects are more intense when the organization is also being restructured. The first side effect is ambivalent authority, with leaders vacillating between authoritarian behaviors that are familiar and new behaviors that are more collegial. An example is ordering faculty and staff to be empowered. Another common side effect is polarized images, i.e., the tendency to cast the current and desired cultures as all-bad or all-good. Those who are uncertain about the culture shift or who wish to preserve the present may consider all proposed culture changes as bad or injurious to the mission; the most zealous champions of change may take a position that the current culture is bad, and the new unquestionably good.

In reality, of course, any culture has elements that are vitally important to the mission and others that may hinder or even preclude responsiveness to altered circumstances. This side effect is best countered by honest, open, and frequent discussion about the elements of current culture that must be maintained and the potential problems associated with the desired change, acknowledging, for example, that employees cannot be expected to take more responsibility without appropriate boundaries, information, and skills.

The third unwanted side effect is disappointment and blame, a prevalent pattern that tends to escalate with uncertainty. There is a tendency to blame faculty for the lack of truly progressive curriculum change when they are usually only responding to traditional reward systems that elevate scholarship more than the creation of new learning experiences or the sensitive, cost-effective care of patients. Avoiding labels such as "resistance" or "opposition" and using tools such as the "ladder of inference" to increase awareness can modulate blaming.

The fourth side effect is "behavioral inversion," a term that Gilmore et al. use to describe the slip back into old behaviors that occurs during transition, especially when uncertainty or anxiety are high. For instance, a vice president may exhort deans and department chairs to take more personal responsibility for fund-raising yet insist that any contact with major donors be preapproved. This approach signals mistrust and desire for control. To promote accountability, the vice president could instead set some boundaries for solicitation and ask to be promptly informed of any donor contact.

Behavioral inversions often stem from the fact that very few people holding top positions in organizations have much actual experience living and leading in the culture they propose. The leaders are learning new behaviors along with the rest of the organization's members.

## LINKING INSTITUTIONAL AND
## CULTURAL VARIABLES

*A house divided against itself cannot stand . . . Our cause must be intrusted to, and conducted by its own undoubted friends—whose hands are free, whose hearts are in the work—who do care for the result.*

—Abraham Lincoln

The work of leaders is to create the movement that represents change, while supporting managers who keep operations running. Whether the leader can be effective in this endeavor depends on his or her attitudes about people and the ability to lead "by the pull of inspiring values" (O'Toole 1995). Change always pushes against beliefs and assumptions that people hold. Major changes such as restructuring, continuous quality improvement, and the promotion of diversity and community outreach also challenge core values. Thus, the connection between change and culture must be considered in any change initiative.

The culture of an organization consists of the shared integrating norms, values, behavior patterns, beliefs, rituals, and traditions that give it structural stability, with the emphasis on "shared." The greater the degree of shared values and beliefs, the more stable the culture. Too much stability, too many shared beliefs, however, may restrict the organization's ability to welcome different talent, to look outward, to see the future, to challenge its own assumptions, to change. Today, the needed changes are of such magnitude that they will have no chance of succeeding without simultaneous and prolonged interventions to reshape institutional cultures. The culture, in turn, is linked back to leadership. Schein (1992) explains the relationship as mutual reinforcement: "Culture and leadership are two sides of the same coin in that leaders first create cultures when they create groups and organizations. Once the cultures exist, they determine the criteria for leadership and thus determine who will or will not be a leader."

Schein argues that creating and managing culture is the most important work for the top leaders of any organization and that, consequently, the ability to understand and work with culture is a key competency for anyone who seeks or holds a position of leadership. When the times require culture shift, there is a predictable mismatch between culture and leadership. The prevailing culture includes a model of leadership, complete with boundaries for acceptable behavior. Yet the magnitude of culture shift necessary today demands leaders who can break out from the old boundaries and model different ways of interacting, people who can move the organization beyond problem solving and fixing to transformation. Behaviors essential to transformation may be deemed unacceptable by those who cling to the old culture. Unless university administration and governance recognize and support culture shift and change, the leaders may be in peril. For sustainable culture change, the leaders must survive the period of transformation, and systems must be institutionalized to nurture and reward people and behaviors necessary to maintain the core values of the transformed organization.

## CONCLUSION

Six guidelines are recommended to those who seek to lead successful organizational change:

1. Nothing is more important than demonstrating respect for others. This does not mean politeness, but a deep respect that opens the leader's mind to different views and prompts him or her to reject paternalism and blaming.

2. One can never communicate too much. People need to hear over and over the rationale for, the details of, and the possible consequences of change. They also need opportunities to voice their feelings and concerns. The leader's communication should follow the 80-20 rule: 80 percent listening and 20 percent talking. And the talk should be clear, honest, and consistent.

3. Keep looking for ways to translate the environmental reality and the desired future in terms that speak to people: how might it look and feel and what might it mean for the individual in terms of gains and losses. Stories and analogy can be particularly useful in helping people link the change to their own lives.

4. Set aside regular time for silent reflection. Leading "by the pull of inspiring values" depends on awareness of one's own values, where they come from, and how they guide daily action.

5. Take time to maintain health and personal balance in body, mind, spirit, and relationships. The rewards of leadership are often intangible and deferred, and the risks are great. If health is compromised in

the effort to lead change, the leader's ability to continue the work is diminished.

6. Finally, keep it—all of it—in perspective. Regardless of the course of institutional change, the world will still turn, the sun will still rise and set, people and creatures will still be born and die, and nature will still be awesome and terrifying.

## WORK CITED

Bridges, W. 1991. *Managing Transitions: Making the Most of Change.* Reading, MA: Addison-Wesley.

Conger, J. 1997. How generational shifts will transform organizational life. In *The Organization of the Future,* eds. F. Hesselbein, M. Goldsmith, and R. Beckhard. San Francisco: Jossey-Bass.

Daniel, J.J. 1997. Why universities need technology strategies. *Change* 29 (July/August).

Drucker, P.F. 1993. Post-Capitalist Society. New York: HarperBusiness.

Gilmore T.N., G.P. Shea, and M. Useem. 1997. Side effects of corporate cultural transformations. *Journal of Applied Behavioral Science* 33(2).

Guskin, A.E. 1996. Facing the future: The change process in restructuring universities. *Change* 28 (July/August).

Hacker, A. 1997. *Money: Who Has What and Why.* New York: Scribner.

Kotter, J. 1990. *A Force for Change: How Leadership Differs from Management.* New York: Free Press.

Kouzes, J.M., and B.Z. Posner. 1992. *Credibility.* San Francisco: Jossey-Bass.

Lerner, J., ed. 1997. *Anatomy of a Merger.* San Francisco: Barrett-Koehler.

Martin, J. 1992. *Cultures in Organizations: Three Perspectives.* New York: Oxford University Press.

McFarland, L.J., L.E. Senn, and J.R. Childress. 1993. *Dialogues with 100 Top Leaders.* Long Beach, CA: Leadership Press.

Medical education in the United States 1976–77. 1977 *Journal of American Medical Association* 238:2761–2799.

Medical education in the United States 1986–87. 1987 *Journal of American Medical Association* 258:1005–1030.

Medical education in the United States 1995–96. 1997 *Journal of American Medical Association* 276:667–750.

Nair, K. 1994. *A Higher Standard of Leadership.* San Francisco: Barrett-Koehler.

O'Toole, J. 1995. *Leading Change.* San Francisco: Jossey-Bass.

Robbins, H., and M. Finley. 1996. *Why Change Doesn't Work: Why Initiatives Go Wrong and How to Try Again—and Succeed.* Princeton: Peterson's.

Schein, E.H. 1992. *Organizational Culture and Leadership* 2d ed. San Francisco: Jossey-Bass.

Smith, J.W., and A. Clurman. 1997. *Rocking the Ages: The Yankelovich Report on Generational Marketing.* New York: HarperBusiness.

Vanselow, N. 1986. Academic health centers: Can they survive? *Issues in Science and Technology* (Summer).

Wilson, M. 1984. *Leadership and Management in Academic Medicine.* San Francisco: Jossey-Bass.

Zemsky, R., and W.F. Massey. 1995. Toward an understanding of our current predicaments. *Change* 27 (November/December).

# LEADERSHIP AMID CHANGE: THE CHALLENGE TO ACADEMIC HEALTH CENTERS

*Gregory L. Eastwood, MD*

> *Nature knows no pause in progress and development and attaches her curse on all inaction.*
>
> —Johann Wolfgang von Goethe

THE WORRIED WISDOM OF HALLWAY CONVERSAtion, reinforced by the pronouncements of recognized experts, informs us at academic health centers that those who can't or won't change will not survive. Or perhaps worse, that those who do not change will be condemned to live out their careers in an atmosphere of increasing mediocrity.

There is an opportunity now for those academic health centers that are willing to change to emerge strengthened from the challenges we confront today. If we position our institutions well for the future, while preserving the values that we cherish, our institutions will not only survive but they will also thrive. To do this takes leadership.

Leadership defies precise definition, but we all think we know it when we see it. Clearly, it comes in many forms. One size does not fit all academic health

*Dr. Eastwood is the president of the State University of New York Health Science Center at Syracuse.*

centers. In the following paper, I review the challenges to leadership at academic health centers today. Then I explore some of the dimensions of leadership, distinguishing between leadership and management and indicating the kinds of people who can best assume leadership roles. Finally, I discuss some of the personal attributes and abilities of effective leaders, all the while recognizing that precise characterization of leadership is not possible.*

## LEADERSHIP FOR THE FUTURE IN
## ACADEMIC HEALTH CENTERS

*The viability of academic medical centers is threatened. These institutions have flourished since the 1960s, even managing to survive the shift toward prospective payment over the past decade, but many now are in danger of becoming severely compromised.*

—Jerome P. Kassirer, MD (1994)

The concept of the academic health center as an entity comprising a college of medicine, a teaching hospital, and usually one or more other health professional schools, is largely a creature of the post-World War II era in the United States (Eastwood 1994). Certainly, the past fifty years have seen academic health centers grow and thrive as a consequence of the remarkable developments in science, education, and health care that have occurred in this nation.

Although academic health centers are relative newcomers to academe, they trace their origins from two longstanding and venerable traditions: the university and the healing arts. The university began about a thousand years ago in medieval cities of Europe clustered around libraries. Its essence is the pursuit of truth, and with this pursuit of truth comes intellectual honesty, scholarship, and the commitment to the missions of learning, research, and service that we express today. The tradition of the healing arts has its origins in ancient times; it is one of compassion and caring for fellow humans.

We who are in academic health centers integrate these two traditions—

---

*Caveat lector. Although I have been bold enough to take on the task of writing about leadership in academic health centers, and thus might be presumed not only to be an expert but to also embody most of the qualities of leadership that I discuss, the reader must remember that it is much easier to write about a subject than to live it. I would be the first to admit that my own leadership repertoire may be deficient.

one, the pursuit of truth and scholarship, and the other, compassion and caring. This is so even as we confront the realities of what it takes for an academic health center to function: the competition for research dollars, the struggle to secure resources for student and other educational programs, and the imperative to create appropriate clinical services and alliances. Add to this mix the need to nurture individual careers; to understand and apply good business principles; to deal effectively with vexing ethical and moral issues; and to accommodate the interests of an endless array of loyal constituents, including students, faculty, patients, trustees, elected officials, and benefactors, and we have the remarkably complex, challenging, and consuming, but exciting and fulfilling, arena of the academic health center.

## Preserving Academic Missions and Values

*To many people, the environment is exceedingly unfriendly: the ground is unstable, and a storm has been stirring for some time, promising to get worse. Virtually every aspect of the health sciences is affected.*

—Gregory L. Eastwood, MD

Remarks to the graduating class
SUNY Health Science Center at Syracuse
May 16, 1993

Even as we attempt to build the clinical programs and relationships required of contemporary academic health centers, clinical science faculty are complaining that patient care demands do not allow them enough time to pursue scholarly and research activities. This situation is not only demoralizing, but it also jeopardizes the faculty's opportunities for promotion and tenure. Basic science and teaching faculty feel similar pressures, citing insufficient institutional support for research and education and the perception that the clinical mission is all that matters anyway. Inevitably, faculty criticize leaders for not allocating institutional resources properly and selling out to the god of clinical commerce.

The interdependence of the educational, research, and service missions is evident to most academic health center leaders. One of the responsibilities of leadership is to remind all interested parties that the interdependence of the missions is real and necessary. It is also to demonstrate that the teaching of students is informed by the clinical context and the discovery of new knowledge, that research thrives in a place that takes care of patients and teaches students, that the creative spirit energizes all activities, including the clinical programs, and that the expansion of the clinical enterprise at this time is meant to enable all purposes of the modern academic health center to prosper.

Linking the missions of academic health centers offers special challenges to leaders as we develop new clinical programs; form strategic alliances, partnerships, and mergers; and expand our clinical base through satellites, management service organizations (MSOs), independent physicians associations (IPAs), and the like. Among the questions that face us: Where do the students fit in? Who should have a faculty appointment and for what reason? What are the opportunities for clinical and outcomes research?

## Accommodating the Business Culture

One of our most vexing challenges at the academic health center has to do with a perceived clash between the values of business and the values of medical academia. E. John Rosenwald, Jr., an investment banker currently vice chairman of Bear, Stearns, & Co., observed, "The most important difference between business and academia is this: In business everything is dog eat dog. In academia it's just the reverse."

Although we appreciate the ring of truth to this statement, we also know that there are some basic differences in culture and values between business and academia. It seems to me that the essential difference is this: In business, the fundamental purpose is to make money. A clothing company's purpose is not to serve the public need for clothing; it is to make money by selling clothes. The fundamental purpose of an academic health center is to fulfill its educational, research, and service missions; money allows those missions to be fulfilled. In business, the product or service is a means of generating money. In academic health centers, money is the fuel that runs the programs that enable missions to be achieved.

Unquestionably, the current health care environment requires that the two cultures and their respective value systems work together. No one argues against the need to apply good business principles to running our academic health centers. Many people are deeply concerned, however, when they see the products of academic health centers regarded as commodities and any savings achieved at the expense of jobs and programs funneled away from the support of education, research, and clinical care, sometimes to meet the expectations of shareholders. The highly publicized, generous salaries of managed care executives have served to inflame this issue. Although these salaries represent a small portion of the total profits, the value system that produces them cannot be overlooked. Perhaps businesses of all sorts, including the new business of for-profit health care, can learn from E. Edwards Deming, the well-known management theorist, who advocates a new definition of the role of a company, namely, rather than making money, it is to stay in business and provide jobs through research, innovation, constant improvement, and maintenance (Walton 1986).

## Decision Making, Reorganizing, and Communicating

Academic health centers are feeling squeezed by both the need to do more with less resources and the demand to make decisions in a coherent, expeditious manner so the institution can compete successfully in the health care marketplace. Successful centers have reorganized to focus authority in a few people who set priorities, provide clear direction, and make decisions.

This approach is an enormous challenge to leadership because it is perceived as a threat to the traditional freedoms and prerogatives of the faculty and department chairs. Faculty usually have been selected, in part, for their independence of thought and action. Furthermore, departments and their chairs traditionally have enjoyed a great deal of independence. But managed care companies have little patience for a decision-making process that requires approval of every detail at all levels of the organization. Prolonged debate and "a thousand points of veto" is a sure path to failure in today's health care marketplace. Leaders must develop an organizational structure that includes a small decision-making body acting when appropriate on behalf of the entire academic health center, while at the same time maintaining communication with faculty and staff, both to solicit input and to disseminate information.

## Developing Partnerships and Alliances

Mergers, acquisitions, partnerships, alliances, affiliations, and networks entered into by hospitals, physician groups, and other health care entities have become a part of the daily agenda at most academic health centers. Although merger mania has been criticized (Andreopoulos 1997), such activities will probably continue. Leaders in academic health centers, therefore, need to know how to develop relationships with other organizations and how to deal with the consequences of those relationships. Partnerships and alliances, almost by definition, delineate those who are to be treated as friends and those who are to be regarded as the competition. These lines of demarcation, however, sometimes get blurred when it becomes necessary to develop agreements with a competitor in order to offer certain services or continue established programs.

When evaluating opportunities for partnership, the following advice seems sound:

1. The resources and skills of the partners should be complementary.
2. The partners should share similar values.
3. The partnership should further the vision and missions of the organizations.
4. The market effects of the anticipated partnership should be analyzed carefully. (Usually the term "market" is used in the context of the health care environment, but it also could apply to the potential pool of students or research programs (Ridky and Sheldon 1993).
5. The partners should like each other. Successful partnerships, like a marriage, are characterized by good personal rapport over time (Marszalek-Gaucher and Coffey 1990).
6. The partners should have a clear understanding at the beginning of the relationship of how to exit the partnership (Third Harvard Conference April 1997).

## THE DIMENSIONS OF LEADERSHIP

*Leadership is an essentially moral act.*

—A. Bartlett Giamatti

### Leadership vs Management

Leaders are people who provide a vision, articulate the vision to the people they are leading, and turn the dream into a reality. Leaders must be able to explain how each person fits into the plan, that is, what role he or she has in the fulfillment of the vision. Leaders are dissatisfied with the status quo; they see new areas that can be explored in more intuitive ways, they can excite people with their visions of the future, they shape ideas rather than respond to them (Ridky and Sheldon 1993; Marszalek-Gaucher and Coffey 1990).

Managers, on the other hand, maintain the status quo, making sure that the operations are running smoothly. They plan, organize, allocate, and oversee, working within the established framework. Managers are important in carrying out the plan for the organization and certainly are necessary to fulfill the vision articulated by leadership.

In practice, leaders, despite their high calling as ethereal visionaries, must have good management skills when they go about the day-to-day responsibilities of leadership. Leaders also often find themselves in the roles of coach and mediator. Clearly, the effective leader today is a blend of visionary, prophet, analyst, manager, coach, and mediator, with skills informed by practical knowledge and experience.

## Who Is a Leader?

"Being president of a university is no way for an adult to make a living," said A. Bartlett Giamatti (1990), former president of Yale University. This sentiment also may hold for chief executive officers of contemporary academic health centers. Academic health centers are complex, vital, and challenging places to work, and they offer exciting and fulfilling opportunities for leadership.

### Anyone Can Be Called On To Lead

Leaders in academic health centers certainly include the CEO (whether that person carries the title of president, chancellor, or vice president) along with vice presidents, provosts, deans, department chairs, directors, and the like. The fact is that almost anyone could be called on, under appropriate circumstances, to exert leadership. The skills and personal attributes of leaders are not the exclusive domain of people with high-ranking titles. In fact, for those leaders with administrative titles to be most effective, they must be able to bring about the synergy resulting from the rank and file—faculty, staff, and students—working together.

### Going Inside or Outside?

The question often posed in seeking new leadership is: Do we need an outside person or should we ask an insider to do the job? Outsiders typically bring fresh perspective and no baggage to their tasks. But they may need a period of acculturation, and their ultimate performance in the new environment is less certain because they are an unknown quantity. Insiders, on the other hand, know the organization, its people, and the issues they face; thus, their performance is more predictable. Their perspective, however, also may be predictable, and they may be burdened by preconceived notions others carry about them and the scars of past conflicts. Clearly, the answer to whether or not to bring in an outsider is situational and depends on the specific needs of the organization, the characteristics of the candidates, and the assessment of the fit between the people in the organization and the prospective leader.

## Preparation for Leadership

How do people become leaders in academic health centers? The traditional route to leadership for faculty with either an MD or PhD degree has been via academic achievement and reputation rather than by virtue of any particular training in finance or administration. On-the-job training has frequently been the answer to lack of experience in negotiating, managing people and money, or dealing with the press and other publics. This situation contrasts with the career path taken in business or even hospital administration, in which individuals usually receive formal training in management. Some leaders in academic health centers who have taken advanced degrees in business (MBA) or public health (MPH), and nearly all who have reached their positions after pursuing an academic career, find it useful to attend programs in management and administration for presidents, vice presidents, deans, department chairs, and other administrators offered by some universities and professional societies, such as those sponsored by the Association of American Medical Colleges.

## Characteristics of a Leader

Experience tells us there is no single formula for leadership. Leaders come in a large variety of sizes, shapes, colors, and ages; from different career stages, geographic origins, social standings; and with varying personal styles. They include a complex mix of personal attributes and abilities that, in those who have achieved success, seems right for them but may not work for anyone else. What are some of the characteristics that leaders often have and may improve on to do their jobs better?

## Motivation

Leaders usually are strongly motivated to do what they are doing. Sometimes the driving power is an ideal, sometimes a specific goal; sometimes the motivation is difficult to articulate. The motivating force provides direction, sustains the leader, lends credibility, and may in the final analysis be a raison d'etre. Although getting their way is important to most leaders, they are apt to agree with Cyrano de Bergerac who said, "A man does not fight merely to win."

## Energy

Most leaders have a great deal of energy and seem to be energized by what they are doing. Clearly, motivation and energy are related. But someone's energy level has little to do with someone's personality. Described in the simplest terms, energy can be said to describe a person's physical ability to express his or her motivation, which is perhaps a kind of internal energy. Whether a leader is flamboyant or reserved, talkative or reflective, tense or relaxed, he or she needs the energy to work hard and the stamina to sustain the level of activity required of most leaders in contemporary academic health centers.

## 'Know Thyself'

For the people in the business of leading others, it is helpful to know themselves: What motivates them? Why do they think and behave in certain ways? How do they think and behave? An understanding of life experiences, from childhood to the present, is often important. Insights into their own personalities—such as that afforded by the Meyers-Briggs personality types test (Briggs 1993)—allow them to understand their own preferences when dealing with situations and people. Do they renew themselves internally or by interaction with others? Do they take in information through the five senses or do they use a sixth sense, that is, their intuition? Do they make decisions in a logical, objective manner or in a personal, value-oriented way? Do they like life to be organized and predictable or spontaneous and flexible?

It is helpful for leaders to understand their own preferences and be able to behave in nonpreferential ways or compensate in some appropriate manner as situations require. For example, leaders typically have to interact with many other individuals professionally and socially; in other words, to be effective, a leader must be outward directed much of the time. Someone who is re-energized by the internal landscape may need to schedule time for reflection or limit interaction to a few close friends. Or a leader who thinks in broad concepts and sees the big picture but tends to neglect detail may need to pay more attention to the fine points when appropriate and, for good measure, select associates who can complement his or her abilities.

Effective leaders need to have some understanding of how they are perceived by others. A certain amount of reality testing is essential to maintain credibility and know how to deal with others.

> O wad some power the giftie gie us/To see ourselves as ithers see us!
> —Robert Burns, "To a Louse"

## Self-Confidence

Effective leaders typically are confident in their own abilities. That does not mean they are arrogant or foolhardy. It does not mean that they do not have normal anxieties and uncertainties. But it does mean that they not only understand themselves, but are also confident that they have the basic equipment to deal with almost anything within their purview. It also means that leaders, at some essential level, must be comfortable with themselves. If a person does not like or respect him- or herself, others will know it.

## Broad Perspective

Leaders are in a unique position to see the larger dimensions of an issue, and effective leaders use that perspective to advantage. They understand how the parts fit together to make something larger and how some of the parts can be aligned or rearranged to achieve certain purposes. They connect people and programs for the good of individual people and also to achieve the goals of the institution.

Leaders anticipate that an action over here can affect something over there. Because they see consequences of an action that others may not see, or may ignore, and they know that they ultimately may be responsible for the actions of others, they are inclined to think through the second- and third-order consequences of decisions. Effective leaders use their perspective to rise above parochial interests, balancing the needs of individuals and the prerogatives of the institution. Leaders must know their own capabilities, personalities, and limits.

## Integrity

Leaders convey to their constituents, by their actions and words, "You can count on me. What I say I will do to the best of my understanding and ability. I am truthful and trustworthy." At a recent Harvard Conference on Strategic Alliances in the Evolving Healthcare Marketplace, a panel of executive recruiters were asked to identify the characteristics of the ideal health care leader. They cited history of accomplishment, wise use of power, intelligence, and aggressiveness. Later, a group of physicians, uninformed by that discussion, responded to the same question by saying that the most highly valued qualities are integrity, honesty, trustworthiness, and truthfulness. From these conclusions we can surmise that academic health centers are best served by leaders who are aggressive, smart, honest, have accomplished a great deal, know how to use power, can be trusted, tell the truth, and leap over all obstacles in a single bound.

## Other-Directedness

The respect that most effective leaders have for others is evident in their speech and actions. They also have an understanding of other people and become skillful at assessing the abilities and motivations of others. Attention to such nonverbal cues as style of interaction, habits, punctuality, demeanor, mood, and dress helps them understand and work with other people.

Academic health centers, of course, intentionally attract bright, accomplished individuals who have a great interest in their own success. (Some are perceived as having big egos.) Leaders have every reason to respect such people and try to support them. However, in my experience, an ego that is perceived as big is sometimes actually a fragile ego protecting itself by some mechanisms its owner has found useful for success; these include such traits as aggressiveness, dominance, and the ability to establish turf. But the owners of these traits may in fact be a little insecure. What one might expect from a big ego in the literal psychological sense—magnanimity, tolerance, self-confidence, constructive use of power—may not be evident or may disappear once the walls of the fortress are threatened. The big egos inside an organization like an academic health center provide some of the greatest challenges to leaders, largely because the big egos contribute in great measure to the success of the organization and, in fact, are widespread among its leaders. As Pogo Possum said, "We have met the enemy and they is us."

## Ability to Communicate

The key to success in any leadership position is the ability to communicate in several different contexts. A leader must not only articulate his or her vision, but also be able to make sense of it to all concerned. Furthermore, the leader will need to articulate reality, and to do so repeatedly, often in the context of "getting things moving." Sometimes the leader must be able to understand that the reality is actually better than how it is perceived by others, and will need to point out this more optimistic state of affairs.

In today's competitive and threatening environment, it is easy for faculty and staff to become demoralized. Actually, most academic health centers have taken meaningful steps to deal with the threats, but sometimes the very steps have exacted their toll on staff. However, a careful analysis of the situation often identifies a number of objective measurements of successes that were achieved, such as improvement in hospital and ambulatory facility use rates, establishment of a reliable practice income, development of clinical networks, growth in extramural funding, a good reputation for research and educational programs, success in attracting high quality students and faculty, and regional and national recognition accorded to deserving individuals. It is important to remind people that the pain is for a purpose and, when you can, demonstrate the successes.

Leaders can find themselves in many different situations that require communication skills. They will have to address large audiences, lead or participate in smaller groups and committees, and meet with one or more individuals. Some situations will be scheduled; some will be spontaneous. Some will be professional; some will be social. The constituents can be endless—faculty, students, staff, alumni, friends, elected and appointed officials, local and national leaders. Some will be supportive; some will not.

Good communication implies a two-way relationship. Leaders need to develop lines of communication that allow them to tell others what they are planning and doing and also allow others to provide appropriate input. This two-way communication is an enormous challenge in large organizations. The trickle-down effect is not reliable. Discussions within the higher committees and boards of an institution do not assure that each member of the board will take the message to his or her constituents. Most effective leaders have developed a number of methods of communication that respect the lines of authority but still provide direct communication with all constituents. They include open fora, newsletters and other publications, retreats, leadership by "walking around," and simply being available to talk. Development of appropriate methods of communication is not the exclusive responsibility of the leader (whether the CEO, a vice president, a dean, or a department chair), but the leader must be visible and at the center of any existing institutional, school, or departmental channels of communication.

## Ability to Listen

The ability to listen, really a subset of the ability to communicate, deserves special mention. Clearly, the roles of listener and speaker change in any conversation, but leaders often find themselves in situations in which they are expected mostly to listen. Good listening requires the ability to focus and pay attention. Some leaders are naturally interested in what other people have to say; others will need to work on that skill. Listening is of value to both the sender and the receiver. People want to be certain that their point of view is heard by someone who is in authority and who cares. They may want something to be done or to be able to contribute to the decision-making process. The listener also benefits. Listening is one way to gather a great deal of information. Often good listening enables one to see a more complete picture. Good listeners must resist the temptation to interrupt and preempt the speaker; a listener won't learn much when he or she does all the talking. However, good listening skills do include good interviewing skills; sometimes, the listener may need to guide the conversation. Experienced listeners learn to watch for nonverbal communications, and they know that important information often comes at the end of a conversation.

## Ability to Organize

Good leaders are usually good organizers. Academic health centers have had to reorganize recently to become more efficient, focus authority in fewer individuals, and bring its structures closer to its functions. Along with these organizational changes have come changes in the traditional roles of some of the leaders. For example, the role of an academic department chair has moved from one with virtual autonomy to that of a team member who integrates the needs of departmental constituents with the direction in which the institution is moving.

Leaders have to understand these phenomena and learn to respond to them. But, in addition to a good sense of institutional organization, they also must be able to organize their own lives reasonably well. The former ability is important for the institution; the latter is important for the leader. And both are important if the leader and the people of the institution are to work together to accomplish something.

## Ability to Select Good People

Related to the talent for good organization is the ability of a leader to develop a senior leadership team that is effective. Most people in leadership positions quickly develop an eye for the talent they are seeking, either right at the home institution or imported from outside. Members of the team need to share the same values but have different perspectives and abilities that complement each other. Leaders should select people who see the future as they, the leaders, do, then lay out clear expectations for them, and give them the space to work effectively. Good leaders are not threatened by colleagues of superior talent; they understand that someone else's achievement reflects well on them. In the changing environment of health care, stability in the leadership team is a clear asset, and instability can be a competitive disadvantage. The leader must make every effort to develop a team in which members work well together, respect one another, and believe in the worth of what they are doing.

## Ability to Handle Uncertainty

In John LeCarre's novel *Tinker, Tailor, Soldier, Spy*, one of the characters says, "An artist is a bloke who can hold two fundamentally opposing views and still function," thereby paraphrasing a statement attributed to the writer F. Scott

Fitzgerald and applying it to the spy business. Many of us feel that leaders in academic health centers also are blokes who can hold at least two—and even more—views and still function. There is a great deal of uncertainty in our business these days, and leaders must be able to function despite this uncertainty. Many leaders in academic health centers are physicians. Although physicians frequently are criticized for not having good business sense, they are trained to deal with a high level of uncertainty and complexity when assessing and managing illness. Does this training make physicians better or less well prepared to deal with the specific issues of the current health care environment? You decide.

## Ability to Handle Praise and Criticism

Ralph Waldo Emerson's observation, "To be great is to be misunderstood," is unquestionably hyperbolic when applied to most of us in leadership positions; each leader at one time or another undoubtedly feels this way. Leaders are the focus for both praise and criticism, some deserving, some not. It is helpful to remember that both praise and criticism often reflect on the other person's need. Because leaders are in positions of authority and represent something larger than themselves, they may receive praise because of their position. Also, a certain amount of integumentary hypertrophy undoubtedly is a requirement for leadership positions in academic health centers. "If you can meet with triumph and disaster/And treat those two imposters just the same," wrote Rudyard Kipling, you will probably do okay in a leadership position.

## Ability to Act and Take Risk

Leaders must be able to act when appropriate and take measured risk, perhaps taking on more risk than may have been comfortable in the past. We act for the purpose of protecting or enhancing the missions of academic health centers, not for the primary purpose of competing. Competition is a reality of contemporary life and can be a consequence of our actions, but being driven solely by competitive pressures seems unwise.

Actions and risk-taking certainly apply to the directions the institution chooses to take, but they also apply to the personal risk of the leader. Leaders in academic health centers are vulnerable because they usually hold their positions at the pleasure of a board of trustees, a president, a dean, or someone else in power. A leader's standing can change very quickly, sometimes for reasons that are not always under his or her control. Nevertheless, a leader must always be capable of acting with forethought, although the action may also be a risk both to the institution and to the leader.

## Ability to Use Power

I believe that one aspect of power is the ability to accomplish what you want to accomplish. The power of the leader varies with the person in the leadership position and with circumstances. The ingredients of power include personal persuasion, credibility, and respect; control over the giving and taking of space, positions, and resources; and the ability to hire, fire, promote, reward, reorganize, or otherwise affect the fortunes of others. In the use of power, it is wise to keep something in reserve. It is rarely necessary to pull out all the stops and play the organ full blast.

## Ability to Make Difficult Decisions

A person who does not get some satisfaction in dealing with vexing, difficult issues, probably should consider something other than a leadership position in an academic health center. Decisions regarding hiring, dismissal, retrenchment, reorganization, and redeployment of resources are daily fare for most leaders. Most times, those decisions profoundly affect the lives of individuals. And the leader is likely to bear the ultimate responsibility for many of these decisions, whether or not a decision has different consequences than initially perceived. Thus, a leader must approach the process of making difficult decisions carefully but, if necessary, expeditiously. I have found that most decisions that I perceived as being difficult actually become relatively easy after I had learned as much as I could about the issue and applied sufficient cerebration to it.

A special word about firing: If one is going to reorganize and develop an effective team to get the job done, it is inevitable that some people have to be hired and regrettable that some will need to be fired. The hiring usually is the fun part. Firing someone is perhaps the most uncomfortable action a leader is required to take. Nearly all decisions a leader makes involve balancing the interests of individuals and the interests of the institution; this also applies to the decision to fire. When push comes to shove, however, the interests of the institution must prevail. A principle attributed to Dr. Eugene Stead, "A faculty member has to be worth the trouble he causes," applies to nearly all personnel in an academic health center. When, after careful consideration (it may take a few hours or it may take months), the decision is made that someone is not worth the trouble he or she causes, then it is time to let this person go, and to do so as humanely and expeditiously as possible.

The advice of Sun Tzu, the third century B.C. Chinese military strategist and putative author of *The Art of War*, applies to dealing with individuals being dismissed. Says Sun Tzu, "A surrounded army must be given a way out," and "When people are desperate, they will fight to the death." In other words, give the person being dismissed as much choice as possible, but make certain that he or she understands that what is not negotiable is the dismissal.

I have found the comment of a distinguished senior administrator reassuring when I must contemplate such personnel matters. "I never regretted firing someone," he said. "However, I have regretted not firing someone."

## Personal Style

*Be wiser than other people if you can, but do not tell them so.*

—Lord Chesterfield

Personal style is so unique and variable that it would be foolish to prescribe any one style, or even a menu of styles, that a leader should have. One's style includes the expression of personal attributes and abilities. But the style and skills of a leader may differ according to the needs and culture of the organization. One institution may need an established leader, another a more entrepreneurial one; one may need a leader who inculcates his or her ideas throughout the institution without much fanfare; another organization may need a leader with a more flamboyant personality.

Regardless of a leader's personal style, however, I believe that leaders are well served to adopt the following elements of style:

1. Try to treat everyone with respect, regardless of the other person's point of view, attitude, or capabilities.
2. Try to be approachable. Being approachable has more to do with a sense that people develop about you from explicit and implicit cues than a matter of what your calendar allows you to do.

3. Try to make others feel valued. Be known as someone who gives credit. If someone else got the job done using your idea, that's okay; the job got done. Running an academic health center is a team sport.

## A PARTING NOTE

Although most leaders derive a great deal of personal satisfaction and fulfillment from what they do, occasionally the responsibilities of leadership can seem unduly burdensome. At such times, I find it reassuring to remember a message that was transmitted to me by Rabbi Milton Elefant during my inauguration as president of the SUNY Health Science Center at Syracuse several years ago. The message: "Do not feel totally, irrevocably responsible for everything. That is my job. Love, God."

## REFERENCES

Andreopoulos, S. 1997. The folly of teaching-hospital mergers. *New England Journal of Medicine* 336.

Birnbaum, R. 1992. *How Academic Leadership Works. Understanding Success and Failure in the College Presidency.* San Francisco: Jossey-Bass.

Briggs, I.B. 1993. *Introduction to Type.* 5th ed. Palo Alto: Consulting Psychologists.

Commission on the Academic Presidency. 1996. *Renewing the Academic Presidency. Stronger Leadership for Tougher Times.* Washington: Association of Governing Boards of Universities and Colleges.

Eastwood, G.L. 1994. The health science university and the new order in health care. In *Academic Health Centers: Missions, Markets, and Paradigms for the Next Century.* Edited by J.P. Howe III, M. Osterweis, and E.R. Rubin. Washington: Association of Academic Health Centers.

Giamatti, A.B. 1990. *A Free and Ordered Space. The Real World of the University.* New York: Norton.

Kassirer, J.P. 1994. Academic medical centers under seige. *New England Journal of Medicine* 331.

Marszalek-Gaucher, E., and R.J. Coffey. 1990. *Transforming Healthcare Organizations. How to Achieve and Sustain Organizational Excellence.* San Francisco: Jossey-Bass.

Ridky, J., and G.F. Sheldon, eds. 1993. Leadership in academic health centers. In *Managing in Academics. A Health Center Model.* St. Louis: Quality Medical.

Walton, M. 1986. *The Deming Management Method.* New York: Dodd, Mead.

# CONFRONTING THE REALITIES OF CREATING AN INSTITUTIONAL CULTURE

*Jane E. Henney, MD*

ONE OF THE MOST CRITICAL FACTORS INVOLVED in changing or reinforcing a culture is the leadership. It is the leader who reflects what is going on—or is going to go on—in the organization by setting a clear strategic direction, making certain that what he or she does reflects what he or she says, and reinforcing the rites and rituals of the organization that affirm leadership commitment to cultural change or affirmation.

Sometimes it means that the leadership must be very visible; sometimes it means working a bit offstage. But at all times it means that the leadership has a high degree of involvement everywhere success can happen. It means having a leader with a value system that is seen to be both ethically and legally sensitive by all members of the organization. It also means not expecting people to walk in lock-step but giving them a chance to become committed to the new strategic direction. If people cannot make this commitment, leave them behind, either through the attrition process or by not rewarding them in the system.

*Dr. Henney is vice president for health sciences at The University of New Mexico Health Sciences Center. This paper is excerpted from her remarks at the Annual Meeting of the Association of Academic Health Centers, Indian Wells, California, September 26, 1997.*

## ESTABLISHING A HEALTH SCIENCES
## CENTER

How did we do this at the University of New Mexico when we set out to create a new structure for our Health Sciences Center in July 1994 as a result of the vision of the university's Board of Regents. The regents were motivated by our risky position in the new, competitive health care environment, the potential onslaught of national health care reform, and the desire for more interdisciplinary activities among all the health components at the university. They really pushed the senior administration of the university, and then the health components, to organize together as a health sciences center with an administrator who would hold the title of vice president for health sciences. The regents saw the need for a more unified approach to the health sciences, a view not shared by all the colleges on the campus.

Each component of the academic health center, both clinical and academic, clearly has its own history and culture. In the clinical arena of our health sciences center, we now have the university hospital, the children's psychiatric hospital, a mental health center, a cancer center, and a children's rehabilitation hospital. Among the academic components are the School of Medicine, College of Nursing, and College of Pharmacy. All of the allied health instruction is done by linkage to the School of Medicine. We have a master's in public health program and we have a graduate biomedical program.

Creating a health sciences culture meant that we had to recognize all the values of the existing components, not by destroying those that were good but by overlaying them with a unifying mechanism. They all are relatively young, especially our School of Medicine. We had our traditions, and clearly we were interested in changing some of them. It became quite a feat to extend what we thought was beneficial and to leave behind others.

The School of Medicine is known for its creative, innovative, and energetic faculty. Many of the staff came out of the Indian Health Service, the Public Health Service, and the Peace Corps and have a very strong commitment to public service. And they have been pioneers of educational reform. Much of the student-based, problem-based, and interdisciplinary-based learning being done in the community came from this wellspring of community commitment.

The College of Pharmacy brought real strengths in curricular reform, and the College of Nursing brought real strengths in distance learning. I think the College of Pharmacy was very interested in becoming a part of the health sciences campus. They had not felt well-treated on the main campus, and saw many opportunities for research and academic alliance with the School of Medicine. But the College of Nursing had always reported to the Main Campus. Now they had to report to us. They were very uneasy about the whole notion of being attacked by the 800-pound gorilla of the School of Medicine and only reluctantly became a part of the Health Sciences Center. I believe that over time they have come to share a different view of the alliance.

Our university hospital's origins were as an Indian hospital, and we have the strong commitment and legacy of a public hospital: caring for a diverse and often indigent clientele. However, over the years, our services have become very reflective of an academic institution; they are now highly developed in tertiary care services not just for the county but also for the state.

Two issues drove a lot of what we have ended up doing.

One, we wanted to foster the faculty's tradition of being involved in innovation and change. The downside of a faculty willing to take on a new curriculum at a moment's notice is the difficulty in keeping them focused on follow-through. For example, we would create one curriculum. Six months later, a group would come in and say, "I don't think we are doing this the right way. We ought to change."

Two, we wanted to respect our strong commitment to the state and the health of its citizens, particularly in the rural communities. We have a saying at our institution that we are not bound by the buildings that we live in, but we are bound by the borders of our state.

## STRENGTHENING COMMITMENTS AND ADDING INITIATIVES

We established a leadership council made up of the deans and the CEOs of the clinical components. At a series of retreats attended by faculty and staff members, we established seven strategic directions. These strategies were taken back to the whole organization. In brief, they commit us to (1) stay involved in rural health; (2) expand academic primary care initiatives; (3) look for opportunities for interdisciplinary initiatives in both the education and the clinical arena;

(4) look at research that is more programmatically driven and that could truly benefit the health of the people of New Mexico (we had a portfolio that was largely driven by RO1 research); (5) look at issues that would drive our development of a model academic health care delivery system for our state; (6) look at all of our operating systems; and (7) look at all of our information systems. These last two strategies concern the infrastructure, but if you do not get them right, you cannot do anything else.

We identified managers for each of the strategies. Each undertaking was co-chaired by faculty and staff, with membership in these groups open to anyone who wanted to attend the meetings. One example: Our rural health group meets every Monday at 7 in the morning. They started out meeting in a sort of an expanded broom closet. Now the meetings cannot be contained in some of our largest conference rooms. People come from all over the state, from outside the institution, from the Department of Health, and from schools across the campus to meet every two weeks to look at the way we are designing initiatives in rural health.

The groups are truly wide open because we did not want to marginalize any of the activities. The strategies must be able to cross-cut the entire organization and be very fluid. They also must have strong leadership from the top so that they will always be moving ahead. To assure this kind of leadership, we appointed members from the leadership council to meet with each group—not as leaders—but as advocates to help them with problem-solving. If the groups need help and guidance along the way, they can also come back to the leadership council. After three years, we are starting to institutionalize many of these activities.

Along the way, we have paid a lot of attention to communicating what we are trying to do through a number of mechanisms, ranging from a biweekly newsletter, to quarterly briefings, to retreats. And we are involving all levels of the organization whenever system changes are about to take place.

Nurturing creativity has also been very important to us. In studying businesses who fail the year after they were most successful, I find that the failure appears to coincide with a lot of creative people leaving the company. These people may well have become the organization's center of discontent or disruption because they did not necessarily want to stick with what was going on. The lesson here is that we must capture the creativity that is going on; we must not lose hold of it. We must feed it and foster it. But we must not let it take over what we are trying to do within our normal line of business. This is our strategy at the Health Sciences Center in terms of educational reforms.

We have also established within our culture an ability to have fun and to interact outside of the workplace. We want to be sure that when our work offers us great challenges, we all know each other in different ways than just from butting heads over issues across the table. We have all kinds of social activities, including weekly concerts, picnics, and celebrations of significant achievement, thus creating environments in which people can get along in different ways.

We had always lived in a very heavily managed care market, but this year we went to a managed care market that was very capitated. Less than 10 percent of our business had been capitated in the past; we are now 60 percent capitated within one year. Now we use many of the strategies we learned by working together internally to try to cope with our external environment.

## CULTURAL CHANGE IN ACTION

Twenty-six task forces have been formed. A hard-driving clinical chair is in charge of coordinating our overall efforts. Faculty and staff are involved as co-equals. All of the health professions are included in this driving effort to totally change our system almost overnight. And, in the end, the outcome will all boil down to the kind of leadership we can exert.

# REFINING THE MISSION OF ACADEMIC HEALTH CENTERS

# THE CHANGING NATURE
# OF HEALTH PROFESSIONS
# EDUCATION

*John Naughton, MD*

OR MOST OF THE TWENTIETH CENTURY, HEALTH professions education has experienced unprecedented growth, development, expansion, importance, influence, and acceptance in America.

As we entered the second decade of the century, for example, medical schools started to evolve from proprietary teaching institutions into complex structures responsible for the education of medical students, graduate biomedical scientists, and graduate medical education (GME) trainees; the conduct of biomedical research; and direct involvement in patient care and community health. Most medical schools became colleges in universities that either owned or were affiliated with hospitals.

Then, with the end of World War II, the relationships of a medical school to its teaching hospitals, community, and university changed gradually, but dramatically. Many medical and health professions schools are now aggregated around the common theme of health education and organized as academic health centers.

Today, medical and other health professions education must deal with the

*Dr. Naughton is professor of medicine, physiology, social and preventive medicine, and rehabilitation medicine in the School of Medicine and Biomedical Sciences at the State University of New York at Buffalo. This paper was supported in part by The Robert Wood Johnson Foundation Grant: The Generalist Physician Initiative, No. 024254.*

dilemma posed by an excellent and superb medical education and health care system that exists side by side with a society that desires increased access to health care, reasonable cost of care, and a high level of consumer satisfaction.

Academic health centers include, at a minimum, a medical school and one or more other health professions schools and one or more teaching hospitals. A recent report by Blumenthal (1997) on the role of academic health centers in providing public goods indicates that 125 centers have met these minimum criteria. More typically, however, an academic health center comprises a number of associated health professions schools that work collaboratively with each other and with hospital and ambulatory facilities to conduct clinical training.

Table 1 reflects the diversity of health professions schools among members of the Association of Academic Health Centers (AHC). In addition to medical schools, approximately one-half of the academic health centers also have schools of nursing, allied health, graduate studies, and dental medicine; almost one-quarter have schools of pharmacy and public health; and less than one-twentieth have a school of social work, veterinary medicine, optometry, or law. Approximately one-half of the academic health centers own or apparently control a teaching hospital; those remaining are affiliated only with one or more hospitals or health care systems. Sixty-seven are affiliated with a major Veterans Administration Health Center (VAHC). Approximately 100 VAHCs, in turn, are affiliated with one or more of the nation's allopathic medical schools.

**Table 1**

**ACADEMIC UNITS BY SCHOOLS OF AHC MEMBERS (1996)**

| Academic Unit | AHC Member With Academic Unit |
| --- | --- |
| Medical | 105 |
| Allopathic (99) | |
| Osteopathic (6) | |
| Nursing | 64 |
| Allied health | 57 |
| Graduate studies | 50 |
| Dental medicine | 45 |
| Pharmacy | 30 |
| Public health | 24 |
| Social work | 4 |
| Veterinary medicine | 4 |
| Optometry | 2 |

The important role played by academic health centers in our nation was clearly recognized during the recent health care reform debate (Clinton 1994) when the Administration recommended universal, unified health care financing for the United States. Critics of the proposal suggested that the Administration's proposed amendment to the Health Security Act did not sufficiently appreciate the intricate dependence of health science schools and teaching hospitals on

Federal funding to support and conduct health-related education and research. Because major cost-shifting across multiple institutions occurs in any academic health center, the case presented to the President and Congress for fiscal support was often made under the guise of academic health centers, in general, rather than for individual schools or other health care organizations.

The failure of the amendments to the Health Security Act dramatically changed the situation for academic health centers. Rather than develop a national health care system that was both more regulated and also limited to one universal payor, as proposed by the President, the nation chose to maintain optimal autonomy and choice, with health care financing and education determined by competitive market forces.

This paper summarizes the activities reflecting the nation's support and commitment to advances in health professions education during the period 1910–1994, sometimes known as The Golden Era, and the changing health care scene since 1994. In the paper, I also speculate on health care changes that most medical and health professions schools will experience with the coming of the twenty-first century. Although it is too early to conclude unequivocally, it appears that a trend is emerging for Federal and state governments to purchase increased amounts of health care through commercial insurers. Under this approach, the share of funds allocated to health care is negotiated competitively through contracts between the public and private sectors with the providers of care.

An additional major approach to medical care that will become widespread before the Year 2000 is that of managed care, a mechanism designed to manage and reduce the cost of health care. Its introduction, combined with the effects of Medicaid, Medicare, and welfare reform, already reflects an acceleration in hospital mergers, the formation of integrated vertical systems of care, the onset of medical school mergers, and the start of downsizing the number of medical school enrollees and graduate medical education trainees.

## THE GOLDEN ERA (1910–1994)

The modern era of medical education has its roots in the Flexner Report (1910). This scathing document condemned the dominance of proprietary medical schools and an excess in the number of physicians, most with minimal for-

Table 2
EXAMPLES OF FLEXNER'S RECOMMENDATIONS
FOR REDUCING ALLOPATHIC MEDICAL SCHOOLS
COMPARED WITH CURRENT SITUATION

| | Number of schools | | |
|---|---|---|---|
| State | In 1910 | Recommended by Flexner | In 1997 |
| California | 9.0 (1 half) | 1.0 (1 half) | 7.0 |
| Illinois | 14.0 | 7.0 | 7.0 |
| Indiana | 1.0 (2 half) | 1.0 (1 half) | 1.0 |
| New York | 11.0 | 2.0 | 12.0 |
| Pennsylvania | 9.0 | 2.0 | 6.0 |

Note: In addition, California, Illinois, New York, and Pennsylvania have a total of five osteopathic medical schools.

mal education, and recommended a reduction in the number of proprietary medical schools as part of an approach to planned obsolescence. Table 2 summarizes the number of medical schools that were operating in California, Illinois, Indiana, New York, and Pennsylvania in 1910, together with the number Flexner recommended as ideal for 1910 and the number in existence in 1997. (Note that at the time of the Flexner Report, a half school was one limited to preclinical education. Two states, New York and Illinois, each had four postgraduate schools, probably the forerunners of today's graduate medical education.) California, Illinois, and Pennsylvania had fewer full schools in 1997 than they did in 1910; Indiana had the same number; and New York had more.

The nation in 1910 apparently was ready for the Flexner Report because, in short order, extensive changes took place. They included the following events:

- Approximately two-thirds of existing medical schools merged or closed.
- Commercial (proprietary) allopathic medical schools became unacceptable to the profession and the public.
- States established accreditation and licensing standards.
- Medical education became more standardized and access to medical education became highly competitive.
- The quality and status of the medical profession were enhanced.
- Medical schools either became intrinsic units within a university or closely aligned to a university. (Even in 1910, universities were willing to include medical schools, but unwilling to commit many resources to finance them.)

The Flexner Report reflected attitudes still relevant for contemporary educational and societal concerns. Flexner, for example, emp[hasized that a quality medical education required students to be well educated in the sciences basic to medicine. A strong scientific faculty did not yet exist. Although Flexner's interest was education, not research per se, subsequent generations of faculty did go on to help medical schools become more research intensive, especially as the post-World War II partnership developed between the National Institutes of Health (NIH) and the nation's universities and medical schools.

## Women in Medicine

Flexner did not see a need to establish medical schools solely to serve women, as three schools were then doing. His conclusion that, in general, access for women to medical careers need not be a concern, based on an enrollment in the years 1904 through 1909 of 1,264 women (5.7 percent), turned out to be faulty because it failed to perceive the important role that women could and would later contribute to the profession.

In addition, the Flexner Report evaluated the seven traditionally black medical schools. Total enrollment from 1904 through 1909 was 750 medical students. Flexner concluded that these graduates would remain in the South to treat African-Americans living primarily in rural environments. He recommended that five of the seven schools be closed, which did take place, and that two, Meharry and Howard Universities, remain open and be upgraded. Despite the socioeconomic and cultural issues that faced African-Americans in 1910, he thought two schools sufficient to attract qualified African-American students to serve the South's minority population. He was apparently unaware of a need for minority physicians in the North.

Influenced by the Johns Hopkins Medical School, Flexner also stated unequivocally that every medical school must control at least one hospital. Ultimately, Flexner's report achieved the Carnegie Foundation's intent to move medical education, the medical profession, and health care to a standard previously not achieved in society. Those aspects of the report that served school and university interests, especially the improvement of education and developing research programs, were successfully implemented; those that were not implemented remain largely unattended even to this day.

## Transformation (1910–1945)

The period from 1910 through 1945 can be described as one of significant transformation for the medical profession. The American Medical Association (AMA) and the Association of American Medical Colleges (AAMC) fostered medical school accreditation. Medical schools required collegiate preparation for medical education and became more selective in accepting students. Licensure boards were established in every state, national standardized examinations evolved, and formal approval of internships was implemented (AMA 1923). Ultimately, every allopathic physician performed at least one year of internship after graduation before entering medical practice. Medical schools, with rare exception, continued a mission limited to educating students prepared to practice clinical medicine. Although a limited number of outstanding hospitals initiated additional training opportunities, the expansion of graduate medical education began in earnest only after World War II. In the first list of approved residencies, published by the American Medical Association (1928), the ratio of interns to residents was 3 to 1.

The impact of World War II on medical schools and the medical profession was tremendous. The entire nation was mobilized for the war effort, with all medical students expected to enter military service after graduation. Education for the medical student was compressed to three consecutive calendar years compared with four years in the past. A large proportion of the existing practicing physician base was called to military service. These physicians, together with the recent medical school graduates, built on their experience in battlefield situations to expand the professional capacity and skill of the medical profession on a scale never before achieved.

## The Postwar Years (1945–1960)

Medical education experienced numerous profound changes in the postwar years. These included increases in the number of applicants to medical school; many, as veterans of the war, were, of course, older and more mature than applicants in the past. However, medical school enrollments increased from 6,000 students per graduating class in 1945 to only 7,300 in 1964 (Coggeshall 1965), even though the nation's population had increased rapidly in number.

By 1960 new missions and increased professional opportunities, which limited the size of a medical practice as each new scientific and technological advance came on the scene, resulted in a trend to the increased specialization and fragmentation of education and the profession. Thus, the number of medical school graduates available to enter general practice was gradually and consistently depleted.

In addition, in contrast to 1910, the nation now had too few medical schools and too few physicians. The Federal and state governments responded by providing funds to construct additional medical schools and provide incentives, leading to an increase in annual class enrollments from 7,500 to more than 16,000 students. Once this goal was achieved, the number of publicly supported schools exceeded that of private schools. But direct government involvement in medical education and health care was limited to supporting the Veterans Administration Health System (VAHS), the Public Health Service, the Department of Defense, the NIH, and a few other smaller Federal programs.

## Increased Government Involvement (1960–present)

The Federal government became increasingly involved in all aspects of medical education and health care from 1960 on. The VAHS had been formed in 1929. Until the end of World War II, its mission was limited to serving the medical and health care needs of veterans. Dr. William Middleton, who served as chief medical director from 1955 to 1963, advocated increased VAHS involvement in biomedical and rehabilitation research, and Congress formally approved the VAHS role in medical and health professions education in 1955. By 1996, the system was supporting 8,910 approved residency training positions, or 12 percent of the nation's pool of the Accreditation Council of Graduate Medical Education (ACGME) (Knapp 1997).

The Ransdell Act of 1930 had formally established the National Institutes of Health, which had its origins on Staten Island, New York, in 1889. In 1960, the Omnibus Medical Research Act mandated that NIH establish disease-related institutes and fund research grants to medical schools and universities. The impact of this legislation was the development by medical schools of a cadre of outstanding basic science and clinical investigators, most of whom were faculty members who also taught medical and graduate students. The NIH made the United States the unchallenged leader in biomedical research throughout the world and achieved a number of enunciated national priorities, especially the eradication of numerous preventable diseases.

Selected governmental involvements in the areas of medical and health professions education, biomedical research, and health care are summarized in table 3. Each legislative initiative had a major purpose and focus, and the integration of the intended activities into health education and health care facilitated the development of academic health centers.

At least nine major laws provided increased funding to medical schools from 1958 through 1976. These early initiatives encouraged an increase in medical student enrollments and in the number of medical schools, particularly in the South and West, the two regions in the United States rapidly gaining population. The Health Professions Educational Assistance Act of 1963 provided funds specifically to support other health professions, especially nursing and dental medicine; offered financial assistance to students in need; and established a loan forgiveness program for students whose debt levels exceeded a capacity to repay loans in a timely fashion.

The Health Professions Educational Assistance Act of 1976 provided special incentives to medical schools in the form of capitation related to the continued promulgation of needed public goods. Particular emphasis was again placed on encouraging more medical students to enter primary care, and funds were appropriated to construct educational ambulatory care centers.

Termination in 1973 of special appropriations to schools was accompanied, as could have been predicted, by annual escalations in tuition fees paid by students enrolled in these and other privately supported schools. In discontinuing the distress financing, the assumption was that medical students could assume higher debt levels because their professional incomes would be sufficiently high to repay them. Unforeseen was the possibility that the continued rise in physician income could cease (which, indeed, it has), thus limiting the rate at which students' loans could be repaid. As a result, students with large debts often choose more lucrative, higher-paying specialties in preference to a generalist career (Colwill 1992). An even greater concern is that many highly indebted students may bring an attitude of personal deprivation and professional unhappiness to the practice of medicine that can interfere with developing an optimal physician-patient relationship.

## Table 3
**FEDERAL INITIATIVES DESIGNED TO EFFECT CHANGE IN THE NATION'S HEALTH THROUGH MEDICAL RESEARCH AND EDUCATION**

| Year | Initiative | Recommendation |
|------|-----------|----------------|
| 1930 | Executive Order 53-95 | Reorganize three agencies to establish national network for veterans' health care |
| 1930 | Ransdell Act | Fund National Institutes of Health |
| 1958 | Bayne-Jones Report | Increase physician output; increase number of medical schools; advance medical research and education |
| 1959 | Bayne Report | Increase physician output; institute Federal program of student financial aid |
| 1960 | Omnibus Medical Research Act | Provide Federal support for biomedical sciences |
| 1960 | Boisfiuillet Jones Report | Increase Federal support of medical research; provide direct Federal support to medical schools and medical education |
| 1962 | Kerr-Mills Act | Fund health care for elderly poor |
| 1963 | Health Professions Educational Assistance Act | Expand enrollment in medical, dental, and other health professions schools by funding construction of medical schools and grants for school loans |
| 1965 | Medicare and Medicaid | Fund graduate medical education |
| 1966 | Health Professions Educational Assistance Amendments | Support construction for new medical schools; provide special grants to improve curricula and provide loan forgiveness |
| 1968 | Health Manpower Act | Continue to expand medical schools; assist schools in financial distress |
| 1970 | Health Training Improvement Act | Offer special project grants; provide emergency assistance to medical schools in financial distress |
| 1971 | Comprehensive Health Manpower Training Act | Provide capitation grants; continue and expand medical school construction; expand enrollment; support GME in family medicine |
| 1971 | National Cancer Act | Establish National Cancer Institute; provide funds to support free-standing comprehensive cancer centers |
| 1976 | Health Professions Educational Assistance Act | Fund capitation in relation to number of primary care residents; increase third-year enrollment to accommodate American students enrolled in foreign schools; construct ambulatory care and primary care teaching facilities; expand primary care training grants |
| 1983 | Tax Equity and Fiscal Responsibility Act | Change Medicare to prospective payment system; help teaching hospitals meet costs of complex health care; indirectly fund medical education costs |
| 1994 | White House health care reform proposal (fails) | Move toward less government funding and control of health care; encourage market forces and negotiated rates |

The Kerr-Mills Act of 1962, enactment of Medicare and Medicaid in 1965, and subsequent revised Medicare legislation in 1984 appear in table 3 even though the principal focus of these legislative acts was providing patient care. Kerr-Mills, the forerunner of Medicaid, provided funds for the elderly poor. Califano (1993) has reported that despite this intent, the vast majority of the funds were absorbed by five states with lower-than-average numbers of the elderly population. Medicaid succeeded Kerr-Mills and extended coverage to more of America's poor and to nursing homes. In terms of medical education, the enactment of Medicare was most significant because it provided funds to support supervising physicians in teaching hospitals and for GME. In 1983, according to reports prepared for the House Ways and Means Committee and the Senate Finance Committee, the Medicare legislation changed the reimbursement system from a cost-plus methodology to a prospective payment system; it also added a source of reimbursement—indirect medical education (IME) reimbursement—to help teaching hospitals absorb the costs related to providing the complex medical and health care typical of teaching hospitals. (The actual costs for education were not determined.) Today, the combined budget for Medicare's share of GME support approximates 6.6 billion dollars annually, one-third to support supervising physicians and residents and two-thirds for IME.

This movement toward providing health care financing for the nation's poor and elderly provided medical schools with additional resources for funding medical education and full-time faculty. The new influx of money to teaching hospitals to support patient care and graduate medical education provided the impetus for schools to become directly involved in patient care and to develop faculty practice plans.

Thus, over a span of more than fifty years, Congress enacted major legislation that, in the aggregate, gradually enunciated a comprehensive, multifaceted public policy in support of medical and health professions education, biomedical research, and health care for the nation's poor, veterans, and elderly. Medical schools, universities, teaching hospitals, and academic health centers benefited significantly from these important developments.

## Diversity in Funding

The diverse activities required to support a modern-day health professions school places a tremendous burden on its leaders to develop a cohesive strategy that protects its primary mission—education. Table 4 depicts the sources of mean funds, by category, that support the expanded missions of 125 allopathic medical schools in 1996 (AAMC 1995), 54 dental schools in 1994 (ADA 1995), and 63 academic health center-related nursing schools in 1992 (AACN 1993). State-appropriated funds primarily flow to publicly supported schools for educational programs. Hospital funds are developed through the allocations that support GME, from direct operating funds to other institutional resources. Grants and contracts flow primarily from NIH and the National Science Foundation (NSF), pharmaceutical organizations, and private industry to faculty investigators. Faculty practice funds are generated through direct patient care and consultations. Of the 54 dental schools, 35 are publicly supported, 13 are private, and 6 are state assisted.

The data also give an indication of the importance of research grants, contracts, and faculty practice plans to the current operational support of medical and dental schools. If budgetary allocations are related to an institution's mission, it is important for institutional administrators to determine how the research and service missions relate to a primary mission of education and what boundaries (if any) should be placed on developing these resources in relation to the funds necessary to provide an outstanding educational experience. The clinic revenue includes fees generated by faculty practice and the rendering of care by supervised students. The item "other" includes gifts and other sources of dental education support. Clearly, most dental schools are more dependent on tuition and state-appropriated funds than are medical schools.

Table 4
**SOURCES OF MEAN FUNDS CURRENTLY SUPPORTING
ALLOPATHIC MEDICAL, DENTAL, AND NURSING SCHOOLS**

| Funding Source | Medical School (1996) $000 (mean) | % | Dental School (1994) $000s (mean) | % | Nursing School (1992) $000s (mean) | % |
|---|---|---|---|---|---|---|
| Tuition | 9.2 | 5.6 | 56.2 | 30.5 | – | – |
| State | 22.6 | 13.3 | 76.2 | 40.4 | 2.9 | 81.0 |
| Hospital | 31.7 | 14.1 | – | – | – | – |
| Grants, contracts | 50.2 | 18.5 | 3.4 | 1.6 | 0.7 | 19.0 |
| Faculty practice | 78.2 | 32.0 | 43.4 | 23.8* | – | – |
| Other | 32.0 | 16.5 | 6.9 | 3.7 | – | – |
| Total | 235.0 | 100.0 | 186.1 | 100.0 | 3.6 | 100.0 |

*Also reflects clinical income earned from student supervision and teaching.

In contrast, nursing schools are supported primarily by institutional funds. The American Association of Colleges of Nursing (AACN) classifies 63 of its members as academic health center-related and 165 as nonrelated. In 1992, AACN reports, academic health center-related schools had a median annual budget approximately fourfold that of nonacademic health center-related nursing schools. The specific distribution of research funds was not reported, but an extrapolation of the information available suggests that the median for an academic health center school was approximately $690,000. A total of 255 schools, 63 academic health center-related and 192 nonrelated, permit nurses to earn additional salary through faculty practice. No fiscal data were available to evaluate the impact of practice revenue on the conduct of the educational programs (AACN 1993).

## Significant Reports on Medical Education

The increased participation of the Federal government in biomedical research, medical schools, and medical and health care since 1960 was stimulated by the interests of educational advocates, their representative organizations, and the perceived needs of the American public. Three major reports, published in the mid- to late-1960s, for example, provided direction to academic medicine. They were the reports of the Citizens Commission on Graduate Medical Education for the AMA (Millis 1966); the Planning for Medical Progress Through Education Report (Coggeshall 1965); and the report on the Role of the University in Graduate Medical Education published by the AAMC's Council on Academic Societies (Smythe et al. 1968).

*The Millis Report.* The AMA's Citizens Commission was made up of ten prominent members from the public and professional sectors, three of whom were physicians. Among AMA's charges to the commission were two particularly pertinent to academic health centers. One was "the preponderance of the narrow specialty viewpoint in decisions affecting the pattern of graduate medical education." The other was that "the general nature of graduate medical education is based largely on the same fundamental concepts that determined the essential characteristics of graduate training programs as initially devised more than thirty years ago."

The commission forwarded fourteen recommendations to the AMA

Board of Trustees. In so doing, the commission:

- Recognized the interaction between medical education and patient care that was required for GME to be successful, and recommended that GME be treated as a corporate, not a programmatic, responsibility.
- Acknowledged the important role of medical specialty societies and residency review committees, but saw a need for a single national accreditation organization comparable to the Liaison Committee on Medical Education (LCME).
- Expressed concern about the erosion of primary care medicine, and emphasized the need to nurture and encourage generalism.

The commission also forwarded additional recommendations supporting the following objectives:

- Termination of rotating and mixed internships and establishment of specialty residencies that medical school graduates can enter immediately after graduation from medical school.
- Provision by medical schools of the necessary foundation to be generalists.
- Involvement in—but not control of—the GME process.

Had all of the commission's recommendations been implemented, the existing situation with medical student and graduate medical education might be vastly different. Although a national consensus is gradually evolving that GME be governed corporately, it was not until 1980 that the ACGME (1982) promulgated guidelines requiring a sponsoring institution for programs conducted in multi-institutional settings. The recommendation that rotating and mixed internships be discontinued was readily implemented even though it was inconsistent with the two charges involving academic health centers presented to the commission by the AMA. Predictably, the commission's recommendations served to strengthen and accelerate the increased specialization and fragmentation that continue to erode generalism as a value in education and health care.

*The Council of Academic Societies.* In 1968, the Council of Academic Societies sponsored a conference on medical education. The core leadership committee included a dozen major academic leaders; the working conference was attended by approximately 155 other academic leaders (Council of Academic

Societies 1968). Its recommendations on two matters differed considerably from those of the Millis Report, as follows:

- University medical school faculty should provide the same leadership for GME that it provides to medical student education.
- Universities should be encouraged to introduce educational innovations in GME.

The report also emphasized the need for a single accreditation organization, but did not explore in detail the issues of generalism and specialization.

*The Coggeshall Report.* The Coggeshall Report should be required reading for every academic leader and policymaker. Developed by the AAMC executive council, it is cohesive, inclusive, and visionary. Indeed, it largely accounts for the events that subsequently transpired in medical education and health care. However, the AAMC moved in a different direction. Rather than move more closely to the university, as recommended by the executive council, AAMC added two other units, the Council of Teaching Hospitals and the Council of Academic Societies, to its organization.

Coggeshall grouped the vast array of social change occurring in the United States and estimated the future impact of such change on medical education and health care. Table 5 shows the arbitrary level of importance that the Coggeshall report accords to social changes and the implications for medical education in 1965, and the level of importance accorded by the author of this paper on the 1995 implications. The greater the number of plus signs, the more important the change. "Scientific growth," for example, receives three pluses for 1965 and two for 1995. The differences in these two ratings do not suggest that growth would not occur in 1995, or that science was less important in that year. The rating system does indicate, however, that in 1965 the knowledge explosion was in its fundamental stages of growth and that scientific advance was developing rapidly. This same degree of change was not anticipated to occur in 1995 and beyond.

The nation's academic health centers have done an admirable job of educating more and better-prepared physicians and other health professionals. The number of physicians in 1995 and projected for the future will probably decrease to a yet undetermined level. However, as the health care industry continues to grow, personnel requirements will call for more people with less, rather than more, professional education. The immediate impact is on medical education,

Table 5.
## IMPLICATIONS OF EMERGING SOCIAL CHANGES FOR MEDICAL EDUCATION IN 1965 AND 1995

| Changes | Relevance* 1965 | 1995 | Implications | Relevance* 1965 | 1995 |
|---|---|---|---|---|---|
| 1. Scientific growth | +++ | ++ | 1. Scientific growth | + | +++ |
| 2. Population changes | ++ | +++ | 2. Population changes | +++ | +++ |
| 3. Individual expectations for health | + | ++ | 3. Individual expectations for health | + | +++ |
| 4. Increased demand for health care | + | ++ | 4. Increased demand for health care | + | +++ |
| 5. Increased specialization | + | +++ | 5. Increased specialization | + | +++ |
| 6. Technological achievement | + | +++ | 6. Technological achievement | + | +++ |
| 7. Institutionalization of health care | ++ | + | 7. Institutionalization of health care | + | + |
| 8. Team approach for health care | + | +++ | | | |
| 9. Increased number of physicians | +++ | + | | | |
| 10. Increased number of health personnel | + | +++ | | | |
| 11. Expanded government role | +++ | + | | | |
| 12. Rising costs | + | +++ | | | |

* Coggeshall (1965)

but over a period of a few years, the need for other highly educated health professions will also diminish.

Of special note is the council's emphasis on medical schools devoting more attention to the nation's needs. In many ways, helping meet the nation's needs should be regarded as an as-yet unmet goal, and one to which academic health centers and their professional organizations must give increased emphasis.

In 1965, the AAMC was the sole organization speaking on behalf of academic medicine. Thus, Coggeshall's vision appeared realistic and achievable. It is regrettable that organized medicine today, especially its academic components, often does not speak with a single voice. There is reason to be optimistic that this situation might change; in 1997, for example—and for the first time in recent history—six major professional organizations signed a joint letter to the House Ways and Means Committee supporting the Institute of Medicine's position on the establishing a GME Trust Fund. The six organizations are the AMA, AAMC,

AHC (Association of Academic Health Centers), AOA (American Osteopathic Association), AACOM, and the National Medical Association.

*Medical schools and health manpower.* Medical education is always at the core of discussions on the development of medical and health professions manpower. Even in the early 1960s, many skeptics were expressing concern that the nation's efforts to increase medical personnel were overzealous. In recent years, a number of studies have consistently indicated that by the Year 2000 there will be a substantial excess of physicians. The Graduate Medical Education National Advisory Committee (GMENAC 1980) has estimated the excess at 145,000, Weiner (1994) projects an excess of 163,000, and the Federal Council on Graduate Medical Education has estimated the surplus at 105,000. In general, there was not sufficient information to predict the effect of managed care; if such estimates could have been made, the surpluses would have been much larger.

Most health-policy experts agree that, to improve the health care system, the nation should be educating more generalists and fewer specialists. Whitcomb (1995) and Cooper (1994) have alerted the medical-education community to the fact that the projected physician excess is not limited solely to an excess number of specialists but to a projected excess of all types of physicians; the actual depletion in the number of available generalists will be less than originally projected by health analysts. However, Cohen and Whitcomb (1997) indicate that despite earlier projections, the emphasis on educating an increased number of generalists per graduating class must continue well into the next century.

*The Pew Report.* The Pew Health Professions Commission Report (1995) also addressed critical challenges to revitalizing the health professions for the twenty-first century. The Commission recommended the following actions:

- Decrease the number of medical student enrollees by 20 to 25 percent by the year 2005.
- Close some medical schools.
- Reduce the number of ACGME-approved resident positions to 110 percent of the number of American medical student graduates (the Canadian model).
- Distribute GME positions: fifty percent to generalist disciplines and fifty percent to specialty disciplines.
- Conduct at least twenty-five percent of the training experience at off-site locations.

- Develop an all-payor system to finance GME.

*The Institute of Medicine Report.* The recommendations of the Pew Commission were further amplified by the Institute of Medicine's (IOM 1997) report submitted to the House Ways and Means Committee. This report contained the following recommendations:

- Stop establishing new allopathic medical schools. (The report is mute on the issue of closing existing schools and the roles of osteopathic medical schools.)
- Do not increase medical school enrollment. (It was mute about the possibility of reductions in enrollment.)
- Reduce the number of funded GME positions provided that substitution funds are available to support alternative care providers.
- Improve career advice for medical students and GME trainees.
- Determine the relationship of physician supply to other workforce issues.
- Expand the definition of GME fields.

## ON TO THE 21ST CENTURY

As health professions educators enter the twenty-first century, the need to restructure most educational programs will grow. The task will be more challenging and difficult than it was in 1910. Medical student education and GME do not relate to, and interdigitate with, one another as well as many people seem to believe. A recommendation to decrease the number of medical students and to close or merge medical schools precipitously may aggravate rather than solve the GME problem.

At present, almost 16,000 students are enrolled in allopathic medical schools, and approximately 2,000 students in osteopathic medical schools. In 1995, there were 84,968 ACGME-approved residents funded in the United States (table 6) or about 12,000 to 14,000 more trainees per year than graduate from American allopathic and osteopathic medical schools (ACGME 1982). The excess numbers of GME trainees either represent American students enrolled in foreign medical schools or immigrants to the United States. Of the latter, approximately half immigrate from India, Pakistan, or the Philippines. Any public policy that is developed must relate the GME pool to the production of future

## Table 6
## NUMBER OF PROGRAMS AND RESIDENTS, 1981 AND 1995,
## COMPARED TO WHITE HOUSE GOALS FOR 1997

|  | 1981 | | 1995 | | Projected 1997 | |
|---|---|---|---|---|---|---|
|  | Programs | Residents | Programs | Residents | Programs | Residents |
| Allergy and immunology | 73 | 203 | 84 | 254 | 50 | 166 |
| Anesthesiology | 161 | 2,930 | 154 | 4,681 | 92 | 3,128 |
| Colon and rectal | 26 | 40 | 31 | 53 | 17 | 31 |
| Dermatology | 99 | 814 | 105 | 850 | 60 | 508 |
| Emergency medicine (1982) | 63 | 885 | 112 | 2,812 | 56 | 1,249 |
| Family medicine | 385 | 7,004 | 455 | 9,261 | 551 | 9,783 |
| Internal medicine | 443 | 17,537 | 416 | 21,071 | 585 | 26,916 |
| Neurology | 123 | 1,236 | 122 | 1,536 | 71 | 772 |
| Neurosurgery | 93 | 608 | 99 | 846 | 57 | 415 |
| Nuclear medicine | 93 | 197 | 82 | 154 | 50 | 111 |
| Obstetrics-Gynecology | 304 | 4,705 | 272 | 5,007 | 383 | 6,793 |
| Opthalmology | 155 | 1,543 | 137 | 1,602 | 80 | 935 |
| Orthopaedics | 180 | 2,667 | 158 | 2,872 | 95 | 1,679 |
| Otolaryngology | 112 | 995 | 108 | 1,211 | 62 | 632 |
| Pathology | 314 | 2,413 | 185 | 2,788 | 113 | 1,428 |
| Pediatrics | 245 | 5,961 | 215 | 7,354 | 300 | 9,369 |
| Physical medicine and rehabilitation | 65 | 605 | 81 | 1,129 | 44 | 573 |
| Plastic surgery | 105 | 389 | 101 | 461 | 60 | 260 |
| Preventive medicine | 33 | 166 | 89 | 434 | 15 | 69 |
| Psychiatry | 223 | 4,336 | 201 | 4,919 | 116 | 2,881 |
| Radiation oncology (1988) | 85 | 470 | 83 | 506 | 48 | 288 |
| Radiology | 221 | 3,135 | 206 | 4,090 | 122 | 2,365 |
| Surgery | 331 | 8,105 | 269 | 8,221 | 161 | 4,721 |
| Thoracic surgery | 98 | 281 | 92 | 346 | 54 | 186 |
| Urology | 153 | 1,027 | 122 | 1,094 | 74 | 592 |
| Transitional year (1983) | 197 | 1,377 | 167 | 1,416 | 101 | 861 |
| TOTALS | 4,380 | 69,629 | 4146 | 84,968 | 3,417 | 76,711 |

physicians by American medical schools. The public-policy community and the medical-education community must work cooperatively and constructively to determine whether GME should continue to be a surrogate for the care of the poor as well as the final professionalization phase of a physician's education.

Medicine and other health professions remain attractive careers for many of the nation's brightest and most creative youngsters. We should have learned a valuable lesson in the 1970s when alternative solutions were developed for qualified students who couldn't gain access to American medical schools. Medical education and policymakers may understand the relationship of medical education to physician personnel, but it is of utmost importance that we take into account the political and public confusion that people have about these issues. Most citizens simply don't understand the rationale for maintaining medical school enrollments at levels almost 35 percent below the number of available ACGME-approved GME positions. At some point, medical school enrollments and GME programs must be reconciled and coordinated, replacing the disparate efforts of today. Throughout the nineteenth century, even when GME was not related intrinsically to basic medical education and licensure, there were an excess of GME positions. In 1964, for example, 60 percent of all GME trainees in New York City were of foreign origin (DHHS 1997).

The Federal government, through the Council on Graduate Medical Education, has attempted to analyze the complex issues surrounding medical and health professions education, health personnel issues, and the availability of health care. Many states have developed advisory bodies devoted to GME, and leadership on this concern has emerged from organizations such as AHC and AAMC. Still, a sufficiently coordinated and cohesive approach has yet to evolve. Although a single all-payer system at the Federal level may not come into being, it is conceivable that, if they so desire, individual states might be able to achieve this goal on their own.

As the twenty-first century approaches, public attitudes toward medical and health professions education will probably change greatly. The age of unfunded mandates will be replaced by voluntary choices made at regional or state levels. More important, political and economic forces will coalesce to prevent the seemingly paradoxical behaviors characterized by differences in the stances taken by Congress, professional societies, medical schools, and teaching hospitals.

Medical and health professions education exert important influences on many aspects of American life that earn academic health centers and their professionals enormous credibility, acceptance, and respect for their leadership and contributions to the well-being of society. The largesse provided to academic health centers by many different programs and agencies has helped develop a world-renowned infrastructure.

Can academic health centers redefine and restructure themselves as individual institutions tied into a network of academic health centers still valuable to American society? A few years ago, economist Eli Ginzberg (1995) and the Macy Foundation conducted a conference to determine how medical schools and academic health centers planned to respond to changes.

At the Macy Conference, held in the midst of the health care reform debate in 1994, participants believed that a universal payor system and increased Federal regulation would become the law of the land. Whatever the outcome of the ongoing debate on health care, however, conference participants held that the perpetuation of fee-for-service medical practice would diminish and be replaced by a system of managed care designed to negotiate rates based on community health outcomes rather than episodic care rendered to individual patients.

To determine both the current status of fiscal support and the outlook for the future if this scenario came to pass, case statements for twelve representative medical schools from throughout the United States (eleven allopathic and one osteopathic) were presented. The assumptions were as follows:

- Public fiscal support of medical and health sciences education, GME, biomedical research, and patient care will decrease.
- Fiscal control for the above functions will be shared by the Federal government, state governments, and the business community.
- Physicians, hospitals, health insurance payers, and large investors will vie for control of health care.
- Academic health centers, through their unique roles related to provision of patient-related services, will begin to work more directly with payors in addition to the affiliated teaching hospitals.

Three schools were heavily dependent on practice plan income. Three were using a public hospital as the principal teaching hospital. Three had a major research program. Three had a predominantly regional role. Regardless of classification and current resource base, each school saw its major future strategy to be that of securing of larger and larger amounts of patient revenue.

In analyzing the twelve case statements, conference participants were impressed by the lack of attention the institutions had directed to their core missions and functions. Accordingly, the Macy Commission recommended that medical schools give the highest priority to strategic plans that reexamine and redefine the institution's missions, and align activities to support the mission.

An institutional mission statement, by definition, must reflect the mission's individual sense of being and worth. But it must also emphasize its relationship to patients and community. It is here that institutions have the opportunity to establish a charter that aligns an institution's spirit to the needs of the nation as well as to other constituents and consumers. In today's chaotic situation, the charter should define the institution's relevance and commitment to the concept that education is a required public good: It helps people become independent thinkers and learners, and more important, to become servers of society. The mission can also be an instrument that defines its providers and elucidates what students, patients, and community represent its consumers.

Mission statements become meaningless and ineffective unless accompanied by a statement of values that represent the commitment to attaining the mission and a statement of vision that can empower, and define the role of, its leadership. And, of course, the institution, at all levels, must lay out an annual work plan designed to meet mission, vision, and value.

In his review of thirty operational multidisciplinary GME consortia for the Council on Graduate Medical Education (COGME), Cox (1997) recognized that many of these organizations were conducting operational affairs unrelated to their mission statements. Such incongruity may exist in many other academic health centers in the United States.

In *Academic Medicine as a Public Trust* (Schroeder et al. 1989), the authors recognized the significant contributions of academic medicine to scientific discovery, new knowledge, medical technology and pharmaceuticals, and decreased death rates, particularly those from cardiovascular disease and stroke. However, the authors suggest that academic medicine was not fulfilling one of its missions, namely, to improve the health of the public. They single out five areas of failure, as follows:

- Failure to influence a reduction in cost of medical care.
- Failure to eradicate the nation's substandard indexes of public health.
- Failure to eliminate the maldistribution of the uneven quality of care among our citizens.
- Failure to help correct the unfavorable geographic and specialty distribution of physicians.
- Failure to minimize needless disability from long-term medical and psychiatric problems.

Ginzberg and Schroeder each emphasize that academic medicine is the beneficiary of very generous amounts of public funding, given in part to carry out a mission that benefits society, expended with an extraordinary degree of institutional autonomy.

## Meeting the Nation's Needs

Throughout the past fifty years, the nation, through Congress and multiple commissions, has consistently and repeatedly identified a common set of national needs and expectations. Some of these needs and expectations have been identified by Schroeder et al. (1989); others are identified according to Congressional intent. At least three of these show how a disconnect can occur among the intent of providers, the stated mission of an academic health center, and the values and vision necessary to implement the missions. The disconnect occurs with the need to (1) promote increased commitments to generalism, (2) join basic science and clinical education with preventive medicine and community health, and (3) ensure increased access, retention, and graduation of students from underrepresented and socially disadvantaged populations.

- Generalism—The nation has expressed its need for generalist physicians consistently and repeatedly since 1960. The rationale was affirmed by the Coggeshall Report of 1965, the Millis Report of 1966, and numerous subsequent reports. The Federal government and many state governments provide generous fiscal incentives to encourage medical schools, GME programs, and teaching hospitals to support generalism. The advent and pervasiveness of managed care organizations in recent years is a new stimulus that heightens the need.

Despite the emphasis placed on developing more generalists, in 1997, 8 of the 125 allopathic medical schools in the AAMC still do not offer a required clerkship or its equivalent in Family Medicine. Three of these schools are in New York City, a region with the largest ratio of physicians and medical specialists to population in the United States (and perhaps with the largest proportion of medically underserved consumers).

Twenty-two medical schools require a clerkship in Primary Care, but not in Family Medicine. Although a Primary Care clerkship may fulfill some of the desired elements of generalism, one should not assume this is always the case. In the Millis Report, the assumption was made that medical schools would provide an integrated experience in generalism that would spawn several disciplines— simultaneously, it was hoped but, more important, in a coordinated manner.

In many schools, a Primary Care clerkship may be limited to one of the identified primary care specialties, and fail to integrate the many desired elements suggested in the Millis Report and the report by the New York State Council on Graduate Medical Education. Seven medical schools require an educational experience in Ambulatory Care but not in Family Medicine. A broad-based, comprehensive Ambulatory Medicine clerkship that requires continuity of care may be a preferable educational experience to one limited to a single primary care discipline, depending on its organization and curricular content.

The findings suggest that the value system necessary to implement a mission of generalism effectively does not yet exist in many of the nation's academic health centers.

• Preventive medicine—Another area in which there is likelihood for incongruity between mission and value is that of preventive medicine and community health. Institutions that do not nurture generalism are the least likely to support these efforts. Because preventive care and community health are identifiable national priorities for providing alternative forms of care and improving the health status of communities, academic health centers must work more closely with other health professional programs such as those in schools of public health.

• Educational opportunities for the socially disadvantaged— Unfortunately, Flexner missed an important opportunity to report correctly on the status of medical education for minority and socially underrepresented citizens in 1910. The important matter was not addressed further until the civil rights movement of the 1960s. Despite tremendous social and fiscal support to increase the access for a growing minority population, medical schools still do not enroll sufficient numbers of minority students. This problem provides an example of how an academic health center's commitment to an educational mission must be extended to work with primary and secondary schools and community groups in a way that promotes the flow into and through the educational pipeline. It also illustrates how leaders in GME, in particular, must work to secure a continuum of academic growth and development for a defined constituency. Ginzberg has concluded that a serious dilemma for medical schools in the future will be the need to reduce faculty size and student enrollments while, at the same time, providing opportunities for faculty and students from socially disadvantaged populations.

In the changing world, where accountability and negotiation will determine the availability of fiscal support and stability for academic health centers, new concepts of evaluation will be required to implement viable strategies. Well-defined missions, vision, and value statements are vital. But there also must be a process to determine to which constituents an institution is of value. Table 7 illustrates the concept of value for a hypothetical academic health center. The value of each academic health center function for each constituent group is stated, with 1 representing a high score and 5 a minimal, or low, score.

Looking at Ginzberg's analysis of the four groups of medical schools that served as case studies at the 1994 Macy Conference, it appears that the schools with major research programs should achieve a higher value score to the nation than a school largely dependent on faculty practice revenues for research. On the other hand, the latter school should be of higher value to the more immediate constituents for functions such as education, patient care, and community service. It seems feasible to suggest that this evaluation can help academic health centers reconcile missions, vision, and values with operations, and further define how their resources should be consistently allocated. It can also be used by departments and other program units as well as academic health centers.

## Relevant Models for Academic Health Centers

The past fifty years have witnessed the development of large centers in which the functions of education, research, and patient care were coordinated. This concept promulgated the perception that all of the needs of medical and

Table 7
**HOW MUCH DO CONSTITUENTS VALUE ACADEMIC HEALTH CENTERS?**

| Major functions | Students, families, parents | Parent university | Region | State | Nation |
|---|---|---|---|---|---|
| Education | 1 | 1 | 1 | 1 | 3 |
| Research | 1 | 1 | 1 | 3 | 4 |
| Patient care | 2 | 1 | 2 | 5 | 5 |
| Leadership | 2 | 1 | 1 | 2 | 4 |
| Public service | 3 | 3 | 2 | 1 | 3 |

Note: Rated on a scale of 1 to 5, with 5 the lowest rating.

health professions education could be met in such centers. Because health education is so closely related to health care and health service delivery, the formation of centers to which all required sources would flow was eventually subject to change. In the past decade, hospitals have come to realize a need to expand beyond existing structures and locations and to form systems of care rather than centers of care.

It is obvious that medical and health systems education must now move from a centralized to a systems approach. Under this scenario, tertiary patient care would remain in a limited number of highly technically specialized facilities while basic science research would be concentrated around expensive, technically oriented laboratory settings. All other elements of care would be provided throughout the community and region. Although masked under the concept of "managed care," the real goal would be to manage the cost of care, make access to care easier and more efficient, and promote the concept of comprehensive, continuous care. It is imperative that health science education be reformed so it can adapt to a new learning environment.

Although it is foolhardy to think that any academic health center has yet accommodated to the required changes, we can evaluate some relevant models to determine how each center might position itself to cope more readily to changes that will continue to occur. Some examples follow:

*Indiana.* The University of Indiana had one complete medical school in 1910; its current model maintains a single medical school rather than a number of additional independent schools. (Its neighbor, Ohio, has seven allopathic and one osteopathic medical schools, having added the allopathic schools during the expansionist period.) When Indiana increased its medical school enrollment, it developed a program in which preclinical education was conducted at a number of university and college campuses throughout the state, and clinical education was conducted at facilities in Indianapolis and in the physician and hospital community throughout the state. As the years went on, the relationships between the University of Indiana and Purdue University strengthened to the point where an educational consortium was formed to provide a seamless education for all of its students at the two institutions.

*Washington, Alaska, Montana, and Idaho.* A novel situation exists in the relationship between these partner states and the University of Washington to form the four-state program known as WAMI. In this model, these four components serve as an interstate educational organization managed by the university. Educational activities extend into the partner states. Despite the wide range of educational responsibility, the university continues to also be a major national leader in biomedical research.

*Illinois.* The University of Illinois at Chicago has always had a relatively large number of medical schools. Its response to the era of expansion was to develop a single new public medical school, the Southern Illinois University Medical School. The University of Illinois medical school, located in Chicago, developed an expanded single institution with additional campuses in Urbana, Peoria, Rockford, and Champaign-Urbana.

*Texas.* A more ambitious model is one developed by Texas Tech University in Lubbock. Representing a regional health professions education institution serving West Texas, its program extends northward from Lubbock to Amarillo and southward to El Paso; programs are also located in the Permian Basin region, which includes Midland and Odessa.

*New York.* The educational network of the New York Medical College located in Valhalla (Westchester County), New York, includes approximately thirty-five hospitals and other training sites extending south to Staten Island, New York, and to its north to Kingston, New York.

*Oklahoma, Kansas, New York, and Florida (clinical campuses).* Several states have opted to maintain a single centralized health science campus joined to clinical campus training sites at distant locations. They include the University of Oklahoma with a clinical campus in Tulsa; the University of Kansas in Wichita; the SUNY Upstate Medical Center in Binghamton, New York; and the University of Florida in Jacksonville. Grafting clinical campuses onto the well-established medical schools mentioned above proved to be more of a challenge than did the models developed in Indiana, Washington, and Illinois.

*New York, Tennessee, Illinois, and Ohio (GME consortia).* A recently introduced alternative model for the governance of GME that could be extended to include other components of academic health centers educational programs is that created through the establishment of consortia. This type of organization falls midway between an educational program operated by multiple, independent organizations, on the one hand, and a program operating as a single, merged fiduciary entity. As such, a consortium provides the unique opportunity to manage and coordinate merged institutional interests without a need to surrender total institutional integrity and autonomy. Today, there are thirty identifiable multidisciplinary GME consortia in the United States. A recent report by Malcolm Cox (1997) on behalf of the Federal COGME, indicates that consortia have the following attributes:

- They are better positioned than any national organization to deal with local or regional GME training needs.
- They provide a framework for examining GME from the perspective of all interested constituencies.
- They possess the inherent flexibility and potential for inclusiveness needed to organize a fragmented GME system.
- They can be effective when given appropriate levels of authority.
- They can focus on the content and quality of programs.
- They can serve as models of shared governance.

The prospect for consortial governance has been evaluated by a number of organizations. In New York State, both the state's Commission on Graduate Medical Education and its successor, the Council on Graduate Medical Education, encouraged the development of GME consortia. The Macy Foundation (Morris and Sirica 1993) also encouraged GME governance by consortia. Cox's report strongly recommended that educational consortia become the coordinators and facilitators for medical student education and GME.

The most comprehensive GME Consortium developed thus far is in Buffalo, New York (Rosenthal et al. 1997). This organization was formed in response to the revised standards promulgated by the ACGME in 1980 (GMENAC 1980). Its members include a medical and dental school, nine teaching hospitals, and a representative for each residency program. The organization also joined the views recommended in the reports by Millis and the Council on Academic Societies Reports in 1965 and 1968, respectively. It has fostered and implemented changes in residency and medical student education (ACGME 1982) and served as an important catalyst for institutional cooperation and collaboration.

New York State's recently enacted Health Reform Act, which neither mandates nor denigrates the potential value of consortia, allocates $54 million per year for regional distribution, and encourages teaching hospitals and academic health centers to develop cooperative plans designed to achieve a specific set of public goods. Included are (1) a decrease in the number of GME positions; (2) an increase in the number of primary care resident positions and a concomitant decrease in the number of specialty GME positions; (3) an increase in representation of minority and other socially underrepresented constituents; and (4) development of GME consortia.

The state of Tennessee was the first state to secure a Medicaid Managed Care Waiver. Initially, the rapid change that ensued placed the medical educational system at risk. The four medical schools—East Tennessee State University, Meharry Medical College, Vanderbilt University, and the University of Tennessee (Memphis)—have now formed a single statewide GME consortia. Its effectiveness will not be known for several more years, but it could become another important model to emulate.

An alternative form of educational consortia is being developed by osteopathic medical schools. Osteopathic schools may be fortunate when they develop this model because each one has more management flexibility and is not as tightly joined to health delivery organizations as the allopathic schools. Some examples of approaches undertaken by osteopathic schools follow.

- The New York College of Osteopathic Medicine provides the educational umbrella for its graduates who train in AOA-approved GME programs throughout New York State.
- The Midwestern University School of Osteopathic Medicine in Chicago has added a new school in Phoenix.
- The Ohio University of the College of Osteopathic Medicine and the Michigan State University College of Osteopathic Medicine each has developed statewide GME consortia.

*Federal government.* The Uniform Services University of the Health Sciences is a relatively new academic health center that could serve as an ideal model for future organizational structures. The only health science school owned and operated by the Federal government, its affiliates are the well-respected Walter Reed Army Medical Center; the Naval Medical Center in Bethesda, Maryland; the Malcolm Grow Air Force Medical Center; and the Wilford Hall Air Force Medical Center. It is conceivable that, as the Federal government is downsized and reorganized, a broader health education enterprise allied with the Public Health Service and NIH could evolve from this academic health center.

## REINVENTING HEALTH PROFESSIONS EDUCATION

Flexner emphasized the need for a sound fundamental educational preparation for physicians that includes the sciences related to medicine. Today, medical schools require not only the basic biomedical sciences but also those sciences related to prevention of disease, behavioral medicine, and community health. It was the need for this type of broader education that led Flexner to believe that medical schools must be intimately joined to universities. Coggeshall also recognized the importance of other academic disciplines to medicine that are not part of the usual biomedical science array.

There are some very relevant priorities that every academic health center should reaffirm with the approach of the new millennium. They are:

- The primary function of a medical and health professions school is to educate the physicians and health professionals of the future.
- Conducting research is important to the development of new knowledge and biotechnical advances, excellence in rendering care, and the proper inculcation of the values of medical practice. In a school, it also serves the needs of the student consumer by providing a proper education that includes breadth of knowledge and fosters curiosity and self-learning, as well as depth of knowledge.
- The focus of a health science education is the patient and the community, not a science or a single specialty. Thus, "the patient" must be returned to medical education and the importance of the health of a community to the well-being of society must be appreciated in proper detail.

Education's importance has been devalued by the tremendous expansion that has occurred in the past half-century and by the relative dominance of the engrafted research and patient care missions. The viability, excitement, and mass of these latter missions have overwhelmed the educational mission to the point where education's professional value and importance are often not recognizable. Abrahamson (1996) ascribed the problem to the enhancement and expansion of the research entrepreneur and the clinical entrepreneur. This assessment is probably correct; increased numbers of faculty are indeed expected to risk their livelihoods through the securing of research grants or practice income, or both. Although this behavior and need probably will not change, they must be seen as tasks that properly value and nourish the educational missions; in addition, all faculty should be rewarded for performance and achievement rather than for the sole ability to generate fiscal resources.

The devaluation of education is evidenced further by at least two observations. The AAMC Survey Report (McInturff 1996), for example, found that the average citizen did not appreciate the role of education in academic health centers but did clearly value the research and patient care missions. And, writes Dr. Edwin Rosinski in a personal communication to this author, when he interviewed medical school deans and other leaders in medical education to determine their perception of advocacy for medical education in America, he found to his surprise that neither the AAMC nor the AHC are recognized as effective advocates for the importance of education.

## Future Educational Needs

An academic health center must consider the specific learning objectives for each of its student constituencies. Most important, it must separate the differences required for graduate trainees from students seeking a primary degree.

The needs of today's students are vastly different than those of their predecessors. As Coggeshall indicated, this situation is largely due to social change. The United States is now populated by a healthier, wealthier, older population whose medical and health care needs are different from those in the past. Physicians and health care professionals must be better prepared to deal with preventive health care and chronic rather than acute illness and with a larger proportion of people who will live into their nineties. Most important, health professionals must adapt to an environment in which patients will help determine the kind of care desired, and care will be rendered less frequently in hospitals and more often in a decentralized but coordinated manner in ambulatory care sites and other community facilities.

Under the above assumptions, medical and health professions education will also be distributed throughout regions and include utilization of professionals and facilities with little previous involvement in academic health centers. How can academic health centers cope with this situation in which previous defined centers of learning become systems of education?

- Many faculty will develop into facilitators of education rather than functioning solely as teachers.
- Students will be expected to gain more information through self-learning strategies, problem-based learning techniques, simulation, experience with standardized patients, and computerized technologies.
- Curricula will be restructured to facilitate more small-group learning experiences, include measured emphasis on preventive and community health, and better integrate basic science and patient care education.
- Reliance on the hospital setting will be reduced, and use of ambulatory and urban and community sites increased.
- Formal classroom instruction will be reduced, with more emphasis directed toward program development and evaluation, self-learning, and use of technology. The educational center will be a resource for all components of a region's educational partners.
- Educational materials will be distributed through an educational information network with materials available to consumers online twenty-four hours a day. The National Library of Medicine will continue to grow as a major resource.

The Buffalo Consortium has worked cooperatively and collaboratively with New York Telephone (NYNEX) to develop fiber optic connection and routing among its ten partners as inexpensively as possible. The university's Health Science Library and its hospital consortium of libraries provides online transmission of bibliographic, journal, and textbook materials to 7,000 users. The network serves thirty-five to forty organizations that include ambulatory teaching sites and health insurers. This system, HUBNET, will form the foundation for an eventual health information network.

It seems apparent that health science libraries and computer information systems will become the backbone and infrastructure for the conduct of education. If this does indeed occur, the Association of Academic Health Centers should determine if health science libraries should not be more prominently represented and involved.

Distance learning and regional teleconferencing capacity will continue to be developed. They are of particular importance to those educational programs that will be conducted in multiple distant sites and as a decentralized effort.

The community, in addition to the teaching hospital, will be utilized as another classroom. Already, education programs are increasingly being operated outside the teaching hospital in urban, suburban, and rural areas. Accordingly, the education center will have to develop adequate evaluation methodologies for the trainees located in remote, less standard environments. The adequacy of the environments will also have to be evaluated.

## Financing Health Professions Education

Future strategies to finance very expensive forms of medical and health professions education remain to be determined. It is apparent that the actual costs must be determined and isolated from budgetary strategies that permit cost-shifting. During the past twenty years, two principal sources have been used to replace other sources of insufficient or lost revenues, namely, research funds and faculty practice plans.

Although these sources can be incremented, it is unlikely that the magnitude will sustain the current enterprise. The strategies being developed by the Federal and state governments and by the business community are designed to reduce expenditures in these areas. The 1994 Macy Conference recommended that the Federal government develop and implement a national workforce plan and provide direct financial support to academic health centers in the form of incentives that will address national needs. Such possibilities still exist, but they are unlikely to occur unless these centers individually and collectively agree to take additional fiscal risks, be held accountable, and demonstrate that their productivity is effective in meeting the specified national needs.

## CONCLUSION

In a span of less than one hundred years, health professions education moved from a cottage industry to a very sophisticated, complex organization manifesting itself as the academic health center. Today, this concept of maintaining centralized centers that can be perceived as self-reliant is being challenged. The nation has rebelled against the concept of government regulation for health care and, for the next generation, control will be shared by the Federal and state governments and the business community. Competition, driven by cost-reduction and efficiency, quality, and consumer satisfaction will be the major path to success.

The nation's academic health centers are expert at competing with one another to achieve excellence in education, research, and patient care. However, they are not particularly adept at being cost conscious or efficient or at restructuring their organizations to become smaller, leaner, and meaner. However, given their importance to society, there is little doubt that most, if not all, academic health centers will make necessary adjustments to compete and serve society's fulfilled role. However, many treacherous forces can serve to detract academic health centers from their principal missions. Each academic health center, therefore, must select its strategies wisely and make certain they are in keeping with its stated purposes. Perhaps the greatest threat to the future would be to view the new competitive environment as an end rather than a means. The competitive forces that have been unleashed will surely thrive on a profit incentive. Furthermore, when this initial period has passed, competition may have attained the results previously attempted through regulations, and have done so more rapidly. However, the results of the profit incentive may bring about more pain, disruption, and chaos than the regulatory approach. Thus, academic health center leadership must focus on its missions constantly, make appropriate midcourse adaptations, and enunciate those values held important and immutable to the students, faculty, patients, and community.

Academic health centers will continue to provide students with a sound scientific foundation while nurturing values of compassion, caring, and generosity. Another major conflict for many academic health centers will be that of idealism versus reality. The former must be held in high esteem in order to promote the most altruistic health professionals possible. The latter, of course, reflects a restructured environment in which being the best, most productive competitor may be viewed as more important and relevant. Medical professionals in particular are already experiencing a loss of professional autonomy and control of patient care. It is at this interface that the academic health centers must structure new educational strategies designed to prepare their graduates for a vastly different reward system, one in which entrepreneurial behavior is more valued than professional stature. And in this respect, the influence of role models will be even more important than was the situation in the past.

## WORK CITED

Abrahamson, S. 1996. Time to return medical schools to their primary purpose: Education. Academic Medicine 71(4).

ACGME (Accreditation Council on Graduate Medical Education). 1996. *Accreditation Alert.* Chicago: ACGME.

————. 1982. *Institutional Responsibility for Graduate Medical Education—The New General Requirements for Residency Training.* Chicago: ACGME.

AACN (American Association of Colleges of Nursing). 1993. *Institutional Resources and Budgets in Baccalaureate and Graduate Programs in Nursing 1992–93.* Washington: AACN.

AAMC (Association of American Medical Colleges). 1995. *Institutional Profile Annual Report 1994–95.* Washington: AAMC.

————. 1997. *Directory of American Medical Education 1996–1997.* Washington: AAMC.

ADA (American Dental Association). 1995. *Survey Center Report.* Chicago: ADA.

AMA (American Medical Association). 1923. *Principles Regarding Graduate Medical Education.* Chicago: AMA.

————. 1928. *Essentials of Approved Residencies and Fellowships.* Chicago: AMA.

Blumenthal, D. 1997. Understanding the social missions of academic health centers. *Report of the Commonwealth Fund Task Force on Academic Health Centers.* New York.

Califano, Jr., J.A. 1993. The last time we reinvented health care we made a mess of it. *Buffalo Evening News* 7(April).

Coggeshall, L.T. 1965. *Planning for Medical Progress Through Education.* Evanston, IL: AAMC.

Cohen, J.J., and M.E. Whitcomb. 1997. Are the recommendations of the AAMC's task force on the generalist physician still valid? *Academic Medicine* 72.

Colwill, J.M. 1992. Where have all the primary care applicants gone? *New England Journal of Medicine* 326(6).

Cooper, R.A. 1994. Seeking a balanced physician workforce for the 21st century. *Journal of the American Medical Association* 272.

Council of Academic Societies. The role of the university in graduate medical education. Washington: October 2–5, 1968.

Cox, M. 1997. Graduate medical education consortia: Changing the governance of graduate medical education to achieve physician workforce objectives. Final Report from the University of Pennsylvania Health System to the National Council on Graduate Medical Education (COGME). Washington: U.S. Department of Health and Human Services.

DHHS (Department of Health and Human Services). 1997. (News release) Letter to the editor re appointment of task force (COGME). May 30.

Flexner, A. 1910. *The Flexner Report*. Washington: Carnegie Foundation for the Advancement of Teaching.

Ginzberg, E. 1995. *The Financing of Medical Schools in an Era of Health Care Reform*. New York: Josiah Macy Jr. Foundation.

GMENAC (Graduate Medical Education National Advisory Committee). 1980. *Summary Report to the Secretary, Department of Health and Human Services*. (vol. 1) Washington: GMENAC.

*Health Security. The President's Report to the Public. 1994*. Washington: U.S. General Accounting Office.

*Indirect medical education funds*. 1983. (Report prepared for House Ways and Means Committee, no. 98-25.)

———. 1983. (Report prepared for Senate Finance Committee, no. 98-23.)

IOM (Institute of Medicine). 1997. *Implementing a National Graduate Medical Education Trust Fund*. Washington: National Academy.

Knapp, R.M. 1997. Medical school GRR's with a VA affiliation. (memorandum) Washington: AAMC.

McInturff, W.D. 1996. What Americans say about the nation's medical schools and teaching hospitals. *Final Report on Public Opinion Research to the Association of American Medical Schools*. Washington: AAMC.

Millis, J.S. 1966. *Citizens Commission on Graduate Medical Education*. Chicago: AMA.

Morris T.Q., and C.M. Sirica (eds). 1993. *Taking Charge of Graduate Medical Education. To Meet the Nation's Needs in the 21st Century*. New York: Josiah Macy Jr. Foundation.

Pew Health Professions Commission. 1995. *Critical Challenges: Revitalizing the Health Professions of the Twenty-first Century*. San Francisco: Pew Health Professions Commission.

Rosenthal, T., R. Berger, M. Noe, and J. Naughton. 1997. A consortium, graduate medical education, and Buffalo: Defining a common ground. *Family Medicine* 29(7).

Schroeder, S.A., J.S. Zones, and J.A. Showstack. 1989. Academic medicine as a public trust. *Journal of the American Medical Association* 262.

Smythe, C. McC., T.D. Kinney, and M.H. Littlemeyer. 1968. *The Role of the University in Graduate Medical Education*. (Proceedings of the 1968 conference) Washington: AAMC.

Weiner, J.P. 1994. Forecasting the effects of health reform on U.S. physician workforce requirements. *Journal of the American Medical Association* 272.

Whitcomb, M.E. 1995. A cross-national comparison of generalist physician workforce data. *Journal of the American Medical Association* 274.

# WEAVING A TAPESTRY OF CHANGE: QUALITY AND VALUES IN EDUCATION

*Paul B. Batalden, MD; John P. Evans, PhD; and Jeanne C. Ryer, MS*

L IFE IN ACADEMIC HEALTH CENTERS SEEMS CHAOTIC today. The messages are many and sometimes even appear to be contradictory:

"Get smaller."

"Use less money."

"Improve outcomes."

"Stabilize community-based service-delivery relationships to assure a better learning experience."

"Build partnerships."

"The new health plan contract eliminates the university health care providers because of the costs."

"Moody's wants to lower the university's overall bond rating as a result of the performance of the health sciences."

In the wake of all these messages, how can the leaders of academic health

---

*Dr. Batalden is director of health care improvement leadership development at Dartmouth Medical School. Dr. Evans is a professor at the Kenan-Flagler Business School, University of North Carolina-Chapel Hill. Ms. Ryer is a principal with Ryer Associates.*

centers manage change even as they are managing daily operations? All face similar underlying questions: Is this change for the good? Should we dig in our heels and resist this or that change—not throw out decades of tradition that brought us excellence? How do we know where to draw the line? What is missing from what we teach and the behaviors we model to others? What do we teach and model that limits student functioning in new circumstances? What current organizational habits limit our performance in a rapidly changing environment?

The next academic health center will emerge from what we did yesterday and what we are doing today, much like a tapestry eventually emerges from threads woven today and those that will be woven tomorrow. The picture may not be entirely clear or complete at this time, but the work goes on.

Academic health centers face three levels of imperative change in the way they are delivering health care today.

- The health care they offer patients, families, and communities must be of good value, given the reality of alternatives now available to them and the kinds of information about health and health care they are getting from many sources.

- The development of health professionals must prepare them to help design and lead innovation in and improvement of health care in complex organizational settings of health care today. Such preparation for students means that there must also be opportunities for the development of faculty.

- Given the social expectations about the pace of change, the academic health center organization itself must become more agile in responding to change.

These challenges are concurrent and assume that the basic biologic research mission of academic health centers will remain strong and vital and will require its own path of development.

In response to these three challenges, this paper attempts to provide leaders with greater understanding of the health care environment. Specifically, it offers:

1. Some helpful disciplines to teach, learn, and use in health care work as that work must change faster and more effectively.

2. An example of new higher education partnerships between professional schools and application settings that are facing fundamental

changes in the way they produce quality products and services that are competitive.

3. An approach for organizations to use to help provoke a more agile, adaptable work environment.

## CHANGING REALITIES

Helen called Dr. Andrew's office and talked to Peter Angelis, Dr. Andrew's office nurse, about her recurrent symptoms of painful urination and increased urinary frequency. Peter said Helen should drop off a urine specimen and pick up the antibiotic prescription that would be waiting for her at the pharmacy. Helen thanked him. After she hung up, she mused at how different it was now to get treated for this pesky problem. A year ago, she had to make an appointment to see Dr. Andrew and produce a urine culture specimen before she was treated. The appointment was always a bit of a hassle. Although the office staff tried hard not to keep her waiting, the office visit and treatment usually took up half a day of her time. Helen really appreciated the new way that she was treated—recognizing her knowledge of her own symptoms, the degree of her discomfort, and the value of her time.

Helen's clinical contact was with Peter, the nurse, but who made the change in the care? Dr. Andrew practiced in a fairly large multispecialty group practice, working every day with two other general internists in the same set of offices. They practiced with an adult nurse practitioner and two office nurses. They shared a receptionist-scheduler, and all used the same information system.

Some time back, the clinicians decided they could improve the process by which they cared for the otherwise healthy women in their practice who had recurrent cystitis. It was a sizable group of patients—about fifty women. They had heard about a clinical protocol that changed the role of the physician, the office nurse, and the patient and that employed a new urinary dipstick screening test for bacteriuria. To make the change relevant to their setting, all the clinicians had to agree, and the new roles for everyone had to be identified and defined consistent with state health professional practice regulations. The preferred clinical flow was determined. The designation of patient eligibility for this new care method and reminders for follow-up had to be programmed into the information system. The evaluation of the change was carried out, and the change was established. This was the same way that the clinical providers worked on nearly everything that they changed because they shared so much of the daily care responsibilities. The clinicians realized they had to regularly reserve some of their scheduled time so they could work on changing and improving what they usually did.

The image of the caregiver that dominates professional education today "pretends" that an earlier reality still exists, that is, health care is the sum of each discipline working alongside one another and within its own subject-matter domain to maximize the application of the total disciplinary knowledge-base to the patient's needs. However, the assumption that professionals from different professional disciplines are engaged in a task that is the *sum* of their individual efforts, rather than the *product* of their interactive work, may not be as helpful as it once seemed to be. From the patient's perspective today, clinical care is given by one clinical person who "represents" the providers. The patient assumes that, as a local functioning group, the clinical providers are in general agreement with the approach to treatment. When their lack of general agreement is evident to the patient, it limits what that patient feels he or she can do alone and adds to the patient's frustration.

When the health professionals described started to work together to change their practices, they had little idea about what was involved in making complex organizations work and change. The improvement and change in care required the entire front-line team to work together; they shared the clinical policy and procedures for the population of patients regularly receiving care from them. This "micro-unit" of the complex health care organization in which they worked consisted of

- the patient and family;
- the physician providers who regularly worked together;
- the midlevel practitioner and the nursing and other support personnel;
- the shared purpose for which they came together;
- the information technology that supported their work; and
- the administrative support and decision-making structure for their unit.

These micro-units can be thought of as the functional units—the core building blocks—for many of the very complex organizations in which most of today's, and probably tomorrow's, patients regularly get or will get health care. But these units, particularly their interdependent functioning and improvement, were not part of the professional preparation of the health professionals involved. The leadership and improvement of their work *together* had not been a part of their professional preparation. Further, the larger debate about "accountability" seemed to focus on individual measures of performance—as if the individual could use that information in isolation to improve, and as if the performance of the individual could be isolated from the contribution of the setting and the micro-organization in which the professional worked.

The knowledge that most successful service enterprises eventually focus on similar micro or "minimum replicable units" had not even been mentioned during their basic or graduate professional study (Quinn 1992). The "pods" or "panels" or "firms" that were referred to in their managed-care setting rotations seemed to be unrelated to what they—as professionals—were supposed to learn (Batalden et al. 1997). Training did not prepare them for understanding the connection between individual- and population-based care. It is the situation that White (1991) referred to as the need for "healing the schism between personal and population health" even though managed care rotations provided clear examples of giving individual care for patients in the context of an explicit, defined population of patients and could have provided great examples of applying epidemiologic knowledge to the design of care.

Does it matter? After all, you can't cover everything in six or seven years' training. However, the service-delivery settings where initial professional preparation happens *must* make these changes in their care for patients. To survive in a marketplace where people have choices, they need to regularly produce grateful patients like Helen.

## IDENTIFYING NEW KNOWLEDGE AND SKILLS

Identifying the content of a knowledge base and skill set that is helpful (but not yet commonly acquired in the usual professional education venues) for managing, improving, and leading front-line health care has been difficult (Shugars et al. 1991; Batalden and Stotlz 1993; Berwick 1991). A growing literature is emerging about useful knowledge and skills, and organizations who hire new graduates are becoming more explicit about what they need (Lurie 1996; Moore 1993; Batalden and Headrick 1996; Ludden 1993). Using those frameworks, it is possible to identify gaps in current knowledge and skills.

A common starting list of "new knowledge and skills" might include

- Health care as a process and a system (Batalden et al. 1997; Mohr et al. 1995).

- Patient preferences (Flood et al. 1996).

- Temporal variation in process, outcomes of care (Berwick 1991).

- Cooperative work, project team membership, and leadership (Ferguson et al. 1993).

- Measurement of biological, functional, satisfaction, and cost outcomes (Nelson et al. 1996).

- Design and leadership change in processes and systems (Langley et al. 1996; Gustafson et al. 1993; Kotter 1996; Batalden and Headrick 1996).

- Reflective practice and learning—personal improvement (Schon 1983; Roberts 1994).

It is helpful to begin by creating a model for understanding the care for patients—outcomes, processes, and systems. Common to understanding the outcomes of care for patients is a concern for

- Clinical parameters, measures of morbidity, mortality, and a return to biological homeostasis.

- Role function in society and a return to "functional homeostasis."

- Patient and family satisfaction with the care that was given.

- Costs—both direct and indirect—incurred in the episode of caregiving.

**Figure 1**
**CLINICAL VALUE COMPASS**

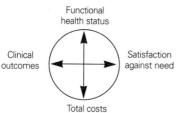

Nelson et al. (1996) have arrayed these outcome domains in a graphic they call a "value compass." In figure 1, this model has been adapted to illustrate the outcome domains in a clinical setting.

Figure 2 represents the core process of clinical care. Together, figures 1 and 2 represent a basic episode of care consisting of

**Figure 2**
**CORE PROCESS FOR CLINICAL CARE**

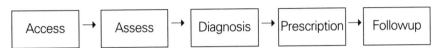

Access → Assess → Diagnosis → Prescription → Followup

process and result.

The care for an explicitly defined population (the minimum-size repeating unit of general medical care) is represented as a series of connected processes in the white background of figure 3. These processes can be called "managing care from the inside out."

The collection of activities performed external to the basic model are represented in the shaded area of figure 3 and can be called "managing care from the outside in."

Such models offer a basic orientation to the system of daily work of the front-line caregiving team in a complex health care organization and a visual representation of the work facing health professionals trying to change and improve

**Figure 3**
**'INSIDE OUT, OUTSIDE IN' IN MANAGEMENT OF CARE**

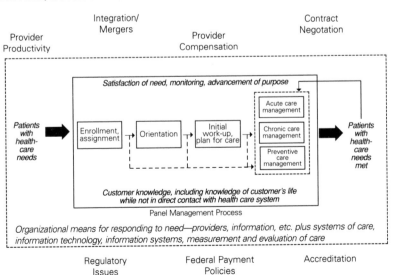

the care for patients like the woman in our story.

W. Edwards Deming (1993) and Batalden and Stoltz (1993) showed that combining professional knowledge (subject, discipline, and values)and improvement knowledge (system, variation, psychology, and the theory of knowledge) leads to innovation and continual improvement.

When the two types of knowledge are combined, new results are possible. Uncountable numbers of tools and techniques exist to help speed the application of this knowledge to the work of change in complex organizations. Several reviews of these tools and methods are available (Plsek 1992; Scholtes 1988; Reynard 1996; Nelson et al. 1997).

Identifying the knowledge and tools needed to effect useful change is not the difficult part. Using them regularly and strategically in busy daily health care practice is. Nonetheless, most manufacturing and many service-sector businesses have been able to incorporate these disciplines into their daily work.

Can collaboration between the academic community and the communities that hire graduates of academic health centers improve the preparation and performance of graduates to better serve society? Although the health care sector has often been reluctant to take example and instruction from other sectors in health care, we believe we can learn from how another sector of American life reacted to a seemingly insurmountable crisis and developed productive collaboration with the academic community. The example that follows provides a brief look at how one such collaboration evolved.

## PROVIDING QUALITY
## PRODUCTS AND SERVICES

In 1989 the Malcolm Baldrige National Quality Award from the Federal government had just completed its first full cycle, honoring a number of leading U.S. corporations making significant commitments to improving the quality of their products and services. At the time, the international competitive position of U.S. companies was significantly weaker than it had been in the 1970s (and also weaker than today). Xerox Corporation, one of the first Baldrige award winners, had been one of these companies. Once a dominant player in the copier industry, it had seen its market share erode alarmingly by the early 1980s.

By the late 1980s, it had recovered a significant portion of its lost market share through a company-wide quality effort carefully designed and implemented through the systematic delivery of orientation and training, starting with the most senior executives in the corporation.

Leaders at Xerox had decided that all employees needed to know the concepts and tools of improving quality, working in teams across functional boundaries, and focusing on the quality and value provided to customers. Significantly, this major training effort was undertaken because the managers and executives in the company had not gathered these skills and knowledge as a result of their education or experience.

Xerox had hardly been unique. Like other companies, it had made a major investment in developing staff capabilities when the company was first established, but leaders at Xerox sought to avoid having to do the same things for successive generations of employees. And like many others, once they retrained their staff in satisfying customers with quality, they reaped handsome rewards.

In 1989, as a result of the growing interest in quality aroused by the Baldrige Award, David Kearns, CEO of Motorola, Inc., brought together representatives from about twenty graduate business schools and ten corporations to the first of what was to become a series of annual forums devoted to the concept of "total quality." The business school representatives were a mix of faculty and administrators. The corporate representatives were people who had been involved in their company efforts to improve quality and customer satisfaction. Kearns's proposition to the academics may be paraphrased as follows:

> Many corporations have found it necessary to train large numbers of people in the concepts, tools, and skills of quality improvement. Even the most recent graduates of your MBA programs do not have enough of these capabilities in sufficient measure. We want you to revise your curricula to address this challenge.

The discussion that followed was lively. (It is important to note that the corporate people were saying that they were prepared to help the educators, but that they assumed the educators knew best how to manage change in their own environments.) Three themes from the experience are relevant to our purpose.

- Although a number of academics agreed that the topic of "quality" was important, others were unconvinced and were representative of the larger audience in their respective schools.

- Even when there was considerable agreement about the importance of "quality" in the workplace, introduction of this subject area on campus was seen not only as a significant change in professional education curricula, but also as a complex undertaking affecting a large number of schools.

- Just as corporations have found it necessary to provide additional training for employees, adding "quality" to the business curriculum requires appropriate preparation of many faculty members and the development of appropriate teaching materials for both students and faculty.

In 1992, Robert Galvin, chairman of Motorola, Inc., invited university participants in that year's Total Quality Forum who had both a business and engineering school on campus to send up to 100 administrators and faculty members to Motorola for one week in order to learn how Motorola conceptualized and applied the concepts of quality improvement. The response was so great that Galvin sought out other corporations to share the activity of hosting the universities. In the first stage, five corporations hosted administrators and faculty from eight different universities. Over the next few years, more than forty universities had been hosted in some way. The presentations provided concrete examples of quality application and the sequence of successes and stumbles experienced by the corporations. Although there was no standard model for the meetings, they shared a number of characteristics. For example, they all

- Included both school administrators and faculty.
- Explored ways in which the principles of quality improvement were being applied in the host corporations.
- Provided opportunities for the university people to explore specific applications of the quality concept in different corporations.

At this writing, seven Total Quality Forums have followed the first meeting convened by Motorola. Sponsored by twenty corporations and graduate schools, they have over the years provided a venue for valuable and constructive exchanges between representatives of the business and academic communities. Early forums helped to improve the academics' understanding of how various companies were incorporating the disciplines of quality improvement into their daily work. Subsequent forums provided examples of curriculum revision.

More recently, these forums have supported discussion of efforts to transplant and adapt the disciplines of quality improvement into the administration of universities.

As their agendas have evolved, the nature of corporate participation shifted, as well. In the early forums, corporate presentations emphasized the conceptual content of quality improvement and exhorted university representatives to modify curricula to include explanation and exploration of these ideas. More recently, university questions have shifted to concerns with how to incorporate these ideas into curricula and how to apply them effectively in the systematic improvement of universities.

In the early forums, discussion about curriculum change in business schools pointed out that much curriculum change occurs in response to published research results. A considerable body of work existed on the specific tools and techniques of quality improvement (e.g., statistical concepts of variation, mechanisms for measuring customer satisfaction, and approaches to the use of teams and mechanisms for recognition and compensation). Opportunities now exist for research into the issues of managing organization-wide initiatives to institute comprehensive and systematic improvement.

The outgrowth of these discussions was the implementation of a new research initiative involving

- A research program, entitled Transformations to Quality Organizations, administered by the National Science Foundation.
- Research funding that includes Federal funds supplemented by contributions from many leading U.S. corporations and the American Society for Quality Control.
- Research projects that involve collaborations between university researchers and applied contexts from existing corporations.
- A project proposal review process that combines evaluations by both academic and corporate reviewers.

## Leadership Steering Committee

Formed in 1992, the Leadership Steering Committee (LSC) comprises senior executives from the corporate and academic communities that coordinate all of the business-academic collaboration. In the early years, the LSC was led by corporate executives who sought additional corporations to host partnerships and provide administrative mechanisms, financial support for the new research program, and approaches for evaluating progress. More recently, the LSC has evolved into a cochairmanship (a corporate CEO and a university president). The intent is to achieve a truly shared leadership of this business-academic collaboration.

The LSC is supported by an advisory council, which serves in a planning and information-gathering function. In particular, the members of the advisory council reinforce the original purpose at the heart of its activities: improving business- and engineering-school graduates' understanding of the concepts and principles of quality improvement.

## Reflections on the Collaboration

Each of the developments in the evolution of the quality forums has played an important part, not only in facilitating the curricula changes that had been sought initially, but also in building a rich working relationship between a large number of business and university people. For example,

- The business-education partnerships have provided important demon-strations of how businesses have planned and implemented corporate efforts to achieve systematic improvement in the quality of products and services and in the value provided to customers.

- The quality forums have provided a context in which several hundred people from the academic and business communities could come together to discuss issues faced in their respective communities, share experiences at individual universities, and explore what might be needed in order to achieve further progress.

- The research program has become a unique public-private partnership creating funding for a body of research activity that is unlikely to have developed in the absence of a unifying effort to solicit and fund research proposals on the transformation of organizations to meet challenges of the modern competitive marketplace.

- The LSC has provided a vehicle for overall coordination and for gath-ering information that permits an assessment of progress on the orig-inal objective of curriculum change.

The central condition that facilitated the above developments was a willingness on the part of a core group of people from both the academic and business communities to seek constructive steps beyond that first quality forum. The business community leaders who initiated that forum exhibited "constancy of purpose" in their sustained expression of the need for graduates who have the knowledge and skills described in that first forum. Participants from the academic community promoted a discussion with the business community about how to achieve the curriculum change that was desired.

The particular activities—the partnerships, the successive forums, the research program, and even the LSC—simply emerged as the products of these discussions. The most important asset, however, was the succession of constructive discussions that occurred and that—in addition to the specific activities and progress—are still occurring. A valuable working relationship has been created among people and organizations that rarely are engaged in for as long or as consistently.

Critical to this entire experience was the identification of a few key leaders from each of the important constituencies who were willing to seek constructive steps for change. Equally important has been the emergence of a second set of people from the advisory council who could volunteer their time to address specific working issues on behalf of the LSC.

Academic health centers do not face the exact situation that schools of management and engineering confront. Our prospective partners are facing the need to change their practices in these uncertain times. We can offer new learning and professional development for them as they help us understand the demands, frustrations, and joys at the interactions between patients and clinicians. Fortunately, we can "take ourselves to school" as we make similar changes in our own internal service delivery capabilities.

## LEARNING TO LOOK FORWARD TOGETHER

We experience both surprising, novel, messy, costly, recurring, and unpreventable events and feelings of lack of direction, absence of coherence, and loss of meaning . . . [and we are offered] . . . the illusion of technique . . . [as an answer] (Vaill 1996).

Academic health centers seeking a sustainable future as service-delivery providers have no alternative except to increase their capacity for changing and improving the quality and value of the care they offer for defined populations of patients. Academic health centers must often compete in markets with other service delivery providers that are able to change and improve—with some agility—the value of the care they provide.

Leaders in academic health centers are quite sure that technique is not the only answer. Though certain that adding a new technique to their management repertoire or adopting the latest nostrum will not rescue them from the pressures of today or the uncertainties of tomorrow, leaders of academic health centers may not be as sure of their own interpretations and responses to the daily invitations for change.

Leaders of academic health centers recognize that they must create an environment that fosters and mobilizes the cooperative responses to these challenges that—taken together—don't seem to fit a familiar pattern. The temptation under increased pressure for change is to "do more of what we've always done—and do it faster." The problem—and one shared by U.S. businesses in the 1980s—is that "we must get what we've *not* gotten before." Trying to get significantly different results from the same methods of creation and production is an exercise in wishful thinking. At some level, we already realize that. How should we proceed?

## Outdated Planning Models

Given the mental models-in-use, it is sometimes hard to make sense of the current environment. Our earlier planning methods served us in the past; why didn't they prepare us for this eventuality? The limits of the rational planning model are confronting most enterprises today (Mintzberg 1994). The familiar predict-and-control methods of planning work well for organizations when the questions for the future are well defined and when the search is for the one right, preferred answer. We recognize its familiar steps:

- Define the mission, or purpose.
- Conduct an environmental analysis of the strengths, weaknesses, opportunities, and threats.
- Identify and select the option or approach with the highest utility.

- Implement the preferred approach.
- Assess and control the deployment of the preferred option.

Forecasts made in this type of planning became extensions of the past. Simple projections have a certain small utility: You know they are very unlikely to occur (Ackoff 1981). Their principal limitation is that they do not communicate the uncertainty we seem to face today. Fortunately, "formal planning" has limited attractiveness to most health professionals in leadership positions in academic health centers. Again, some lessons from outside the health sector seem pertinent:

- In times of rapid change the large, well-run companies are in particular danger of suffering from strategic failure, caused by a crisis of perception . . . the inability to see an emergent novel reality by being locked inside obsolete assumptions (Wack 1985).
- The problem surfaces when changes in society reduce interest in the organization's main activity and the organization finds that it does not have a rich enough mental model to observe and adjust to signals of evolving needs from the world outside the organization (Van der Heijden 1996).
- If the ultimate aim is to make the organization more adaptable in a changing world, strategy processes must pervade the organization (Van der Heijden 1996).
- Continuous, fundamental changes in the external world—a turbulent business environment—require continuous management for change in the company (De Geus 1997).

David Ingvar (1985), head of neurobiology at University Hospital, Lund, Sweden, has observed that every moment of our lives, we, as individuals, instinctively rehearse plans and actions for the future—anticipating the moment at hand, the next minutes, the emerging hours, the following days, the ongoing weeks, and the anticipated years to come. He called these anticipations, "memories of the future." De Geus (1997) asks if, as individuals, we can and do constantly spin out to the future, why are we not able to do this as groups and as organizations? Often, in organizations, we can see only when a crisis opens our eyes, or we see only what we have already experienced or what is relevant to our personal "movie" of the future. Sometimes, we cannot see what is emotionally difficult to acknowledge. Van der Heijden echoed this observation when he said, "Human beings and organizations do not act in response to reality but to an internally constructed version of reality."

Can creating collective rehearsals of the future allow us to develop more creative actions in times of dramatic change? Can we stimulate the creation of an environment inside academic health centers that is more capable of "agile" responses to major changes in the external environment? Specifically, how can we link the changing assumptions of today's world of health services with some attractive, alternative views of health-professional preparation?

The assumptions that underlie the earlier methods of planning health services and health professional education seem to be changing. We began this century with the idea that personal health-services delivery and the health of the population should pursue separate and distinct paths, and collectively, we have spent most of our energies making that separation operational (White 1991). With capitation financing and the assumption by provider institutions of risk for the provision of health care services for the mainstream of the population, the continued separation of the theory and practice of personal, individual health services and the health of the population is something of an anachronism.

## Scenario-Based Planning

Other economic sectors have faced radically changing assumptions for their work. According to White (1991), an approach that some have found helpful in preparing their leaders for taking different kinds of action is "scenario-based planning." It has the following attributes:

- Aims at examining and considering change in the mental models-in-use of decision makers.
- Deals with the need to understand the relatively predictable and uncertain factors.
- Creates vivid, reframed composite stories of the issues involved, permitting the introduction and engagement of new perspectives.

Scenario-based planning as a tool for strategic thinking and management has been well tested in settings other than health care since the 1970s. Although such planning had been in use by the military since just after World War II, it began to achieve wider notice when Royal Dutch Shell, which had developed a scenario-based planning process as part of its strategic planning, weathered the 1972–73 oil crisis considerably better than its stronger competitors, largely because of decision-making processes and strategies arising out of its scenario-based planning processes (Georgantzas and Acar 1995; Schwartz 1991). Although scenario-based planning is becoming more widely adopted in health care strategic planning, it is still a new process for many (Bezold 1992; Donker and Ogilvy 1994; Gelb and Zentner 1991).

Scenarios are a means of addressing and improving our perceiving skills; they are not forecasts. According to Van der Heijden (1996), scenario-based planning holds that "the less things are predictable, the more attention you have to pay to the strategy process. Uncertainty has the effect of moving the key to success from 'the optimal strategy' to the 'most skillful strategy process.'"

Scenario-based planning assumes that there is "irreducible uncertainty and ambiguity in any situation . . . and that successful strategy can only be developed in full view of this" situation.

Beginning with Herman Kahn of RAND, there have been attempts to separate the predictable, "predetermined" elements from the uncertainties. Separating the inexorables—or "driving forces," as Schwartz (1991) called them—from the uncertainties requires considerable fundamental analysis of causal relationships, maintains Van der Heijden. The uncertainties are allowed to play themselves out differently in the various scenarios. The objectives of scenario-based planning according to Van der Heijden are as follows:

1.  To generate projects and decisions that are more robust under a variety of alternative futures.
2.  To do better thinking about the future.
3.  To increase the perceptual skills of people, allowing them to recognize events as parts of a pattern (often a "new" one), and on this basis, anticipate new implications and possible actions.
4.  To influence a local leader's decisions and actions by "context setting" rather than "direct intervention."

In a recent use of scenario-based planning for health professions leaders and educators, we developed scenarios that we then used to generate discussions, strategic thinking, and conversations in three separate settings: a national forum of health professions educators and other health care leaders, a summer sympo-

**Figure 4**
**THE SCENARIO MATRIX**

|  |  |
|---|---|
| Scenario 4:<br>Within disciplines<br>Community-based | Scenario 1:<br>Within disciplines<br>Academic health center-<br>based |
| Scenario 3:<br>Across disciplines<br>Community-based | Scenario 2:<br>Across disciplines<br>Academic health center-<br>based |

sium for health professions educators who teach regularly about the improvement of health care, and a session of a national conference on health care quality improvement.

The processes for creating scenarios has been described and reviewed by Schwartz and Van der Heijden. We began by identifying two very fundamental themes in health professions education:

- Locus of the education and training in academic health center settings or in community settings.
- Discipline boundaries for the education and training within or across the disciplines.

These themes were used to construct a matrix for developing the scenarios. (See figure 4.)*

First, we identified many of the inexorables:

- Population getting older.
- Continued pressure on costs of care as a percent of the gross domestic product.
- Continued decrease in "unit cost" of technology.
- Continued pressure to "manage" care for increased effect and value.
- Continued evolution of "neighboring" disciplines such as education and social service work.

---

* Information on ordering copies of the scenarios is available from Paul Batalden, MD, Health Care Improvement Leadership Development, Dartmouth Medical School, Hanover, NH 03755.

- Continued existence of "free market" to develop offerings of service and information.
- Increased access to data and information.

We then created stories that brought these "inexorables" together in what we thought were creative, novel ways. We experienced significant frustration with our abilities to succeed at this task, showing real difficulty getting beyond what was already happening somewhere. Nonetheless, the view of the future depends on one's present circumstance, and for many participants, the scenarios were sufficiently different from the current reality to prove challenging.

The three trials of scenario-based planning used different times and formats dependent in large part on the settings. The first, a U.S. Bureau of Health Professions Partnership Forum, included scenario planning in an all-day meeting. The second took place at the intensive summer symposium for health professional educators where we processed the scenarios in shorter discussions over several days. The Institute for Health Improvement Annual Conference used the scenarios in a two-hour workshop.

In all of these sessions, participants were provided with copies of the scenarios and asked to read and reflect on them. They met in small groups with skilled facilitators using a set of tasks and questions to work through the implications of the assigned scenario. Participants were strongly encouraged not to question the scenarios, but to see them as stories of *possible* futures that would free them to think of the future creatively. Even so, some participants found it difficult not to focus on details and on why a particular set of events could never happen. Others found it difficult to let go of the current construct of health care as they lived it and think openly about how that construct might be different even a few years hence.

Format and timing had some impact on how well the groups were able to use the scenarios and the process to develop their own views of the future. (Many health care leaders face considerable and pressing demands on their time and attention and found it difficult to push pressing issues aside.) One use of the scenarios in a time-compressed format was very successful; in this instance, the group comprised people already fully engaged in health care improvement and in thinking about future-oriented issues in a conference setting.

## CONCLUSION

Given the emerging patterns of health care, the actions we take, the plans we propose, the threads that we weave into the tapestry that becomes known as the next academic health center must allow us to confirm that we possess the following attributes.

- We are able to continually change and improve the practices of patient care—both internally in academic health centers and in the health care practices of our community partners.

- We can foster the learning that will be helpful for the health professional students that we develop and offer them a sense of satisfaction and mastery as they progress to roles leading society's responses to the ever-changing environment of health care.

- We have provided the means for the faculty development we need.

- We have increased our agility as organizations to constructively engage the forces that now seem somewhat inimical to our mission.

New partnerships, in the sense of *different* partnerships, between health professions educators and health care service providers and communities will be needed. It is not at all clear that a partnership such as the academic-business collaboration is possible in health care, or even desirable. But it has been done, and it has caused enormous change in educational settings that are quite diverse. Our challenge is to fashion the collaborative relationships that will enable the future of our fundamental and important social mission.

### Acknowledgments

*The authors gratefully acknowledge the assistance of Susan Culp, Creigh Moffatt, and Julie J. Mohr in developing this manuscript and preparing it for publication.*

### REFERENCES

Ackoff, R.L. 1981. *Creating the Corporate Future.* New York: Wiley.

Batalden, P.B., and L.A. Headrick. 1996. Presentation at the Summer Symposium on Building Knowledge for the Leadership of Improvement of Health Care, Woodstock, VT.

Batalden, P.B., and J.J. Mohr. 1997. Building knowledge of health care as a system. *Quality Management in Health Care 5.*

Batalden, P.B., J.J. Mohr, E.C. Nelson, S.K. Plume, G.R. Baker, J.H. Wasson, P.K. Stoltz,

M.E. Splaine, and J.J. Wisniewski. 1997. Continually improving the health and value of health care for a population of patients: The panel management process. *Quality Management in Health Care* 5(3).

Batalden, P.B., S.D. Smith, J.O. Bovender, and C.D. Hardison. 1989. Quality improvement: The role and application of research methods. *Journal of Health Administration Education* 3(7).

Batalden, P.B., and P.K. Stoltz. 1993. Performance improvement in health care organizations. A framework for the continual improvement of health care: Building and applying professional and improvement knowledge to test changes in daily work. *The Joint Commission Journal on Quality Improvement* 19.

Berwick, D.M. 1991. Controlling variation in health care: A consultation from Walter Shewhart. *Medical Care* 29.

———. 1993. TQM: Redefining doctoring. *The Internist* (March).

———., A. Enthoven, and J.P. Bunker. 1992. Quality management in the NHS: The doctor's role. *British Medical Journal* 304.

Bezold, C. 1992. Five futures. *Health Care Forum Journal* 36(6).

Brassard, M., and D. Ritter. 1994. The Memory Jogger II. Methuen, MA: Goal/QFC.

De Geus, A. 1997. *The Living Company*. New York: McGraw-Hill.

Deming, W.E. 1993. *The New Economics for Industry, Education, Government*. Cambridge: MIT Center for Advanced Engineering Study.

Donker, R.B., and J.A. Ogilvy. 1994. The iron triangle and the chrome pentagon. *Health Care Forum Journal* 36(6).

Ferguson, S., T. Howell, and P.B. Batalden. 1993. Knowledge and skills needed for collaborative work. *Quality Management in Health Care* 1.

Flood, A.B., J.E. Wennberg, and R.F. Nease. 1996. The importance of patient preferences in the decision to screen for prostate cancer. *Journal of General Internal Medicine* 11.

Gelb, B.D., and R.D. Zentner. 1991. Scenarios: A planning tool for health care organizations. *Hospital & Health Services Administration* 36(2).

Georgantzas, N.C., and W. Acar. 1995. *Scenario Driven Planning: Learning to Manage Strategic Uncertainty*. Westport, CT: Quorum.

Gustafson, D.H., W.L. Cats-Baril, and F. Alemi. 1993. *Systems to Support Health Policy Analysis*. Ann Arbor: Health Administration.

Ingvar, D.H. 1985. Memory of the future: An essay of the temporal organization of conscious awareness. *Human Neurobiology* 4.

Kotter, J.P. 1996. *Leading Change*. Boston: Harvard Business School.

Langley, G.J., K.M. Nolan, T.W. Nolan, C.L. Norman, and L.P. Provost. 1996. *The Improvement Guide*. San Francisco: Jossey-Bass.

Ludden, J. 1993. Requirements of medical directors for hiring new graduates/residents (panel discussion). Washington: Institute of Medicine.

Lurie, N. 1996. Preparing physicians for practice in managed care environments. *Academic Medicine* 71(10).

Mintzberg, H. 1994. *The Rise and Fall of Strategic Planning*. New York: Free Press.

Mohr, J.J., P.B. Batalden, and E.C. Nelson. 1995. Flowcharting: A guide for depicting a process. Unpublished.

Moore, G.T. 1993. The impact of managed care on the medical education environment. *Report to the Council on Graduate Medical Education.* Rockville, MD: U.S. Health Resources and Services Administration, Bureau of Health Professions.

Nelson, E.C., P.B. Batalden, S.K. Plume, and J.J. Mohr. 1996. Improving health care, part 2: A clinical improvement worksheet and user's manual. *Joint Commission Journal on Quality Improvement* 22.

Nelson, E.C., P.B. Batalden, and J.C. Ryer, eds. 1997. *Clinical Improvement Action Guide.* Oakbrook Terrace, IL: Joint Commission on Accreditation of Health Care Organizations.

Plsek, P.E. 1992. Quality improvement project models. *Quality Management in Health Care* 1.

Quinn, J.B. 1992. *Intelligent Enterprise: A Knowledge and Service Based Paradigm for Industry.* New York: Free Press.

Reynard, S., ed. 1996. *The Team Memory Jogger.* Madison, WI: Joiner Associates.

Roberts, H.V. 1994. A primer on personal quality (essay). Graduate School of Business, University of Chicago.

Scholtes, P.R. 1988. *The Team Handbook.* Madison, WI: Joiner Associates.

Schon, D.A. 1983. *The Reflective Practitioner.* New York: Basic Books.

Schwartz, P. 1991. *The Art of the Long View.* New York: Doubleday.

Shugars, D.A., E.H. O'Neil, and J.D. Bader, eds. 1991. *Healthy America: Practitioners for 2005, an Agenda for Action for U.S. Health Professional Schools.* Durham: Pew Health Professions Commission.

Vaill, P.B. 1996. *Learning as a Way of Being.* San Francisco: Jossey-Bass.

Van der Heijden, K. 1996. *Scenarios: The Art of Strategic Conversation.* West Sussex, England: Wiley.

Wack, P. 1985. Scenarios: Shooting the rapids. Scenarios: Uncharted waters ahead. *Harvard Business Review* 63.

White, K.L. 1991. *Healing the Schism: Epidemiology, Medicine and the Public's Health.* New York: Springer-Verlag.

# THE CASE FOR INTERDISCIPLINARY EDUCATION

*DeWitt C. Baldwin, Jr., MD*

SOCIETY TODAY SEEMS TO SUPPORT THE CASE FOR interdisciplinary education in virtually all fields, demanding from our academic institutions, including academic health centers, greater efficiency and effectiveness—and more important—greater relevance and responsiveness to societal needs and directions. Interdisciplinary education better meets these criteria and better fits the nature of our scientific universe than do our current structures, which were intended for the industrial revolution and are still mired in a Newtonian model of science.

## CLARIFICATION OF TERMS

I believe that the word "interdisciplinary," at least in education, probably ought to be confined to a situation encompassing the mingling of several disciplines traditionally distinct in such a way as to create a unified product: a course, a paper, or even a curriculum. If the result is substantial and gains wide acceptance, a fresh discipline may be established.

However, "the term 'interdisciplinary' is frequently used as a genus for which such other terms as multidisciplinary, crossdisciplinary, transdisciplinary, etc., stand as species" (Scott 1979). Although the terms are frequently used interchangeably, there is a difference between the "multidisciplinary" and "interdis-

---

*Dr. Baldwin is scholar-in-residence and senior associate at the Institute for Ethics of the American Medical Association.*

ciplinary." The difference is crucial.

The first concept limits us to existing formulations and solutions, in other words, to a mix of what is already known; no discipline need change. In education, it implies that the student is exposed to a variety of separate disciplines; little or no integration of learning may take place. One could easily substitute the word "patient" for "student," with some of the same implications.

The second concept implies cooperation to the point of true collaboration. In such a situation, teams not only pool their knowledge and skills to solve complex problems and work in a more fluid, flexible, and egalitarian manner, often with shifting leadership, but also integrate their individual contributions in a manner designed to produce new solutions. In this regard, Peter New's (1968) description of the interdisciplinary approach to problem-solving, which follows, can hardly be improved upon.

1. The problem is big and/or complex enough to require more than one set of skills or knowledge.

2. The amount of relevant knowledge or skills is so great that one person cannot possess them all.

3. Assembling a group or team of professionals with more than one set of knowledge or skills will enhance the solution of the problem.

4. In the solution of such a problem, the possessors of the relevant skills or knowledge are (at least temporarily) considered to be equal or equally important.

5. All of the involved professionals are working for a common goal for which they are willing to sacrifice some professional security.

So let's agree to limit the term "interdisciplinary" largely to the earlier or more academic end of the spectrum and use the word "interprofessional" when referring to clinical forms. In 1975, Rosalie Kane introduced two new terms in her classic monograph on health care teams. These terms, "interprofessional" instead of the more academic "interdisciplinary," and "teamwork" rather than "team," served to clarify (or perhaps complicate) the picture. However, the term "interprofessional" for collaboration at the level of practicing health professions undoubtedly provides a more precise definition than the indiscriminate use of the word "interdisciplinary" for all such efforts. Nevertheless, I think it is important to preserve the term "interdisciplinary" in some situations. Certainly, it applies to modern scientific research, which requires input from and collaboration among a variety of complex. (Witness the epochal Mars landing.) In similar fashion, I believe the term "interdisciplinary" is still useful and appropriate when referring to preprofessional or undergraduate education at the university level. These more academic experiences represent one pole of a spectrum of collaborative educational efforts that also includes students enrolled in schools of the health professions, such as medicine, dentistry, nursing, and pharmacy. At the other end is the educational or team training process involved in preparing practicing health professionals to participate in collaborative team efforts in a variety of clinical sites and formats.

In this paper, I talk more about interdisciplinary education.

## TEAM HEALTH CARE: PRECURSOR OF INTERDISCIPLINARY EDUCATION

The idea of interdisciplinary education for health professions students followed by more than half a century the introduction of practicing interprofessional health care teams. Even before 1900, teams of physicians, nurses, and auxiliaries were delivering care to villages in colonial India (Fendell 1972). By 1920, team delivery of care had been proposed in both the United States and the United Kingdom (Cabot 1915; Davis and Warner 1918; Dawson 1920). Multidisciplinary teams in medicine and surgery took off in the United States during World War II with the advent of specialization and advancing technology that could be applied to complex problems such as rehabilitation. They became even more prominent after the war with treatment of conditions such as cleft palate that called for the skills of multiple specialists. These teams still function effectively with the required mix of cooperating professional and nonprofessional personnel from relevant disciplines and are probably the most common type of team in the health field. (Multidisciplinary teams tend to preserve traditional hierarchical relationships.)

The shift to interdisciplinary practice and thinking began in the late 1940s, with three experiments. Two involved community outreach efforts at Montefiore Hospital in New York City: one initiated by Martin Cherkasky (1949) for the home care of people with chronic illnesses, and the other by George Silver's Family Health Maintenance Project (Silver 1958, 1974). What made these experiments different was not only the continuity of care they provided but also the nature of the team's relationship to the patient and to their colleagues.

As a result of the third experiment—the creation of an interdisciplinary, community-based clinic for the care of children and their families at the Child Health Center at the University of Washington in Seattle (Deisher 1953)—several significant conceptual shifts took place: the emergence of a "health" rather than "medical" model; an emphasis on prevention and health maintenance; and the shift from a multidisciplinary to an interdisciplinary approach to care. The University of Washington project was also the first effort of which I am aware to place students in the health professions together and employ a permanent interdisciplinary faculty from these same professions.

## INTERDISCIPLINARY EDUCATION
## IN THE UNITED STATES

The evolution of interdisciplinary education in education and primary care health-team training in this country can be divided into a number of distinct phases.

Phase 1 encompasses the late 1940s and early 1950s when the pioneering efforts of Cherkasky (1949) and Silver (1958) in interprofessional clinical outreach took place and the early interdisciplinary educational model was developed by Deisher (1953) and Baldwin (1996).

Phase 2 occurred during the mid-to-late 1960s under the aegis of the community health center movement. It was primarily oriented to clinical care, especially primary care (Parker 1972).

Phase 3 took place during the mid-70s when the Office of Interdisciplinary Programs of the Department of Health, Education, and Welfare funded team training of health professions students in about twenty educational institutions and programs.

In 1972, the Institute of Medicine also convened a conference on Education for the Health Team chaired by Edmund Pellegrino (1972). The team's report supported the concept of interdisciplinary education for health science students and proposed that an educational experience could be considered interdisciplinary if there was a mix of disciplines among the students, among the teachers, or both. Thus according to this definition, each of the following situations could be considered interdisciplinary: (1) students from more than one health profession are taught by faculty from one health profession; (2) students in one health profession are taught by faculty from more than one profession; and (3) students from more than one health profession are taught by faculty from more than one profession. At the same time, the Institute for Health Team Development (1974) and the Snowbird Workshop (Baldwin and Rowley 1982) elaborated some early theories and techniques of interdisciplinary health team training.

At the close of the 1970s and the end of Federal funding, interdisciplinary education and team training programs virtually ceased. The exceptions were at institutionalized programs such as those at the University of Kentucky, Ohio State University, and the University of Nevada. At this point, education and training for health care teams might have disappeared had it not been for a rising interest in better meeting the needs of geriatric patients.

Phase 4 was not realized until the early 1980s, when the Veterans Administration (VA) funded the Interdisciplinary Team Training in Geriatrics Program; it provided support for about a dozen VA team projects over a period of several years. (Personal communication from J.H. Feazell, 1995.) They are still in place and have been expanded.

Phase 5 began in 1988 when an initiative for interdisciplinary health team training in rural areas was authorized by the Division of Associated, Dental, and Public Health Professions of the Health Resources and Services Administration (HRSA). It is still in existence, and more than thirty programs have received funding. As of spring of 1994, 1,267 students, 720 preceptors, and 3,749 providers had received training. (Personal communication from R. Merrill, 1995.) The initiative focuses on nonphysician students and collaborates with existing interdisciplinary, community-based programs such as Area Health Education Centers, Health Education and Training Centers, Geriatric Education Centers, Health Career Opportunity Programs, and AIDS Education and Training Centers across the country.

Phase 6, now under way, includes the more recent generalist efforts of the Kellogg Foundation in 1991, Robert Wood Johnson Foundation in 1992, and the Pew Commission in 1995. All emphasize the need for interdisciplinary and interprofessional education and practice among health professions students, as well as greater community input and involvement in designing programs.

An emerging Phase 7 stems from the rapidly expanding interest in continued quality improvement of interdisciplinary teams in education and practice.*

Most prior efforts at interdisciplinary education recognized the importance of two essential methods for creating interdisciplinary learning opportunities. The first was to provide a relevant, task-oriented or problem-based situation or setting that encourages group problem-solving, resulting in learner-ready or real-time learning. The second consisted of enlisting the small-group process to foster interaction, encourage differing role perspectives, dispel stereotypes, and enhance innovative solutions.

In general, experience shows that interdisciplinary student-learning experiences are far more difficult to achieve in traditional, hierarchical, discipline-oriented, academic settings. In the health care arena, they have proved less difficult to achieve when located outside of the tertiary care hospital (where traditional power and status dispositions tend to predominate). The training is probably best achieved in experiences dealing with complex family or community problems that require multiple skills and in underserved areas where no one else cares to go and the team experience poses no threat to any vested establishment.

## THE CURRENT ACADEMIC ENVIRONMENT

Universities today are primarily a product of the Middle Ages. They were formed in response to the need for training students to serve society's growing needs in commerce, law, medicine, and the church. Here is when the concept of the academic discipline was forged. Disciplina originally referred to the instruction of students or disciples who were subordinated to doctrina in a hierarchical system. Such a relationship stultified learning and, by the sixteenth century, the intellectual tradition in Europe passed into the hands of scientific academies, where new knowledge in the developing sciences arose.

Science soon became the province of the specialist, leading in turn to new fields of study and to new disciplines. These newer disciplines then underwent an internal fission into narrower specialties and subspecialties (Rudolph 1962). In

---

*An extensive review of interdisciplinary education in the United States over the last four decades appears in Baldwin (1996).

the health care field, especially, the research and training function eventually fostered the development and proliferation of separate and independent disciplines and specialties in academic health centers under the largesse of the National Institutes of Health (NIH) and the national research enterprise. Such status and independence for the specialities only hardened the disciplinary lines and led to progressive insularity. As a result, education went from one by faculties to one by disciplines, leading to bureaucracies characterized by inertia, self-maintenance, and rule orientation.

Thus, even though we envision students in the health professions as being able to work collaboratively after graduation, for the most part they learn in separate sites from diverse faculties using different curricula. They come to school prepared to think in an interdisciplinary fashion, but once in school, are conditioned to think in narrow, disciplinary ways. In such an environment, do we lose contact with the society we are meant to serve? Have we turned inward, no longer responsive to the changing directions of our science, our industry, and our students? Certainly, business, in general, and managed care organizations, in particular, are sending a clear message that the graduates of these programs are poorly equipped to deal with today's complex problems and work with members from other disciplines in common problem-solving exercises.

Changing this situation will require that the teachers lead, follow, or get out of the way. How do they learn to do this? They learn by working and dialoging together. In any case, it is the leadership of academic health centers who must point the way to interdisciplinary education.

Under the Newtonian model, we have made incredible technological advances. But Margaret Wheatley (1994) maintains that the newer views of the nature of our universe have moved us far beyond the classical Newtonian image, which focused primarily on the structured units of matter. She describes a model, based on the newer findings of quantum physics, chaos theory, and self-organizing systems, that focuses on the relationships between these units of matter and on the nature of energy and information exchange in creativity and innovation.

We live in an age of information. Many organizations have difficulty communicating information. In the Newtonian model information is considered a *thing*, to be transmitted, controlled, managed, and manipulated. We even refer to information as "bits"—limited and quantifiable. In the usual institutional setting, the passing of information is viewed as a one-to-one or one-to-many process. But with the computer revolution, information exchange has become a process of many to many. Formerly a source of power and control in most hierarchical systems, information now is controllable, more fluid, and dynamic—an energy force for change in itself—more and more like the new science that facilitated the process!

We must not only accept the challenge of an open information system, but facilitate it. An anecdote from the Manhattan Project illustrates the pitfalls of a closed system. When the project began, it apparently was considered so secret that scientists were isolated from each other, each one working on separate pieces of the experiment. Progress was disappointingly slow until the project managers brought people together and encouraged them to interact, producing an immediate explosion (if you will pardon the term) of progress.

We in the health field have spent enough years moving pieces around our organizational chess boards, ordering and reordering the design, hoping for innovation but finding disappointing sameness. Many organizations, confirming Wheatley's observations, reflect this mechanistic, reductionist thinking by progressively dissecting knowledge into disciplines and subjects, and further dividing it into isolated, independent structures.

These organizations have rigid rules and protocols about who can talk to whom, and seem afraid to have information flow freely. Fearing disorder, they desperately hang onto order. In the new science, however, order flows from disorder and disorder from order—a veritable ballet of chaos. Growth and creativity arise from adapting to disequilibrium, from seeing new connections between things. Children's play often seems chaotic, for example, and yet that is how they learn.

## ONE INSTITUTION'S EXPERIENCE

My experience at the University of Nevada is one example of how an interdisciplinary program can impact on an institution. Twenty-five years ago with the help of the Robert Wood Johnson Foundation, we introduced an interdisciplinary curriculum, from college entry to graduation, at the University of Nevada for all preprofessional and professional students in about a dozen health-related disciplines (Baldwin and Baldwin 1979). The program consisted of a required core curriculum of interdisciplinary courses in the physical and natural sciences, required courses in a number of knowledge and skill areas common to all the health sciences (including nutrition and bioethics, and this in 1972!), medical terminology, communication and interviewing, growth and development (including aging, death, and dying), health systems, health maintenance, physical and psychological assessment, and team dynamics. The program also consisted of several levels of clinical team experiences supervised by a teaching and practicing interdisciplinary faculty team.

Enrollment in the program increased from about 350 students in 1971 to over 1,000 (nearly one-sixth of the university) by 1974–75. Many of the required courses are still running, with approximately 600 students enrolled annually.

## DO THE NEW APPROACHES WORK?

In an article in the *Journal of Interprofessional Care* (Baldwin 1996), I completely failed to raise the question of whether interdisciplinary education really works! Is interdisciplinary education more likely than traditional disciplinary or professional education to produce students who are more open to, attuned to, interested in, and capable of working together in collaborative team practice relationships?

Unfortunately, the research in this area seems to depend on who wants what answers to which questions in what form and within what time period. Thus, rather than measuring what should be measured, researchers often resort to measuring what can be measured. As a result, nearly all of the literature consists of short-term, descriptive, so-called head-count or satisfaction reports designed to meet the hurry-up demands of administrators, policymakers, and funding agencies.

Those studies on interdisciplinary and multidisciplinary research in the health care field that do exist have been conducted on clinical teams delivering care or service. Here the data show that teamwork benefits patient care and that health care professionals seem to get along with and learn from each other, especially if there has been a team development or team training program. But in the case of interdisciplinary education, we cannot point to much in the way of solid long-term outcomes at this time.

Does multidisciplinary teamwork result in higher costs? There is substantial empirical evidence in many settings outside health care that the introduction of such teamwork can lead to increased effectiveness in the delivery of both quantity and quality of goods or services (West and Poulton 1993). As a result, the concept of teamwork is now a dominant philosophy in the manufacturing and service sectors where demonstrable, positive bottom-line effects are being seen on measures of performance, including employee satisfaction, absenteeism, turnover, efficiency, and quality (Macy and Izumi 1993). From these settings also comes the message that education is not providing the future workforce with the kinds of interdisciplinary and teamwork skills needed in the fast-changing competitive world of business.

Heeding such findings, health care institutions are borrowing the concepts and practices of Continuous Quality Improvement (CQI) teams from industry and business to decrease costs (Headrick et al. 1995). And, noting that it takes a physician six months to a year to learn to team effectively with other health workers in the new cost-conscious settings, managed care organizations in the United States have been supportive of the concept of interdisciplinary education.

In Britain, a major revolution is taking place in the health field. In the interest of efficiency and cost savings, the government has mandated the integration of health and social services, stating that the best and most efficient outcomes for patients and clients are achieved when professionals work together, learn together, engage in the clinical audit of outcomes together, and generate innovation to ensure progress in practice and service (NHSME 1993).

In this country, similar pressures on education and on the academic health center are prevailing, not so much from government as from business and the marketplace, to provide a flexible workforce ready to use a team approach to problem- solving and decision making—in short, a workforce possessing interdisciplinary skills. According to the Council on Graduate Medical Education (COGME), the growth of managed care will magnify the deficiencies of the current educational system but will also provide new and essential educational opportunities to improve physicians training for their future role (COGME 1995). CQI teams, directed both at health professions education and health care appear to be important vehicles for teaching these skills.

Is an interdisciplinary education in the health field more likely than traditional disciplinary or professional education to produce students who are more open to and capable of working collaboratively in team-practice relationships? The research is thin, and the evidence in favor of interdisciplinary health care education is less than convincing. Although short-term changes in knowledge, skills, and attitudes have been demonstrated, I do not know of any reports of significant long-term changes and, perhaps more important, of long-term outcomes in career commitment to and participation in team delivery of care. And given the inevitable problems of limited, sporadic, short-term funding, as well as the generally small numbers of subjects and the lack of proper controls, it seems unlikely that the proposition will meet definitive scientific requirements in the near future. Research has also been difficult to pursue because educators (read "idealists") are often not attuned to or trained in research.

In addition, interdisciplinary efforts are still relatively new and, thus, appear threatening to established disciplines and their existing resources. Professional associations and accrediting bodies fear loss of disciplinary control and identity, and the efforts challenge the traditional status and authority of certain professions, raising issues of egalitarianism that are often frightening. As Brown (1982) and others have pointed out, much of the push for interprofessional teams has come from the have-not, or aspiring, professions, and this ideological flavor has generated its own resistance.

Finally, there are legitimate critics of the idea of interdisciplinary education who believe it to be too early and potentially inimicable to the development of professional identity and competence.

## CONCLUSION

The challenge to the academic health center is to open communication between the different professions, sectors, schools, departments, and disciplines; enunciate a vision of free-form problem-solving; and create the places and spaces for dialogue about common problems and innovative solutions—in short, to adopt a course of interdisciplinary education.

I doubt if our program at the University of Nevada could be easily duplicated today. The situation was unique because, although the program was developed in an established university, it happened coincidentally with the formation of a new community-based medical school that needed the help and resources of other schools and departments—and was humble and realistic enough to ask openly for them. What happened, however, was a ferment of dialogue and discussion that made some amazing things happen twenty years ago!

Mandating interdisciplinary education is not a simple task. Teamwork must be enabled. Teams only work, however, when the goal or task is clear, real, and specific—one of the tasks of leadership—and task and faculty become involved. Much is being written about establishing interdisciplinary education, a concept initiated in the 50s, developed during the 70s and, unfortunately, having to be reinvented during the 90s.* By creating interdisciplinary task forces and crossdisciplinary curriculum committees to communicate the vision, create the atmosphere, and set up the channels of communication and information exchange, the needed changes can be put in place.

Although many assumptions about interdisciplinary education and interprofessional care have not yet been proved scientifically, it frequently takes years to make a scientific case for a worthwhile endeavor. It took years for the Head Start Program to demonstrate significant long-term effects on enhancing learning and social development and reducing school dropout and juvenile delinquency. We all received relief from aspirin long before science understood why. As Carl Deutch stated, "There are three classes of knowledge in the world: great truths, truths, and science. Great truths are those truths the opposite of which are equally true. Truths are truths, the opposite of which are patently false. And science is the art of turning a great truth into a truth." Interdisciplinary education is one of the great truths awaiting scientific confirmation.

## REFERENCES

Baldwin, D.C., Jr. 1996. Some historical notes on interdisciplinary and interprofessional education and practice in health care in the USA. *Journal of Interprofessional Care* 10:173-187.

Baldwin, D.C., Jr., and M.A. Baldwin. 1979. Interdisciplinary education and health team training: A model for learning and service. In *Medical Education since 1960: Marching to a Different Drummer.* A.D. Hunt and L.E. Weeks, eds. East Lansing: Michigan State University Foundation.

Baldwin, D.C., Jr., and B.D. Rowley, eds. 1982. *Interdisciplinary Health Team Training.*

---

*One of the best and most recent books is *The Wisdom of Teams* by Jon Katzenbach and Douglas Smith (1993). Although aimed at business organizations, it looks at what higher management can do to harness the creative potential of teams.

Proceedings of a workshop for the Office of Interdisciplinary Programs, DHEW. (2nd edition). Lexington: Center for Interdisciplinary Education, University of Kentucky,

Brown, T.M. 1982. A historical view of health care teams. *Responsibility in Health Care,* G.J. Agich, ed. Boston: D. Reidel.

Cabot, R. 1915. In *Social Service and the Art of Healing.* New York: Moffat, Yard.

Capra, F. 1983. *The Turning Point: Science, Society, and the Rising Culture.* New York: Bantam.

Cherkasky, M. 1949. The Montefiore Hospital home care program. *American Journal of Public Health* 39:163-166.

COGME (Council on Graduate Medical Education). 1995. Sixth Report. *Managed Health Care: The Physician Workforce and Medical Education.* Washington: COGME.

Davis, M., and A. Warner. 1918. *Dispensaries: Their Management and Development.* New York: MacMillan.

Dawson, Lord. 1920. *Interim Report of the Consultative Council on Future Provision of Medical and Allied Services.* London: Her Majesty's Stationery Office.

Deisher, R.W. 1953. Use of the child health conference in the training of medical students. *Pediatrics* 11:538-543.

Fendell, N.R.E. 1972. *Auxiliaries in Health Care.* Baltimore: Johns Hopkins.

Headrick, L.A., D. Neuhauser, P. Schwab, and D.P. Stevens. 1995. Continuous quality improvement and the education of the generalist physician. *Academic Medicine* 70 (Supp). S104-S109.

Institute for Health Team Development. 1974. Curriculum for Interdisciplinary Faculty Training (mimeo). 3329 Rochambeau Avenue, Bronx, NY 10467

Jantsch, E. 1980. *The Self-Organizing Universe.* Oxford: Pergamon.

Kane, R.A. 1975. *Interprofessional Teamwork.* (Manpower Monograph 8) Syracuse, NY: Division of Continuing Education and Manpower Development, Syracuse University School of Social Work.

Katzenbach, J.R., and D.K. Smith. 1993. *The Wisdom of Teams.* New York: Harper Collins.

Kockelmans, J.J. 1979. *Why interdisciplinary? Interdisciplinary and Higher Education,* J.J. Kockelmans, ed. University Park, PA, and London: Pennsylvania State University Press.

Macy, B.A., and H. Izumi. 1993. Organizational change, design and work innovation: A meta-analysis of 131 North American field studies, 1961–1991. In *Research in Organizational Change and Development,* vol. 7, eds. Richard Wordman and William Pasinore. Greenwich, CT: JAI.

Meadows, D. 1982. Whole earth models and systems. *Co-Evaluation Quarterly.* Summer:98-108.

New, P.K. 1968. An analysis of the concept of teamwork. *Community Mental Health Journal* 4:326-333

NHSME. 1993. *Nursing in Primary Care-New World, New Opportunities.* Leeds: NHSME.

Parker, A.W. 1972. *The Team Approach to Primary Health Care*. Berkeley: University of California.

Pellegrino, E. 1972. *Education for the Health Team*. Washington: National Academy of Sciences.

Rudolph, F. 1962. *The American College and University: A History*. New York: Knoff.

Scott, R.L. 1979. Personal and institutional problems encountered in being interdisciplinary. In *Interdisciplinary and Higher Education*, J.J. Kockelmans, ed. University Park, PA, and London: Pennsylvania State University Press.

Silver, G. 1958. Beyond general practice: The health team. *Yale Journal of Biology and Medicine* 31:29-38.

Silver, G.A. 1974. *Family Medical Care: a Design for Health Maintenance*. Cambridge, MA: Ballinger.

Thayer, L. 1975. On the functions of incompetence. *Perspectives in Biology and Medicine*. Spring:332-344.

Thornton, B.C., E. McCoy, and D.C. Baldwin, Jr. 1979. Role relationships on interdisciplinary health care teams. *Interdisciplinary Health Care Teams in Teaching and Practice*, D.C. Baldwin, Jr., B.D. Rowley, and V.H. Williams, eds. Seattle: New Health Perspectives.

West, M.A. and B.C. Poulton. 1997. A failure of function: Teamwork in primary health care. *Journal of Interprofessional Care* 11:205-216.

Wheatley, M.J. 1994. *Leadership and the New Science*. San Francisco: Berret-Koehler.

# MENTORS, ADVISORS, AND ROLE MODELS IN GRADUATE AND PROFESSIONAL EDUCATION

*Judith P. Swazey, PhD, and Melissa S. Anderson, PhD*

N THE FIELD OF HEALTH, AS IN MOST PROFESSIONS AND occupations, mentors, advisors, and role models are believed to play important roles in stimulating people to pursue a given career path, shaping their training and socialization and providing support and guidance. The importance attached to these roles, however, rests heavily on conventional wisdom rather than on scientific research. Furthermore, mentoring studies in one occupation or profession have often been applied to another without critically examining their applicability; Yoder (1990), for example, points out that much of the nursing literature on mentoring has adopted the attributes of mentors from business and education literature, a deficit being addressed by recent research on nurses' perceptions of mentors (Walsh and Clements 1995). And what research-based literature does exist is almost devoid of studies addressing the various phases of medical education and the early career paths of physicians.

## WHAT'S IN A NAME?

Much of the research conducted to date also fails to distinguish clearly between mentor (both classical and formal), advisor, and role model. These roles,

*Dr. Swazey is president of The Acadia Institute, Bar Harbor, Maine; Dr. Anderson is assistant professor, Department of Educational Policy and Administration, University of Minnesota.* This paper is a shortened version of Mentors, Advisors, and Role Models in Graduate and Professional Education. *Washington: Association of Academic Health Centers, 1996.*

as well as that of preceptor, sponsor, and docent, can have overlapping attributes and functions and should be distinguished from each other.

Indeed, studies of advising and mentoring in doctoral education emphasize the fallacy of assuming that just because a student has an advisor or other person directly responsible for his or her career preparation, it means that the student has a mentor. If this were so, all graduate trainees would have mentors. But "although the ideal model of graduate education includes a great deal of student-faculty interaction" (Baird 1990), studies show that even with faculty whom students consider to be especially supportive, there is little interaction in many aspects that are important components of doctoral training and professional socialization.

The word mentor itself, and the characteristics classically ascribed to the mentoring role, have been handed down from Greek mythology: When Odysseus began his ten-year journey, he entrusted the care of his son Telemachus to his close and loyal friend, Mentor. As epitomized by the parent-like role that Mentor assumed with Telemachus, and in contrast to other faculty-student relationships, mentoring generally encompasses an evolving, long-term, active, and often close personal relationship between a senior person and the person who becomes the protégé (Barondess 1994). The relationship can be highly positive; it can also be deeply toxic (Darling 1986).

Formal mentoring programs, as opposed to the classic mentoring described above, have been initiated in a number of fields including medical education.* The reasons vary, but in general the situation is due to a decreasing availability of senior people who have the time and willingness to invest in the type of long-term, one-on-one relationship that traditional mentoring entails (Tyler 1994, Barondess 1994).

An advisor, in general, performs more narrow technical and formal functions than the mentor. The role can involve relatively little contact with an advisee. (There may be more contact in the sciences because advisors usually also are the principal investigators or laboratory directors for the projects that sup-

---

* Curtis et al. 1995, program for pediatric residents; Gaffney 1995, graduate school mentoring program; Lobeck and Stone 1990, class mentors for medical students; Morzinski et al. 1994, program for junior faculty in academic medicine; and Ricer et al. 1995, program for medical students interested in family practice.

port their advisees and for which students do dissertation research.)

It is from a role model that a student can learn values, attitudes, and behaviors through observing and trying to emulate the admired other, usually an older person (Bandura 1977, Hurley 1978, Kemper 1968). In contrast to the primary functions of the mentor and advisor described above, the role model's function is to play a largely passive role of which she or he may not even be aware. Role models appear to be vital for adult career development (Rakatansky 1994; Speizer 1981), and may or may not be mentors. In terms of professional training, a person may have many role models (Bidwell and Brasler 1989).

## DOCTORAL EDUCATION

The Acadia Institute conducted a retrospective study of 2,000 doctoral students and 2,000 doctoral faculty who had been in the fields of sociology, civil engineering, chemistry, and microbiology during the period July 1985–June 1988. The "good news" is that the great majority of the students who completed our survey report having at least one "particularly supportive" faculty member. However, since all doctoral students have an advisor, who usually also serves as the student's research supervisor, it is troubling that 11 percent of the respondents do not believe that any of their faculty are particularly supportive of them and their work.

## DOCTORAL STUDENT
## EXPERIENCE WITH MENTORING

For those students who say they have a particularly supportive faculty member, the extent of the guidance and help they receive impresses us as limited. In our judgment, the data raise a number of grave concerns about the extent and content of the advising and purported mentoring of a substantial proportion of doctoral students in major research universities. Of the fourteen specific types of faculty support itemized in table 1, more than 50 percent of the students reported receiving "a lot of help" in only one category ("expressing a continuing interest in my progress").

We also found that three-quarters of the faculty surveyed in this study believe that they should have collective responsibility for the professional-ethical conduct of their students. But only about one-quarter said this responsibility was being exercised.

What experiences do doctoral students have with mentoring types of support in the departments where faculty believe strongly in their collective responsibility for their students' ethical conduct? Two major foci of the Acadia study were the transmission and content of professional values and ethical standards and practices. In relation to the rather uneven levels of support that students appear to get from faculty members in their own departments, it is interesting to

Table 1
**PERCENTAGE OF DOCTORAL STUDENTS WHO RECEIVED PARTICULAR KINDS OF HELP FROM A FACULTY MEMBER**

|  | A Lot | Some | None |
|---|---|---|---|
| *Teacher/Coach* | | | |
| Provides information about ongoing research relevant to my work | 39% | 50% | 11% |
| Assists me in writing for presentations/publications | 39 | 42 | 19 |
| Provides helpful criticism on a regular basis | 37 | 58 | 5 |
| Teaches me the details of good research practice | 35 | 48 | 18 |
| Teaches me to write grant and contract proposals | 14 | 34 | 53 |
| Advises me about teaching | 6 | 31 | 63 |
| *Sponsor* | | | |
| Writes letters of recommendation | 47 | 40 | 13 |
| Helps me get financial support | 46 | 35 | 19 |
| Finds support for me to go to professional meetings | 24 | 37 | 40 |
| Helps me develop professional relationships with others in my field | 17 | 50 | 33 |
| Helps me in locating employment opportunities | 16 | 39 | 45 |
| *Counselor* | | | |
| Expresses continuing interest in my progress | 61 | 36 | 3 |
| Provides emotional support when I need it | 28 | 43 | 29 |
| Helps me to learn the art of survival in this field | 23 | 51 | 27 |

Note: Percentages may not add to 100 due to rounding.

learn how faculty rank in comparison to other influences on the education and socialization of doctoral students.

In this respect, the student's advisor/mentor (our only mention of this specific term in the survey) was rated very important by a third of all students, second only to the student's family. Between 21 and 27 percent of students ranked their religious beliefs, other graduate students, friends outside of school, and their undergraduate faculty as very important. There were no significant differences by discipline, gender, citizenship/race, or number of years in the doctoral program.

According to the students, the least influential means for imparting attitudes and knowledge about values and ethical issues in their discipline are other graduate faculty; discussions in courses, labs, and seminars; professional organizations in their fields; and courses dealing specifically with ethical issues. We reason that the low rating of other graduate faculty as a very important influence reflects the fact that most students have relatively little contact with faculty other than their "advisor/mentor" once they have completed course requirements and begun their dissertation research.

The low important ratings given to courses dealing with ethical issues, discussions in other contexts such as labs and seminars, and the role of professional organizations are not encouraging findings for those engaged in efforts to stimulate ethics and values education. Other portions of our survey and interview results, however, support the view that these sources are not unimportant per se, but rather that students have had relatively little exposure to them.

## MEDICAL SCHOOLS AND
## UNDERGRADUATE MEDICAL STUDENTS

A number of medical school programs have explored the use of various types of formally organized programs designed to help students deal with "the faculty forest" (Swanson 1984) and foster closer mentoring types of relationships. The 1984 report of the Project Panel on the General Professional Education of the Physician and College Preparation for Medicine (GPEP) recommended that a faculty member work closely with a small group of medical students throughout the four years of their medical school education (Muller 1984). Several medical schools have experimented with such programs for entire classes or for groups of students, both before and in response to the GPEP report. Reflecting the semantic inconsistencies and role confusion that we have discussed, the faculty involved in these ventures have been variously termed and characterized as mentors, docents, supervisors, preceptors, and role models.

Two such programs are the University of Wisconsin Medical School's "class mentor" program, which began in 1985, and the University of Missouri-Kansas City Medical School (UM-KC) docent program for BA-MD students initiated in 1971.

In the UM-KC program, a "docent unit" consists of a physician faculty member and twelve students (three each in years 3–6 of the six-year program). "According to the school's academic plan, the docent should function as a practitioner of team medicine, a role model, a teacher, a counselor, a curriculum planner, an ombudsman, a parent figure, and an administrator" (Calkins et al. 1986). A descriptive account of the Wisconsin program and a survey-based assessment of the UM-KC program indicate that students and faculty are enthusiastic about them and believe they serve important functions (Calkins et al. 1986, 1987; Lobeck and Stone 1990).

The current resurgence of strategies to increase the supply of generalist physicians includes the development of numerous types of programs for medical students in both the preclinical and clinical years, including formal mentoring programs. Ricer et al. discuss such programs in family medicine and offer basic strategies for creating a program "that will have the best chance of success." They emphasize that "faculty development is a mandatory component of a successful program" (Ricer et al. 1995, Gaffney 1995).

Another area of concern in academic medicine, growing more acute as funding sources diminish, is attracting future MDs to pursue careers as clinical researchers. Baird (1990) supports the idea that recruiting future clinical researchers would be strongly fostered by the early and continuing exposure of medical students to such research and to the faculty who can serve as clinical research preceptors, mentors, and role models.

Neinstein and MacKenzie (1989) recommend that a "graduated experience of research training and exposure" for future clinical research faculty include "early exposure in medical school to participation in clinical research projects...The addition of one-to-one relationships of medical students with clinical research faculty members, who would serve as preceptors, would also encourage increased participation of these students in research."

One effective strategy that could be adapted and tested for medical students is suggested by the Valdez and Duran (1991) study of research-mentorship teams. The teams, composed of university faculty and graduate and undergraduate students, were designed to meet two objectives: (1) to expose undergraduates to research and to graduate students, and (2) to help faculty and graduate students develop mentoring relationships that would increase faculty involvement with students and enhance students' research abilities and their commitment to a research career.

## MEDICAL RESIDENCY AND
## FELLOWSHIP TRAINING

Continuing the powerful socialization experiences of medical education, house officers receive an apprenticeship-like training through which they learn the clinical skills, normative standards, and values of their field from senior house officers, fellows, and clinical faculty (see, for example, Bosk 1979 for an excellent ethnographic study of surgical residency training). As in other areas of health education, there is little empirical research on mentors and role models in graduate and postgraduate training pathways for physicians, or on the newer phenomenon of formal mentoring programs such as that described by Curtis et al. in a pediatric residency program (Blackburn and Fox 1983, Bland and Schmitz 1986, Curtis et al. 1995).

Ahrens (1992) observes that mentors can serve as "useful advisors" during residency training, informing residents about, and exposing them to, either basic or applied patient-oriented clinical research (POR) and POR-training opportunities. Bennett (1992) argues that all trainees in internal medicine, not just those who will pursue clinical research, need a strong didactic curriculum in science. Like Ahrens, he flags the importance of clinical mentors and role models for such scientific education, and emphasizes the need for these figures themselves to be versed in and able to integrate biomedical sciences and clinical medicine.

Neinstein and MacKenzie (1989) recommend that a "graduated experience of research training and exposure" for future clinical research faculty include "early exposure in medical school to participation in clinical research projects....[and that the] addition of one-to-one relationships of medical students with clinical research faculty members, who would serve as preceptors, would also encourage increased participation of these students in research."

## TRAINING FOR CLINICAL RESEARCH

A study of full-time faculty in departments of medicine has found that the presence of a mentor was one of the most important factors leading young academic physicians to pursue postdoctoral research training (Gentile et al. 1989, Levey et al. 1988). Many studies and reports dealing with clinical research training and workforce needs, however, make no reference to the roles of mentors. The 1988 Institute of Medicine report on *Resources for Clinical Investigation*, for example, does not include the roles of advisors, preceptors, or mentors in discussing the components of a "good training program" or the role of faculty in such programs (IOM 1988). A similar absence is found in the brief discussions of research training for physician-scientists in the IOM report on *Funding Health Sciences Research* (IOM 1990).

## TRAINING IN THE RESPONSIBLE
## CONDUCT OF RESEARCH

Another growing body of literature dealing with graduate and postgraduate research training issues for both MDs and PhDs concerns integrity and misconduct in research, including discussions of how ethical standards can best be inculcated during training. Here too, the treatment of mentoring is variable. The IOM (1989) report on *The Responsible Conduct of Research* does briefly note that "the value of mentoring should not be overlooked in institutional efforts to communicate responsible research practices."

The committee, however, recognized two important limitations in the role of mentors. First, institutions must recognize that the absence of support and rewards for mentoring are barriers to its effective occurrence. Second, the "informal communications" and other socialization processes involved in mentoring may not be sufficient to ensure "student awareness of the ethical and professional dimensions of research work." The committee's panel on education and training for research did include a consideration of mentoring relationships in its discussions and developed a number of useful guidelines dealing with the responsibilities of mentors and the expectations (or rights) and responsibilities of students and trainees. But this panel, like the subsequent National Academy of Sciences report (1989), made the questionable assumption that "those persons responsible for conducting research training" are, by definition, mentors.

A number of studies suggest why a growing number of individuals and groups concerned with the responsible conduct of research are convinced that reliance on "transmitting ethical and technically valid research practices 'by example' is not adequate" (Krulwich and Friedman 1993). As the Commission on Research Integrity observed in its 1995 report, "...given the size, complexity, and at times impersonality of many training environments, other mechanisms are also needed to ensure that high scientific practices and ethical standards are clearly and credibly communicated and fostered." For this reason, the commission recommended to the Secretary of Health and Human Services that the 1992 NIH training grant requirement for instruction in the responsible conduct of research "be augmented by an assurance [of ethical standards] applied to all individuals supported by PHS (Public Health Service) research funds" (Commission on Research Integrity 1995).

## CLINICAL FACULTY AS MENTORS

Much of the recent literature dealing with mentors and role models in academic medicine has concentrated on the experiences of women physicians during both their training and their medical careers (see, for example, Adler 1991; Clark and Tolle 1991; Fried et al. 1991; Johns Hopkins 1991; Levinson et al. 1989, 1991; Nadelson 1989; Ochberg et al. 1989; Osborn et al. 1992; Sirridge 1985; and Weilepp 1992).

The research has not clearly established whether mentors of the same gender as their protégés are more effective, by various measures, than those of the opposite sex. Though based on small numbers of respondents, data also indicate that women physicians who report that they have or have had a mentoring type of relationship receive less of the classic types of support and assistance from their mentors than do male physicians. But we do know that higher percentages of male than female physician-faculty consistently report having had a mentor during their training and early years as a faculty member (Kirsling and Kochar

1990, Johns Hopkins 1991, Osborn et al. 1992). And as is true in other career areas, those with mentors report greater work satisfaction and career success than those who have never had a mentoring relationship (Levinson et al. 1989, 1991; Lorber and Ecker 1983).

One reason that significantly fewer female than male physicians report having had a mentor or role model probably relates to the fact that senior faculty most often are mentors or role models for students or junior faculty of the same sex and race as themselves (Blackwell 1989). The paucity of women in more senior positions in academic medicine means that there have been limited numbers of potential same-sex mentors and role models for the growing number of women in medicine. Additionally, younger women physicians have complained "about difficulty with women superiors. Competition, envy, and devaluation often affect the reactions of women toward newcomers in fields largely dominated by men" (Sirridge 1985; see also Brown and Slein 1982).

As is the case for medical students and residents, formal mentoring programs are being developed for new clinical faculty in academic medicine. One program, initiated at the Medical College of Wisconsin in 1991, is designed to "socialize junior faculty" in the Department of Family and Community Medicine for successful careers in academic medicine (Morzinski et al. 1994). The Wisconsin program builds on the work of Bland and her colleagues on professional academic skills, which includes "three essential areas in which faculty new to academic medicine need to be socialized." The areas involve "(1) adopting academic values, (2) managing an academic career, and (3) establishing and maintaining a productive network of colleagues. Success in these three areas is so critical that it appears to predict those faculty who will be high achievers and those who will not" (Morzinski et al. 1994; Bland and Schmitz 1986; Bland et al. 1990).

## BARRIERS TO MENTORING AND ADVISING

In May 1991, several of the most eminent physician-investigators and medical educators from the post-World War II "golden years" of patient-oriented clinical research met for a three-day oral history conference with some of today's senior and younger clinical researchers and medical educators, and several sociologists and historians of medicine. Here they recounted and compared their professional and personal experiences in becoming physician-investigators and in training new generations of physician-investigators (Fox, Swazey and Watkins 1992).

During their extended conversation, the emeritus participants often spoke reverentially about certain "giants" such as Fuller Albright and Soma Weiss, whom they considered to be their mentors or role models even as they went about their work as hands-on teachers, clinicians, and researchers. The physicians also discussed the ways in which their education and training as physician-investigators (including the mentoring they received, and the research, teaching, and mentoring that they in turn did) were fostered by the relatively small number and size and the organizational structure of their medical schools and teaching hospitals.

The accounts provided striking comparisons with the discussions of contemporary affairs and the literature. Together, they depict a variety of barriers to faculty being mentors, serving as the types of clinical role models that embody the "good Samaritan" attributes of physicians (McDermott 1978), and being more than narrowly formal, technical advisors in graduate and postgraduate training.

Some of the most serious obstacles have been created by the increasingly large and complex social organization, the reward system, and the climate of the institutions in which physicians, PhD biomedical researchers, and many other health professionals are trained, including the nature of the demands upon the time and efforts of faculty (Acadia Institute 1996).

One of the most widely discussed substantial barriers is also the fact that there are few rewards in academia for being a dedicated and effective Teacher (with a capital T), the role most closely linked with mentoring in academia.

To ask, as those concerned with higher education often do, "Where are the mentors?" begs the question, "Where are the Teachers?" In contrast to the institutional demands and rewards for successful grantsmanship, publications, and large, revenue-producing patient case loads for clinical faculty, there are few career path rewards and weak institutional support for teaching and serving as an advisor or mentor to graduate or postgraduate students or junior faculty. Even for faculty strongly committed to these roles, the criteria for "success" as a graduate or professional school faculty member mitigate against frequent and close contacts with students (Acadia Institute 1996).

Another factor to which attention is being paid, particularly in biomedical research areas, is the extent to which the size and specialty mix of research groups affects the amount and quality of technical and moral supervision that can be provided by the principal investigator or head of the group (Barinaga 1991; Panel on Scientific Responsibility 1992).

Due to the relative lack of emphasis on teaching roles and the autonomy accorded faculty members, there is also little attention to "training the trainers" in various aspects of teaching, advising, or mentoring, although the need for this sphere of faculty development is beginning to be addressed in many fields, including health professions education by some of the new formal mentoring programs. A policy statement by the Council of Graduate Schools states:

Despite the central importance of [the adviser-advisee] relationship, most universities offer faculty little or no guidance on that role. Expressing a widely shared sentiment, one graduate dean commented only partly in jest, "Generally we feel that faculty members are born with the capacity to supervise dissertation research just as they are born with the skills of teaching".... [However,] there is a growing sense at a number of universities that the graduate school and department should take more deliberate action to strengthen this aspect of graduate education. In a dynamic, changing research environment where fields are becoming more subdivided and specialized...the role of a dissertation adviser in guiding an advisee through the maze acquires new weight. Moreover, graduate students tend to be less sanguine than faculty about the state of dissertation directing (Council of Graduate Schools 1991).

## CONCLUSIONS AND RECOMMENDATIONS

The research findings and other writings reviewed in this paper suggest several key points that should be considered in any efforts to develop or strengthen mentoring and mentor-like programs.

1. The availability of teacher-mentors and the institutional and professional supports to facilitate the development of effective mentoring or mentor-like advising relationships are but two of the many factors shaping the education

and socialization of individuals entering the health professions and their subsequent careers. The weight of available evidence, however, suggests that they are important factors.

2. Faculty and an institution's educational leadership need to understand and clarify the differences among the roles of advisors, counselors, traditional mentors, mentors in formal programs, preceptors, docents, and role models. Although they have commonalities, the terms are not synonymous or interchangeable.

3. Most faculty believe that they are the best vehicle for transmitting ethical standards and practices to their students by example and other informal guidance. But the reluctance to assume responsibility for the professional-ethical conduct of their students is one indication of a significant disparity between beliefs and practices, and speaks to the need for training-the-trainers in the responsible conduct of research.

4. Institutional efforts to foster the roles and functions of mentors and advisors need to recognize and attempt to deal realistically with the many barriers to mentoring and advising. The barriers include the organizational, economic, culture, and climate factors that have greatly diminished the centrality of education as a primary institutional value and mission, particularly in research-intensive universities and academic health centers. At the same time, linkages between teaching and research, and between teaching, research, and patient care in academic medicine, have been weakened. Overall, there are many indicators of what can be thought of as a deinstitutionalization of advising and mentoring in graduate and professional education. If institutions are serious about education as a central mission, they need to support faculty-educators financially and in terms of criteria for recruitment, promotion, and tenure.

5. Institutions and their programs need to undertake major strategic changes, not just tactical maneuvers, if they genuinely want to restore or maintain a central focus on education.* In line with what some schools are attempting to do, for example, the reward system needs to be fundamentally altered by making what the late Ernest L. Boyer defined as "teaching scholarship" a major criterion for appointments, promotion, and tenure for at least a subset of facul-

---

* The National Project on Institutional Priorities and Faculty Rewards is a major effort by a range of disciplines to expand the activities "considered to be a legitimate

ty (Boyer 1990). Strengthening the role of faculty-educators in practice as well as in principle should, in turn, enhance both the amount and quality of mentoring and advising.

6. Training programs and departments that develop formal mentoring programs in an effort to foster more and better faculty-student or faculty-faculty interactions need to define their program's objectives clearly and realistically; carefully plan its implementation, beginning with the recruitment and training of faculty mentors; monitor its progress; and evaluate its short- and long-term outcomes. Valuable guidance concerning the objectives, structure, content, and assessment of such programs can be drawn from a number of diverse mentoring projects underway in university graduate programs. (Gaffney 1995)

7. It is difficult to generate conclusions or detailed programmatic recommendations about mentoring and advising in health professions' education because of the dearth of empirical information that deals specifically with these topics.

Future cross-sectional or longitudinal survey and interview research can provide a better basis for decisions than now available about whether efforts need to be undertaken to increase or improve mentoring and advising (and, if so, what might be the most effective strategies) and illuminate the nature and effects of advising and of traditional and formal mentoring relationships. Such studies also need to look at both the positive and "toxic" effects of advising and mentoring, and assess whether those who work with students are sufficiently knowledgeable about current career options and opportunities in their field. Writes Floyd Bloom (1995) "Our young scientists say one thing loud and clear. Their traditional academic mentors are out of touch with the remarkably altered circumstances of today's job market."

Formal instruction is an essential component of health professional education. But acquiring substantial amounts of the knowledge, techniques, and norms of their discipline through an apprenticeship type of learning and doing

---

scholarly or professional work" for promotion and tenure. The project, based at Syracuse University, has been supported by the Fund for the Improvement of Postsecondary Education, the Lilly Endowment, and the Pew Charitable Trusts. As of May 1994, fifteen professional societies and associations were involved (Diamond 1994).

and through the professional socialization is also an integral part of such training. If further research on this subject is undertaken, those responsible for its design and implementation can benefit from the many lessons, both positive and negative, in the extant literature on mentors, advisors, and role models.

## Acknowledgments

Research for this paper was supported in part by grant numbers 8913159 and 9222889 from the National Science Foundation for the Acadia Institute on Professional Values and Ethical Issues in the Graduate Education of Sciences and Engineers. All opinions, findings, conclusions, and recommendations are those of the authors and do not necessarily reflect the views of the National Science Foundation.

## REFERENCES

Acadia Institute and Medical College of Pennsylvania Project on Undergraduate Medical Education. 1996. *Fulfilling the Mission. Medical Schools and the Education of Medical Students*. Philadelphia: Medical College of Pennsylvania and Hahnemann University.

Adler, N.E. 1991. Women mentors needed in academic medicine. (editorial) *Western Journal of Medicine* 154(April):468-469.

Ahrens, E.H. 1992. *The Crisis in Clinical Research*. New York: Oxford University.

American College of Physicians. 1991. Promotion and tenure of women and minorities on medical school faculties. *Annals of Internal Medicine* 114:63-68.

Baird, L.L. 1969. A factor-analytic study of graduate students. *Journal of Educational Psychology* 60:15-21.

————. 1972. The relation of graduate students' role relations to their state of academic career, employment, and academic success. *Organizational Behavior and Human Performance* 7:428-441.

————.1990. The melancholy of anatomy: The personal and professional development of graduate and professional school students. In *Higher Education: Handbook of Theory and Research*, vol. 6, ed. J.C. Smart. New York: Agathon.

Bandura, A. 1977. *Social Learning Theory*. Englewood Cliffs, NJ: Prentice-Hall.

Barinaga, M. 1991. Labstyles of the famous and well funded. *Science* 252(28 June):1776-1778.

Barondess, J.A. 1994. A brief history of mentoring (President's address). *Transactions of the American Clinical and Climatological Association* 106:1-24.

Bell, R.M. 1987. Presidential address: Of mentors and academic responsibility. *American Journal of Surgery* 154(November):465-470.

Bellflower, D.K. 1982. Developing a mentor relationship. *Roeper Review* 5:45-46.

Bennett, J.C. 1992. Development of a didactic curriculum in science related to internal medicine. *Annals of Internal Medicine* 116(15 June):1088-1090.

Bidwell A.S., and M.L. Brassler. 1989. Role modeling versus mentoring in nursing education. *Image: Journal of Nursing Scholarship* 21(1):23-25.

Blackburn, R.T. 1979. Academic careers: Patterns and possibilities. *Current Issues in Higher Education* 2(September):25-27.

Blackburn, R.T., and T.G. Fox. 1983. Physicians' values and their career stage. *Journal of Vocational Behavior* 22:159-173.

Blackwell, J.E. 1989. Mentoring: An action strategy for increasing minority faculty. *Academe* (September-October):8-14.

Bland C.J., and C.C. Schmitz. 1986. Characteristics of the successful researcher and implications for faculty development. *Journal of Medical Education* 61(January):22-31.

Bland C.J., C.C. Schmitz, F.T. Stritter, et al. 1990. *Successful Faculty in Academic Medicine*. New York: Springer.

Bloom, F.E. 1995. Launching *Science*'s next wave (editorial). *Science* 270(Oct.):11.

Bloom F.E., and M.A. Randolph, eds. 1990. *Funding Health Sciences Research*. A Strategy to Restore Balance. Washington: National Academy.

Blotnick, S. 1984. *The Corporate Steeplechase: Predictable Crises in A Business Career.* New York: Facts on File.

Bosk, C.L. 1979. *Forgive and Remember. Managing Medical Failure.* Chicago: University of Chicago.

Bova, B.M., and R. Phillips. 1984. Mentoring as a learning experience for adults. *Journal of Teacher Education* 35(May-June)16-20.

Boyer, E.L. 1990. *Scholarship Reconsidered. The Priorities of the Professoriate.* Princeton NJ: Carnegie Foundation for the Advancement of Teaching.

Bragg, A.K. 1976. *The Socialization Process in Higher Education. ERIC/Higher Education Research Report No. 7.* Washington: American Association for Higher Education.

Brim, O.G. 1966. Socialization through the life cycle. In *Socialization After Childhood: Two Essays,* O.G. Brim and S. Wheeler, eds. New York: Wiley.

Brown S.L., and R.H. Slein. 1982. Woman-power in the medical hierarchy. *Journal of the American Medical Women's Association* 37:155.

Brown, J.P., J.F. Williams, and M.S. Hoppe. 1995. The role of mentorship in dental graduate education. *Journal of Dental Education* 59(5):573-577.

Bucher, R., and J.G. Stelling. 1977. *Becoming Professional.* Beverly Hills: Sage.

Calkins, E.V., L.M. Arnold, T.L. Willoughby, et al. 1986. Docents' and students' perceptions of the ideal and actual role of the docent. *Journal of Medical Education* 61(September):743-748.

Calkins, E.V., L.M. Arnold, and T.L. Willoughby. 1987. Perceptions of the role of a faculty supervisor or "mentor" at two medical schools. *Assessment and Evaluation in Higher Education* 12(Autumn):202-208.

Cameron, S.W., and R.T. Blackburn. 1981. Sponsorship and academic career success. *Journal of Higher Education* 52:369-377.

Clark, B., and S.W. Tolle. 1991. Mentors and role models for women in academic medicine. *Western Journal of Medicine.* 154:423-426.

Collins, G.C. 1978. Everyone who makes it has a mentor. *Harvard Business Review* 56:89-101.

Collins, N.N. 1983. *Professional Women and Their Mentors.* Englewood Cliffs, NJ: Prentice-Hall.

Commission on Research Integrity. 1995. *Integrity and Misconduct in Research.* Report to the Secretary for Health and Human Services, the House Committee on Commerce, the Senate Committee on Labor and Human Resources.

Council of Graduate Schools. 1991. *The Role and Nature of the Doctoral Dissertation. A Policy Statement.* Washington: Council of Graduate Schools.

Creager, J.A. 1971. *The American Graduate Student: A Normative Description.* American Council on Education Research Report.

Cronan-Hillix, T., L.K. Gensheimer, W.A. Cronan-Hillix, et al. 1986. Students' views of mentors in psychology graduate training. *Teaching of Psychology* 13:123-127.

Curtis, J.A., H. Adam, and S.P. Shelov. 1995. A formal mentoring program in a pediatric residency. *Academic Medicine* 70(5):453-454.

Daloz, L.A. 1983. Mentors: Teachers who make a difference. *Change* 15:24-27.

————. 1986. *Effective Teaching and Mentoring: Realizing the Transformational Power of Adult Learning Experiences.* San Francisco: Jossey-Bass.

Dalton, G.N., P.H. Thompson, and R.L. Price. 1977. The four stages of professional careers. A new look at performance by professionals. *Organizational Dynamics* 6:19-42.

Darling, L.A. 1984. What do nurses want in a mentor? *Journal of Nursing Administration* 14(10):42-44.

————. 1985a. Endings in mentor relationships. *Journal of Nursing Administration* 15(11):40-41.

————. 1985b. Mentor matching. *Journal of Nursing Administration* 15(1):45-46.

————. 1985c. Mentors and mentoring. *Nurse Educator* 10(6):18-19.

————. 1986. What to do about toxic mentors. *Nurse Educator* 11(2):29-30.

Diamond, R.M. 1994. The tough task of reforming the faculty-reward system. *Chronicle of Higher Education* (11 May):B1-3.

Eastwood, S. P. Derish, E. Leash, et al. 1996. Ethical issues in biomedical research: Perceptions and practices of postdoctoral research fellows responding to a survey. *Science and Engineering Ethics* 2(1):89-114.

Evanoski, P.O. 1988. The role of mentoring in higher education. *Community Review* 8(Spring):22-27.

Fowler, D.L. 1982. Mentoring relationship and perceived quality of the academic work environment. *Journal of NAWDAC* 45:27-33.

Fox, R.C. 1990. Training in caring competence in North American medicine: Reforming the reforms. *Humane Medicine* 6(1):15-21.

Fox, R.C., J.P. Swazey, and J.C. Watkins. 1992. *The Study of the Sick.* Proceedings of a Conference on the Development of Clinical Research, May 20-22, 1991.

Philadelphia: Medical College of Pennsylvania and Allegheny-Singer Research Institute.

Fried, L.P., K.M. Carbone, C.A. Francomano, et al. 1991. A report from the task force on women's academic careers in medicine. Baltimore: Johns Hopkins University School of Medicine.

Friedman, N. 1987. *Mentors and Supervisors*. IIE Research Report No. 14. New York: Institute of International Education.

Gaffney, N.A., ed. 1995. *A Conversation About Mentoring: Trends and Models*. Washington: Council of Graduate Schools.

Gentile, N.O., G.S. Levey, P. Jolly P, et al. 1989. Postdoctoral Research Training of Full-Time Faculty in Departments of Medicine. Washington: American Association of Medical Colleges.

George, P., and J. Kummerow. 1981. Mentoring for career women. *Training/HRD* 18:44-99.

Hagerty, B. 1986. A second look at mentors. *Nursing Outlook* 34(1):16-19,24.

Heinrich, K.T. 1991. Loving partnerships: Dealing with sexual attraction and power in doctoral advisement relationships. *Journal of Higher Education* 62 (September-October):514-538.

Heins, M., S.N. Fahey, and L.I. Leiden. 1984. Perceived stress in medical, law, and graduate students. *Journal of Medical Education* 59:169-179.

Heiss, A.M. 1964. *Berkeley Doctoral Students Appraise their Academic Programs*. Berkeley: University of California Center for the Study of Higher Education.

Hennig, M,, and A. Jardim. 1977. *The Managerial Woman*. New York: Doubleday.

Hunt, D.M., and C. Michael. 1983. Mentorship: A career training and development tool. *Academy of Management Review* 8:475-485.

Hurley, B.A. 1978. Socialization for roles. In *Role Theory: Perspectives for Health Professionals*, M.E. Hardy and M.E. Conway, eds. Norwalk, CT: Appleton-Century-Crofts.

IOM (Institute of Medicine). 1988. *Resources for Clinical Investigation*. Report of a Study by a Committee of the Institute of Medicine Division of Health Sciences Policy. Washington: National Academy Press.

———. 1989. *The Responsible Conduct of Research in the Health Sciences*. Washington: National Academy Press.

———. 1990. *Funding Health Sciences Research: A Strategy to Restore Balance*. Washington: National Academy of Sciences.

Johns Hopkins University School of Medicine. 1991. Department of Medicine Task Force on the status of women. Survey data related to mentoring. Unpublished.

Jowers, L.T., and K. Herr. 1990. A review of literature on mentor-protégé relationships. In *Review of Research In Nursing Education*, vol. 3, eds. G.M. Clayton and P.A. Baj. New York: National League for Nursing.

Kalichman, M.N., and P.J. Friedman. 1992. A pilot study of biomedical trainees' perceptions concerning research ethics. *Academic Medicine* 67(11):769-775.

Kapustiak, M., S.M. Capello, and R.L. Hofmeister. 1985. The key to your professional success is you: Networking, mentor-mentee relationships, and negotiation. *Journal of the American Dietetic Association* 85(7):846-848.

Kelley, W.N., and M.A. Randolph, eds. 1994. *Careers in Clinical Research. Obstacles and Opportunities.* Washington: National Academy Press.

Kemper, T. 1968. Reference groups, socialization and achievement. *American Sociological Review* 33:31-45.

Kirsling, R.A., and M.S. Kochar. 1990. Mentors in graduate medical education at the Medical College of Wisconsin. *Academic Medicine* 65:272,273.

Klauss, R. 1981. Formalized mentor relationships for management and executive development programs in the federal government. *Public Administration Review* 41:489-496.

Kram, K.E. 1983. Phases of the mentor relationship. *Academy of Management Journal* 26:608-625.

Krulwich, T.A., and P.J. Friedman. 1993. Integrity in the education of researchers. *Academic Medicine* 68(supplement):S14-S18.

Levey, G.S., C.R. Sherman, N.O. Gentile, et al. 1988. Postdoctoral research training of full-time faculty in academic departments of medicine. *Annals of Internal Medicine* 109(1 Sept.):414-418.

Levinson, D.J., C.N. Darrow, E.B. Klein, et al. 1978. *The Seasons of A Man's Life.* New York: Knopf.

Levinson, W., S. Tolle, and C. Lewis. 1989. Women in academic medicine: Combining career and family. *New England Journal of Medicine* 321:1511-1517.

Levinson W., K. Kaufman, B. Clark, et al. 1991. Mentors and role models for women in academic medicine. *Western Journal of Medicine* 154(April):423-426.

Lobeck, C.C., and H.L. Stone. 1990. Class mentors: A step toward implementing the GPEP report. *Academic Medicine* 65(June):351-354.

Lorber, J., and M. Ecker. 1983. Career development of female and male physicians. *Journal of Medical Education* 58:447-456.

Lough, M.E. 1986. Networking and working with a mentor: Keys to eliciting support for clinical research as a staff nurse. *Heart and Lung* 15:525-527.

Luis, K.S., M.S. Anderson, and L. Rosenberg. Academic misconduct and values: The department's influence. *Review of Higher Education.* 18(4):393-422.

Mateo, M.A., K.T. Kirchoff, and M.G. Schira. 1991. Research skill development. In *Conducting and Using Nursing Research in the Clinical Setting,* M.A. Mateo and K.T. Kirchoff, eds. Baltimore: Williams and Wilkins.

May, K.M., A.L. Meleis, and P. Winstead-Fry. 1982. Mentorship for scholarliness: Opportunities and dilemmas. *Nursing Outlook* 30:22-28.

McDermott, W. 1978. Medicine: The public good and one's own. *Perspectives in Biology and Medicine* 21:167-187.

Merriam S.B., T.K. Thomas, and C.P. Zeph. 1987. Mentoring in higher education: What we know now. *Review of Higher Education* 11(2):199-210.

Morton-Cooper, A., and A. Palmer. 1993. Mentoring and Preceptorship. *A Guide to Support Roles in Clinical Practice.* Oxford: Blackwell.

Morzinski, J.A., D.E. Simpson, D.J. Bower. et al. 1994. Faculty development through formal mentoring. *Academic Medicine* 69(4): 267-269.

Muller, S. 1984. Physicians for the Twenty-First Century. Report of the project panel on the general professional education of the physician and college preparation for medicine. *Journal of Medical Education* 59:Part 2(November).

Nadelson, C.C. 1989. Professional issues for women. *Psychiatric Clinics of North America* 12(March):25-33.

National Academy of Sciences Committee on the Conduct of Science. 1989. *On Being A Scientist.* Washington: National Academy.

Neidle, E.A. 1985. The mentor apprentice program - A modest proposal for alleviating the scarcity of clinical researchers in dentistry. *Journal of Dental Education* 49(5):272-274.

Neinstein, L.S., and R.G. MacKenzie. 1989. Prior training and recommendations for future training of clinical research faculty members. *Academic Medicine* 64(January):32-35.

Ochberg, R.L., G.M. Barton, and A.N. West. 1989. Women physicians and their mentors. *Journal of the American Medical Women's Association* 44(July-August):123-126.

Osborn, E.H., V.L. Ernster, and J.B. Martin. 1992. Women's attitutes toward careers in academic medicine at the University of California, San Francisco. *Academic Medicine* 67(January):59-62.

Panel on Scientific Responsibility and the Conduct of Research, Committee on Science, Engineering, and Public Policy, 1992. *Responsible Science: Ensuring the Integrity of the Research Process,* vol. 1. National Academy of Sciences, National Academy of Engineering, and Institute of Medicine. Washington: National Academy Press.

Phillips-Jones, L. 1982. *Mentors and Protégés.* New York: Arbor House.

Pilette, P.C. 1981. An encounter of the leadership kind. *Nursing Leadership* 3:22-26.

Puetz, B. 1983. *Networking for Nurses.* Rockville, MD: Aspen.

Queralt, M. 1982. The role of the mentor in the career development of university faculty members and academic administrators. Paper presented at the annual meeting of the National Association of Woman Deans, Administrators, and Counselors, 3 April 1982, Indianapolis. ERIC Document Reproduction Service, ED 216 614.

Rakatansky, H. 1994. The role of the role model. *Rhode Island Medicine* 77(10):339,340.

Ricer, R.E., B.C. Fox, and K.E. Miller. 1995. Mentoring for medical students interested in family practice. *Family Medicine* 27(6):360-65.

Schmidt, J.A., and J.S. Wolfe. 1980. The mentor partnership: Discovery of professionalism. *NASPA Journal* 17:45-51.

Scott, M.E. 1992. Designing effective mentoring programs: Historical perspectives and current issues. *Humanistic Educational Development* 30:167-175.

Sirridge, M.S. 1985. The mentor system in medicine — how it works for women. *Journal of the American Medical Women's Association* 40(2):51-53.

Speizer, J.J. 1981. Role models, mentors, and sponsors: The elusive concept. *Signs: Journal of Women in Culture and Society*. 6(4): 692-712.

Swanson, A.G. 1984. The medical school student and the faculty forest. *Bulletin of the New York Academy of Medicine* 60:290-296.

Swazey, J.P. 1993. Teaching ethics: Needs, opportunities, and obstacles. In *Ethics, Values, and the Promise of Science*. Sigma Xi Forum Proceedings, Feb. 25, 26, 1993. Research Triangle Park, NC: Sigma Xi.

————, M.S. Anderson, and K.S. Louis. 1993. Ethical problems in academic research. *American Scientist* 81(6):542-553.

Tyler, J.L. 1994. The death of mentoring. *Hospitals & Health Networks* 68(19):84.

Upham, S. 1995. University of Oregon: Guidelines for good practice in graduate programs. *Communicator* 28(10):10-12.

Valadez, J.R., and R.P. Duran. 1991. Mentoring in higher education. Paper presented at the Annual Meeting of the American Education Research Association, Chicago.

Vance, C. 1982. The mentor connection. *Journal of Nursing Administration* 38:7-13.

Walsh, C.R., and C.A. Clements. 1995. Attributes of mentors as perceived by orthopaedic nurses. *Orthopaedic Nursing* 14(3):49-56.

Weilepp, A.E. 1992. Female mentors in short supply. *Journal of the American Medical Association* 267(5 February):739,742.

Werley, H.H., and B.J. Newcomb. 1983. The research mentor: A missing element in nursing? In *The Nursing Profession: A Time To Speak*, N.L. Chaska, ed. New York: McGraw-Hill.

Williams, R., and R. Blackburn. 1988. Mentoring and junior faculty productivity. *Journal of Nursing Education* 27:204-209.

Yoder, L. 1990. Mentoring: A concept analysis. *Nursing Administration Quarterly* 5(1):9-19.

Zey, M.C. 1984. *The Mentor Connection*. Homewood, IL: Dow Jones-Irwin.

# MAKING SENSE OF
# THE TENURE DEBATE

*Elaine R. Rubin, PhD*

ISTORY REMINDS US POWERFULLY OF THE ways that societal vagaries affect educational institutions and their members. If, indeed, societal views about the scholarly pursuit of knowledge and the role of higher education can be measured by the tenure debate, we must consider the academic health center in a historical context. Public disillusionment with higher education, escalating costs, trendy curriculums, and discontented faculty are evidence of troubled times. As the millennium approaches, society increasingly questions its commitment to granting a privileged status to the pursuit of knowledge in universities. Because tenure, for better or worse, symbolizes the university, calls for changes in the system must be balanced against the potential for damaging both the nature of higher education and the public view of education.

In recent years, the debate over the meaning, function, and relevance of tenure has intensified both within and outside the academic community. But nowhere else on a campus does the question of tenure emerge as boldly as it does at academic health centers, the institutions responsible for a major portion of the nation's health professions education, biomedical research, and patient care. As they seek ways to survive financially, tenure is coming under intense scrutiny, particularly within their schools of medicine. Tenure within academic health cen-

*Dr. Rubin is assistant vice president for program at the Association of Academic Health Centers.*

ters therefore deserves special attention, for what happens in these institutions may be a bellwether for all institutions of higher education.

History becomes an important element in the debate for it calls attention to the connection between tenure and the larger societal, professional, and institutional issues at stake. To some degree, the outcome may be an important proxy for societal views on the place and purpose of academics and the university in the twenty-first century.

Also at issue, and increasingly symbolized by the tenure debate, is the extent to which academic functions are being devalued within academic health centers in the face of the economic exigencies. Modifications to tenure are raising questions about academic health center commitments to academic principles and linkages within the university.

History shows that tenure has evolved in every age, becoming the embodiment of new ideals and new meanings to fit academic environments and changing societies. Over time, it has incrementally become a conglomerate of interrelated elements that for many people defy separation. At issue is whether the modifications now under way are a beneficial response to academe in a new age or whether they represent the beginning of the end of tenure, a bulwark of universities and scholarship.

In short, current visions and models of organizations are today being tested against time-honored university principles and values. Academic health centers are struggling to embrace the cost-cutting disciplines of competition while defending the moral obligation of the teacher, the deliberation of critical issues, and free inquiry in their classrooms. An examination of the issues of tenure at academic health centers can help illuminate and enlarge the debate over tenure in higher education, regardless of the type of academic institution involved.

All face the key question: Can modifications to the tenure system be consistent with a history that has evolved by safeguarding the basic values of scholarly professions and the contributions of universities? Or will overbearing economic considerations require a revolutionary departure from past practices and the demise of the tenure system?

## SOME MOTIVATIONS BEHIND
## TODAY'S DEBATE

Today's debate over tenure has been triggered by recent flare-ups of attitudes and problems that have been part of the university system for centuries. For two hundred years, the driving forces behind attacks on tenure have included widespread economic distress, public resentment, declining budgets, decreased funding for academe, and, more recently, a history of tension on campus. Neil Hamilton (1997), trustees professor of regulatory policy at William Mitchell College of Law, points out that the aftermath of the campus disruptions of the 1960s combined with the economic stress of the early 1970s to produce a serious challenge to tenure on many university campuses. With the long postwar expansion of higher education slowing and jobs becoming scarce, many institutions that had given tenure freely, perhaps even extravagantly, then proclaimed themselves overtenured (Brown and Kurland 1990).

Part of the difficulty in making sense of the tenure debate is that the two sides frame the issues surrounding tenure very differently. Opponents hold that it is a system of privilege for an elite class of workers; it needs to be abolished, or, at the very least, drastically reformed. Societal needs in the 1990s, they note, require productive and efficient organizations. In such settings, tenure is the principal barrier to achieving institutional flexibility and competitive advantage in the marketplace, increased accountability, and enhanced productivity.

Those who defend tenure believe that higher education is using the tenure system as a scapegoat for its economic problems. They say that attacks on tenure violate academic freedom and threaten the nature of professional office and, ultimately, the survival of scholars and academe as we know them. They go on to argue that the attempt to mold universities into a corporate model will do irreparable harm to society.

The professional and social standing of academics also has generated discussion, if not outright resentment, throughout the ages. Hamilton (1996) notes that academics occupy a salient particularly exposed to the lust to censor in the name of higher moralities. He does not find it surprising that periodic waves of zealotry from McCarthyism to the politics of the radical left have affected universities in this century. Some experts find the tenure bashing of the 1990s particularly ominous for it coincides with the restructuring of the U.S. economy and the diminishing respect accorded higher education in American life.

Some observers are troubled that the dismantling of tenure coincides with the moment when, along with the nation's changing demographics, the makeup of the professoriate also is about to change dramatically, according to University of Arizona Professor Annette Kolodny (1996). Although it is sometimes assumed that the growing polemic (particularly by the conservative right) against tenure is intended to dislodge the tenured radicals of the 1960s, Kolodny argues that the dismantling of tenure is aimed at those who have yet to attain a firm foothold within academe but who now seem poised to enter. Many who advocate either restrictions on tenure or abolition of tenure are betting that without the job security afforded by tenure, those from still marginalized groups will find academic employment too uncertain to attract them. And without the academic freedom protections of tenure, even those few who do enter the professoriate will be less likely to challenge the established norms and procedures of their fields.

Tenure is a concept that embodies ideals and principles, represents commitments and obligations of individuals and institutions, and reflects many societal goals and expectations. But because its practice developed over centuries and has been understood differently in different countries and times, the term evades precise definition and its practice defies uniformity.

For the American Association of University Professors (AAUP), tenure is a means to certain ends; specifically (1) freedom of teaching and research and of extramural activities, and (2) a sufficient degree of economic security to make the profession attractive to men and women of ability. Freedom and economic security, hence, tenure, are indispensable to the success of an institution in fulfilling its obligations to its students and to society. A faculty member obtains tenure by passing through an academic review that follows a period of probation, which may vary but is normally seven years. In its landmark 1940 statement, the AAUP (1995) draws attention to societal issues and the common good. Institutions of higher education are conducted for the common good and not to further the interest of either the individual teacher or the institution as a whole. The common good depends upon the free search for truth and its free exposition.

## ORIGINS OF TENURE

The issues surrounding tenure—privilege, prerogatives, academic freedom,

and governance—are rooted in the Middle Ages when scholars in Europe benefited from an array of favors from the monarchs, including exemptions from
taxes and military service, which protected and enhanced both their physical and
material well-being. The hallmark of scholarly privilege in the Middle Ages,
however, was the immunity from monarchical power that scholars obtained
through incorporation.

In this setting, societies or corporations decided the rules to be followed for
functioning within the organization as well as those that forced exclusion from
the fellowship. Medieval scholars had the right to elect their own officers and
representatives, to sue and be sued as a single juristic person, and to enact the
rules and regulations to which they and those who dealt with them had to conform. Self-governance is a significant legacy from this period.

During the sixteenth and seventeenth centuries, English tutors and the fellows who studied under them were members of self-governing corporations and
gained privileges from that membership. These scholars enjoyed unlimited tenure
unless deprived of it by the monarch or their peers (Metzger 1973). On the
European continent itself, professors had expansive administrative powers and
were presumed to hold office during their lifetime, barring serious offense.

In the United States, the autonomy of the corporation was an ideal that
lived on at Harvard and other Colonial colleges. However, American universities
would yield control of their boards of overseers to laypeople, a situation that
largely negated the ideals of corporate governance and disassociated the role of
teaching from governing. This disassociation would transform the relationship
between the faculty and the corporation making it contractual and focused on
the exchange of valued objects. One of the concomitant of a contractual relationship, says Metzger, is that it focuses attention on duration of a relationship
as opposed to a collegial relationship where time is not a critical dimension.
"Tenure" became "time" in this period of American history (Metzger 1973).

In the eighteenth century, the corporation was not only limiting the time
of tutorial appointments but also the time each teacher could spend within that
rank, with the maximum being eight years (Quincy 1840). The alleged purpose
was to prevent incumbencies from being lengthened by reappointments given
out of neglect or sympathy. The "up or out" rule is also traced to this period with
evidence that no limit was set on the total years of trial nor enforcement of the

out (Metzger 1973).

By the nineteenth century in Europe, faculties in German universities enjoyed two forms of academic freedom: lernfreiheit, which guaranteed faculty an absence of administrative coercions in the learning situation, and lehrfreiheit, which guaranteed faculty freedom of teaching and inquiry (Hofstadter and Metzger 1955).

In nineteenth century America, all faculty members at many universities were being appointed for a year, and reappointment occurred only for incumbents who could pass a new test. Governing boards justified such a system on the grounds that legislatures provided funding on a yearly basis, thus making it impossible to make commitments to faculty for longer than the period of funding.

From the mid to late nineteenth century the gulf between administrators and faculty widened. As professors gained more prestige, administrators were increasingly viewed as persons with organizational power and second-class academic skills (Metzger 1973). The complexities of governance issues and the ambiguity of faculty status often resulted in judicial cases that highlighted this emerging gulf between faculty and administrators on tenure and governance. In a tenure case in the late nineteenth century, a Kansas Supreme Court judge wrote that the legislature did not intend to confer upon them [the University of Kansas Board of Trustees] the irresponsible power of trifling with other men's rights. On the other hand, the court noted that "making the regents responsible for their acts does not in the least abridge their powers." Overall, tenure was still a nebulous concept at the beginning of the twentieth century. In 1878 the Board of Regents in Kansas held that indefinite tenure, for example, meant what academics thought it meant, which could be much or little.

University presidents would eventually lead the opposition to the one-year term policy, saying that the efficiency of the university was in jeopardy every year as a result of the nervousness on the part of the faculty. Presidents preferred contracts of varying fixed duration for faculty members in lower ranks and indefinite appointments for the rest. From 1860 to 1914, most institutions moved away from the one-year term. However, ambiguity in the meaning of appointments abounded. It was not unusual for a recipient of an indefinite appointment to expect that, except for gross negligence, it was a lifetime guarantee (Metzger 1973).

## A PROFESSIONAL ORGANIZATION
## TAKES ON TENURE

Faculty concerns over tenure and academic freedom were joined with the institutional and societal interests of the profession with the founding of the AAUP in 1915. The organization sought to undertake "the gradual formulation of general principles respecting tenure of the professional office and the legitimate grounds for the dismissal of professors" (Lovejoy Papers). The AAUP also wanted to establish a representative judicial committee to investigate and report cases in which administrative authorities were alleged to have interfered with freedom or caused injury to the professional standing and opportunities of any professor. The hope was to shape tenure rules to the interest of professors rather than the interest of lay controllers.

A major catalyst for the action of the founding professors was the famous Ross case at Stanford University in 1900, when Edward A. Ross, a new economist, was dismissed for his outspoken economic ideas that ran counter to those of Jane Lathrop Stanford, the sole trustee of the university.

The AAUP founding fathers tried to establish the right of the faculty as a body to judge the fitness of a member when the issue was in dispute. Among the founders, Arthur Lovejoy in particular had been convinced that the peril to modern professors was attacks on academic freedom that were officially disguised as something else.

The founders did not dispute the legal power of university governing boards to review their findings. But they held that those not "trained for a scholar's duties" could not intervene in cases involving the ideas or the expression of ideas "without destroying, to the extent of their intervention, the essential nature of the university" (AAUP 1915). Faculty control would remain integral to tenure and a continuing source of conflict.

By 1940, the AAUP statement on tenure had incorporated an emphasis on job security. Also significant was that the 1940 statement advanced the notion of judicial tenure, that is, all dismissals were to be for cause and all were to be determined through the application of preestablished procedural and due process standards. The expansion of rights and procedural safeguards for civil service employees greatly influenced the emergence of this concept.

## TENURE TODAY: AN AMALGAM
## OF CONCEPTS

The literature on tenure today describes a complex issue, but each discussion tends to focus on only one element of the concept, such as academic freedom or job security. In 1958 in Worzella v. Board of Regents, the Supreme Court of South Dakota observed that the exact meaning and intent of this so-called tenure eludes us. Its vaporous objectives, purposes, and procedures are lost in a fog of nebulous verbiage.

In general, however, most education experts agree that tenure involves three concepts. First, tenure is part of academic freedom, because it frees a faculty member from restraints and pressures that otherwise would inhibit independent thought and action. Second, tenure represents a communal acceptance by one's peers into the professorial guild. And third, tenure is a means for providing job security to promote institutional stability and loyalty and to reward individual service and accomplishment (McHugh 1973).

These interrelated concepts create an environment that encourages the pursuit and advancement of knowledge. At issue in the current debate is whether such an environment can be created and sustained by uncoupling, separating, or abolishing individual elements of tenure.

### Academic Freedom

Academic freedom (which encompasses freedom in research and publication, freedom of discussion in the classroom, and freedom from institutional censorship) is the element of tenure most often contested and least amenable to resolution. According to Hofstadter and Metzger (1955), the modern idea of academic freedom incorporates the intellectual, economic, and political thinking of our age. For example, modern science has contributed ideas about the empirical search for truth verified by objective processes. The free competition of ideas comes from commerce, and the idea of free speech and free press emerged from politics. The spirit of tolerance stems from the religious liberalism of the age.

Perhaps no document better sums up the issues at stake in academic freedom than that of a 1940 AAUP statement regarding tenure. By ensuring freedom to dissent from authority and to criticize one's employer, the principles in the statement ran counter to both the employment law and practice of the period.

The notion that faculties were not subordinated to the state or administrative authorities was quite revolutionary. In the universities, for example, many considered the trustees to hold absolute power. Earlier in the century, after the dismissal of University of Pennsylvania Professor Scott Nearing for advocating laws prohibiting child labor, J. Levering Jones, a trustee of the University of Pennsylvania, had said, "No one has the right to question us" (Finkin 1997). Tenure as contemplated by the 1940 document was intended to change that notion by instituting a model of peer review and shared governance.

Jordan Kurland (1996) of the AAUP holds that in earlier decades, problems of academic freedom were related to broad and impersonal political, economic, and societal issues. He suggests that in the 1990s there has been a shift to issues involving personal expression, and relationships whether artistic, ethical, religious, sexual, racial, or ethnic. Many, however, would argue that tenure has neither contributed to open debate nor protected the jobs of scholars with unorthodox views, opinions, or findings (Tallman and Ward 1997).

For those who say that academic freedom is in little jeopardy, Ernst Benjamin (1995) and other education experts point to scientific issues such as animal experimentation, creationism, recombinant DNA, and fetal-tissue research as areas that create continuing controversy and require protection for scholars. Even if public assaults on academic freedom were rare, argues Benjamin, erosion of the professional and programmatic integrity that academic freedom serves to protect is at risk and a very real concern.

Critics of the need for a special provision to safeguard academic freedom cite the First Amendment as offering scholars any protections they need to speak freely. Dr. C. Peter Magrath, president of the National Association of State Universities and Land-Grant Colleges, has been widely criticized for saying that academic freedom and tenure have been uncoupled, that is, since all persons enjoy the protections of the U.S. Constitution, tenure is not needed to protect academic freedom (Magrath 1997).

Ann Franke (1997), former counsel of the AAUP, says this thinking is false. The first amendment to the Constitution forbids the state from infringing free speech rights, thus ensuring protection for people in state agencies and state colleges and universities. However, a private university may fire a professor for espousing controversial views without violating the First Amendment.

Franke also states that the first amendment protects speech from government interference, but many activities that academic freedom covers (e.g., curriculum design, textbook selection, syllabus preparation, and grading) may not fall into the legal category of speech. Legal experts point out that the Constitution does not shield all pure speech. In 1993, the U.S. Supreme Court limited the first amendment rights of public employees to matters of public concern, thus leaving open to interpretation whether calculus, English, anatomy, molecular biology, or internal medicine fall into this category, too.

## Peer Review and Shared Governance

Deeply embedded in the concept of tenure, and often forgotten or not fully understood, are the role of faculty in governance and the duties of peer review. It is generally assumed that university functions are based on shared governance between administrators, faculty, and trustees, and that faculty have the right to speak on institutional policy. It is also assumed that faculty will carry out their self-governing prerogatives through peer review, the correlative duty that first conditioned the granting of academic freedom to faculty by university employers in 1915 (Hamilton 1997). Hamilton asserts that these correlative duties include faculty enforcement of professional competence and ethical conduct following the granting of tenure.

Many who support tenure have pointed to peer review as a way for faculty to embrace and enforce this professional policing role granted to them throughout history. In 1915, at the time AAUP was founded, its leaders had cautioned that if the profession was unwilling to purge its ranks of the incompetent and unworthy, or to prevent the freedom which it claims from being a shelter for inefficiency, for superficiality, or for uncritical and intemperate partisanship, it is certain that the task will be performed by others (Hamilton 1997).

Tradition and practice frequently have diverged on this issue. Recent data indicate that only approximately 50 de-tenurings occur a year out of more than 300,000 tenures held at 2,200 institutions of higher learning. Thus, the question arises as to whether the professoriate has proven itself willing to purge itself of the incompetent and the unethical (Hamilton 1997). The lack of awareness of these correlative duties is blamed for much of the attack on tenure. Hamilton holds that accountability through effective peer review is the way to resolve the problem.

# Job Security

Dr. Kingman Brewster, Jr., a former president of Yale University, was mindful of the institutional and intellectual environments that require consideration when he cautioned that

> the rationale of academic tenure . . . is somewhat different from job security especially in an institution which wants its teachers to be engaged in pushing forward the frontiers of learning. This lies in the fact that contributions to human knowledge and understanding which add something significant to what has gone before involve a very high risk and a very long-term intellectual investment. This is true especially of those whose life is more devoted to thought, experimentation, and writing than it is to practice. . . . If scholarship is to question assumptions and to take the risk of testing new hypotheses, then it cannot be held to a time-table which demands proof of pay-out to satisfy some review committee (Brewster 1972).

The pursuit of scholarly endeavors and the complex nature of research and discovery cannot be constrained by time or measured by ordinary standards employed in business or industry, agree the advocates of tenure. But Benjamin (1995) and other authorities say that the job-for-life assumption held by many people is false. The tenure of faculty, like the tenure of judges, they hold, protects against undue influence by either influential people or public trends. It therefore assures scholars of sustaining long-term research projects that may challenge established doctrines but hold the promise of leading to exciting breakthroughs. But it does not assure them of employment forever.

## DEADWOOD: A SERIOUS FAILURE OR HYPERBOLE?

Critics of tenure say that permanence of employment diminishes accountability and fosters mediocrity, thus creating deadwood. The result is said to be a situation in which the institution cannot get rid of an incompetent professor (Commission on Academic Tenure 1973). Defenders of tenure say that strict tenure rules make it imperative for an institution to be more careful in selecting its faculty and more courageous in dismissing those who do not measure up (Machlup 1964). Strict tenure, they add, encourages greater quality control and increases the quality of faculty, not the reverse.

Defenders of tenure also argue that the typical probationary period of six years, when the tenure decision is made, is the best indicator of the future work of an individual. Some mistakes can be made, say Machlup and others, but the deadwood problem is more characteristic of institutions not enforcing strict limits to probationary periods than of institutions where limits are strictly observed (Gray 1997).

Deadwood, meaning mediocrity, according to Machlup (1964), is the major issue intertwined in so many tenure arguments. Machlup distinguishes two situations in which mediocrity grows: (1) when an increasing number of mediocre people are appointed or promoted to tenure positions; and (2) when able people, once assured of tenure, lose interest and slide into mediocrity. Many observers agree that it is not uncommon to find faculty members who lack intellectual vitality or who have long since stopped keeping up to date in their fields (Nelson 1997).

A variant of the deadwood argument is probably valid for institutions wanting to raise standards and improve faculty quickly. Tenure does make it difficult to replace mediocre people (e.g., faculty who would be judged as mediocre under new higher standards but who had been acceptable under an older standard). In such a situation, the two options available to institutions are to enlarge departments or wait until people retire. The former is expensive, and the latter defeats the quick fix to change.

Machlup contends that tenure is not to blame but rather the practice of poor selection and evaluation of faculty. "The real responsibility for accumulating mediocrity . . . lies in poor judgment and inertia on the part of those in charge of appointments and promotions," he says. Others point to incompetent hiring, with unqualified faculty members sitting on hiring committees or insecure faculty hiring people who don't threaten them intellectually (Nelson 1997).

William Cotter (1996), president of Colby College in Maine, asserts that quality in faculty performance does not decline after the tenure decision. In virtually every case at Colby, the granting of tenure has liberated that faculty member to become an even more productive and important contributor to the quality of academic and campus life, and her or his finest scholarly work is usually produced after the tenure decision, not before.

Defenders of tenure do admit that some people, probably very few, lose interest over time, but the academic environment or even the leadership of the institution may also be to blame for the loss of enthusiasm. Machlup asks, "Is it really believable that many faculty members, once alert, ambitious, inspiring, and productive, but now lazy and dull, would still be live wires, full of spark, and constantly recharged with new learning, if only they had no assured tenure, if only they had to live in constant fear for their jobs?"

Most significant perhaps, Brown and Kurland (1990) point out, is that the deadwood issue is devoid of anything resembling data about the extent of the blight. Having studied the issue for more than thirty years, they found only one numerical estimate: Dean Rosovsky of Harvard said that "the label deadwood would apply only to under 2 percent of a major university faculty; that is my totally unscientific conclusion." These experts ask, "What is the deadwood index for comparable sectors of the workforce? . . . Is the detriment to society from the existence of unpruned deadwood among civil servants, accountants, bankers, or lawyers . . . more or less severe than the harm caused by sloth among tenured academics?"

The sheer numbers of faculty may account in part for the persistence of the deadwood argument. In fact, some scholars believe that the roots of controversy and change in institutional and professional commitments and values lie in the dramatic expansion of the professoriate that has occurred in the last fifty years. Faculty increased from 147,000 in 1940 to 824,000 in 1990 (NCES 1993). Most of the relative growth in part-time faculty also occurred between 1972 and 1977, a period characterized by increased institutional interest in alternatives to the tenure system (AAUP 1995d).

Recent attacks on tenure have resulted in the formation of two major efforts to address tenure. An AAUP task force is now reassessing tenure, and another of the American Association for Higher Education is seeking to open new dialogues. The pressures for change, societal needs, the protection of historic rights and privileges, proposed revisions to the system, and the role of the university are among the issues under examination.

## THE ACADEMIC HEALTH CENTER CONFRONTS THE ISSUES

Tenure in the medical school, the major component of academic health centers, is a relatively new phenomenon that developed when medical schools became integral to universities in the post-World War II era (AAUP 1996). Yet the compatibility of tenure with the academic health center's tripartite mission has been a concern for some time given that the center's functions are directly connected to the well-being of the public via the delivery of patient care. Nowhere else is this service mission as direct and extensive.

Dr. Jordan Cohen, president of the Association of American Medical Colleges, notes that because of their increased involvement in the real world of health care delivery, medical schools are also linked to the corporate culture, with its brutal devotion to productivity without guarantees of economic security (Cohen 1995). The volatility of this environment has further led to the current reexamination of tenure.

The scrutiny may have far-reaching implications for administration, academic health center-university relationships, higher education, and the public in the years ahead. Economic forces are testing the uniqueness of academic health centers at the same time that the basic conceptual framework of the medical professionals within these institutions is being destabilized (Rabkin 1998). Indeed, nowhere else in the tenure debate have issues been framed so starkly.

## Peer Review and Self-Governance

The role of faculty in decision-making and governance is an increasing concern at academic health centers, in part because the modern medical school has the attributes of a business enterprise with largely individual entrepreneurial activities in both patient care and research. Faculty members are counted on to bring in funds not only to underwrite salaries for supporting personnel, laboratory equipment and supplies, and the indirect costs necessary to maintain the infrastructure of the enterprise. The funds are also used to underwrite faculty salaries, frequently including a portion of the salaries of tenured faculty members (AAUP 1996).

The AAUP has affirmed that the presence of income-generating activities in no way weakens the claim of faculty members in those schools to protections of academic freedom and tenure. And although the award of tenure may not be appropriate for all clinical faculty members, the AAUP argues that such classes of faculty should enjoy academic freedom, including, but not restricted to, the right to speak on institutional policy and protection against the application of unreasonable or capricious sanctions. The AAUP also reaffirms that tenured faculty within the medical school are responsible for ensuring such conditions within the context of a sound system of shared governance (AAUP 1996).

Of interest is the fact that the concerns of faculty have not been as evident recently as the administrative viewpoint in the literature on this debate. Perhaps when institutional economies are strong and modes of health care delivery are not at issue, professional practice can provide all the sense of well-being faculty require.

An antitenure view has been evident in surveys of medical school deans who over the years have shown strong preferences for either the abolition of the system or the modification of the existing one. A 1974 survey of medical school deans by the Association of American Medical Colleges (AAMC), for example, shows that 70 percent of medical school deans indicate a preference for abolition of tenure (Keyes et al. 1975). Although a 1976 survey of deans by Spellman and Meiklejohn (1977) found that respondents strongly favored retaining tenure in some form, only 24 percent endorsed their present tenure system; 59 percent would retain tenure with modifications. More than 60 percent of deans rated tenure as an asset in recruiting faculty of high quality, but 75 percent viewed tenure as encouraging the retention of ineffective faculty. One-half acknowledged that tenure permits faculty to avoid institutional commitments. Dr. Robert Petersdorf (1984), former president of the Association of American Medical Colleges, argues against tenure, asserting that it creates a deadlock on resources, promotes competition among young investigators, and leads to disengagement of older faculty.

Although the nature of the medical enterprise has always been viewed as unique, some changes within the academic health center have mirrored those occurring in other segments of higher education. Increases in the professoriate that occurred during the 1970s were very pronounced in academic health centers. In 1965-66, there were 88 accredited allopathic medical schools, which together employed 17,118 full-time faculty of which 5,671 were preclinical faculty and 11,447 clinical faculty (Jolly and Hudley 1997). In 1975, the number of full-time faculty members in U.S. medical schools reached more than 36,000, with the majority in clinical departments (AMA 1975). This expansion accelerated in the 1980s with full-time clinical faculty reaching 57,183. Almost 10,000 part-time and 127,000 volunteer faculty also joined these faculty (Jonas et al. 1989). In 1995-96 there were 126 accredited allopathic medical schools which together employed 92,239 full-time faculty of which 17,154 were preclinical faculty and 75,085 clinical faculty (Jolly and Hudley 1997). The changes in the numbers and duties of faculty members reflected the expanded involvement of medical schools in patient care activities and corresponding changes in faculty appointment practices (Petersdorf 1997).

## Ongoing Changes in Tenure

Given the amount of data available, the numbers of tenured faculty, and current modifications to the tenure system, the academic health center discussion will center on medical schools. However, we must not overlook the status of faculty in other health professions schools. Here, the numbers of tenured faculty are lower, ranging from approximately 26 percent in medicine to 54 percent in dentistry.

For nursing, the 1997-98 statistics of the American Association of Colleges of Nursing show 551 institutions reporting 9,965 full-time faculty, of which 37 percent are tenured; 26.6 percent on tenure track (not tenured); 28.8 percent on nontenure track. Among these schools, 7.6 percent have no tenure system. These figures show a slight increase over the years, with a 3-percent increase in number of tenured faculty since 1991 (Berlin, Bednash, Scott 1998). The 1997-98 profile of pharmacy faculty shows 1,489 of the 3339 full-time faculty in 79 pharmacy schools are tenured; 773 are on tenure track but nontenured and 1,077 are nontenure track (AACP 1997). For dentistry, 54 dental schools reported the following statistics in 1997: 5,233 full-time faculty of which 1,355 are on a tenure track, and 1,032 already have tenure. Tenured faculty represent about 54 percent of all full-time faculty (AADS 1997). Allied health data reveal that approximately 40 percent of the faculty are tenured.

Discussions on tenure have not reached the same level of intensity as in the medical schools although the American Association of Colleges of Nursing reports that schools are increasingly examining criteria for tenure.

Meanwhile, some major transformations are occurring at medical schools in the United States and Canada. In terms of tenure, statistics from the AAMC provide evidence of a solid tenure system in U.S. and Canadian medical schools.

Of the 125 accredited allopathic medical schools in the United States, 120 have tenure systems. The five schools with no tenure system are Morehouse School of Medicine, Boston University School of Medicine, Mayo Medical School, Universidad Central del Caribe, and Ponce School of Medicine. Another six schools limit the award of tenure to basic science faculty.* No school has abolished tenure (Jones 1993). However, the Association of American Medical Colleges reports that the proportion of full-time faculty with tenure appears to be decreasing (Bickel 1991). And more than 70 percent of chairpersons of basic science departments in academic health centers recently reported that it was becoming increasingly more difficult to attain tenure (Mandel 1997).

The figures, however, do not reveal the challenges facing these institutions and the major change that has occurred over the past two decades. According to a survey of 142 U.S. and Canadian schools in 1983, 77 percent of the close to 10,000 full-time basic science faculty listed on the AAMC Faculty Roster System held appointments in the tenure track stream (i.e., they were either tenured or on track). By 1993, the total number of full-time basic science faculty had grown by 29 percent, with 72 percent of the faculty tenured or on track. From 1983 to 1993, the percentage of tenure track positions for basic science faculty remained relatively constant (Jones and Sanderson 1994). For clinical faculty, however, the situation was quite different. In 1983, 59 percent of the 30,856 clinical faculty were in tenure streams. By 1993, the number of faculty had doubled to 58,607. However, only 47 percent were in tenure streams (Jones and Sanderson 1994). Jones and Sanderson point out that the emergence of special full-time clinical tracks, with such titles as clinical scholar and clinician-educator, has facilitated non-tenure-eligible clinical faculty appointments. As the titles imply, there is a deemphasis on traditional research requirements (Jones and Sanderson 1994).

According to a 1997 survey of U.S. medical schools, nearly three-fourths of schools now have a separate and distinct faculty track for full-time clinical faculty whose primary responsibilities are in patient care and teaching. Eighty-one

---

* The six schools that limit tenure to basic science faculty are Brown University School of Medicine, Loma Linda University School of Medicine, Northeastern Ohio Universities College of Medicine, Tufts University School of Medicine, University of Missouri-Kansas City School of Medicine, and Wright State University School of Medicine. At Brown and Wright, basic science faculty receive tenure through the university, not the medical school (Jones and Gold 1998).

percent of these tracks do not permit faculty to be tenured. Nevertheless, 71 percent of the tracks carry the obligation to provide evidence of scholarship for promotion reviews. A broad definition of scholarship has evolved to include publication of case reports, book chapters, development of learning tools, curricular development activities, presentations to professional groups, and development of clinical service programs (Jones and Gold 1998).

The creation of these classes of faculty has been a major response to the changing environment in which academic health centers have been operating. The variety of positions highlights the segmenting and weighting of faculty functions by teaching, research, and service. The nontenure track positions still remain an issue of concern for the AAUP, particularly when the positions carry the same functions designated by traditional academic titles.

Many observers believe that the growth in nontenure track faculty has eroded the size and influence of the tenured faculty and thus undermined tenure (AAUP 1995d). The growing trend to place research and clinical faculty of the institution on temporary contracts weakens the academic freedom of the professor and, in so doing, also weakens the protection afforded the institution and the public welfare when professors are free to evaluate research in their field candidly. Another consequence of lack of tenure is that academic freedom is more vulnerable to manipulation and suppression.

Finally, according to the AAUP, the quality of education is at risk when curriculum, advising, and instruction are not in control of a faculty to whom the institution has made the kinds of commitments that ensure scholarly development and recognition of performance.

The unique history of medical education makes it difficult to judge the significance of these concerns within academic health centers themselves. Use of volunteer and other clinical faculty has been an integral part of the medical education enterprise not duplicated in other parts of the university. Within the academic health center and the university, a problem with status often emerges with this multitrack system. McHugh (1994) argues that such a system can be a temporary solution to the diversity problem, but it eventually produces strong feelings of discrimination and neglect. Ultimately, an increasing use of nontenurable, full-time as well as part-time faculty, whose main purpose may be to support growing clinical networks emerges as a concern. It raises serious questions about the nature of the education being offered and of the educational institution itself.

*Guaranteed salary.* Significant change has also occurred with regard to financial guarantees that traditionally accompanied tenure in academic health centers; these changes may be fueling perceptions about the abolition of tenure. In large measure, uncertain funding and economic conditions are leading administrators to increasingly disassociate or decrease financial guarantees that come with tenure. The AAUP (1996) has noted that it is not uncommon for a medical school to have tenure guarantees attached to 20 or 30 percent of a faculty member's full-time appointment, with the remainder of the salary dependent on the procurement of external funding.

In 1983, 41 percent of schools in the AAMC survey indicated that tenure guaranteed no more than a continued appointment at a designated rank without salary guarantee (Jones and Sanderson 1994). However, at that time, responses from 29 percent of schools indicated that perhaps there was no clear policy on guarantees. By 1994, policies had become more specific in defining this link between tenure and economic security. At twenty-three schools (17%), tenure guarantees were limited to a continuing appointment without any financial guarantee. At 69 percent of the schools, tenure was uniformly defined to include a financial guarantee (Jones and Sanderson 1994).

Fifty-five percent of schools defined the financial guarantee in terms of (1) the component of salary from university/state funds, or (2) a base salary otherwise defined. For 18 percent of the schools, the financial guarantee was defined as total salary/compensation excluding clinical income (8 schools) or clinical and research grant income (11 schools). Seven percent of the schools guaranteed total salary for basic science faculty, but had very limited or no financial guarantee for clinical faculty (Jones and Sanderson 1994).

In its 1997 survey, the AAMC found that for the basic science faculty, 29 percent of schools that associated tenure with a financial guarantee defined it as total salary/compensation regardless of sources of funding. Another 28 percent of schools guarantee that portion of salary/compensation derived from university or state funds while 19 percent guarantee a base salary, which is variously defined among the schools. The monetary outcomes are very similar regardless of the formula used. In instances where tenure for basic science faculty provides a financial guarantee, the AAMC concluded that guarantee very often covers their total salary or a figure close to it (Jones and Gold 1998).

Again a financial guarantee traditionally not only provided a sense of job security to faculty but also symbolized an institutional commitment to create an environment conducive to intellectual pursuit without constraints. The scaling back of guarantees therefore has produced concerns about job security and aroused debate over the quality of the intellectual environment.

A different picture emerges for clinical faculty. Compensation from clinical earnings is usually exempt from tenure guarantee. The six schools that said tenure guarantees the total salary and compensation of clinical faculty regardless of funding source also said clarification or redefinition of tenure guarantees were under consideration.

An increasing number of schools have moved to what might be called a three-component faculty salary plan, for example: (1) the university base; (2) a merit/market supplement based on the individual faculty members, special contributions to the school in teaching, research, clinical practice, and service; and (3) the revenue-generation incentive that reflects revenue generated by an individual faculty member through clinical practice, sponsored research, or otherwise (Adler 1996).

Given the premise that tenure is linked to a sufficient degree of economic security to make the profession attractive to men and women of ability, major questions have been raised about what the concept means under the conditions that protect only a portion of a faculty member's income. The concern is whether the principles of academic freedom or an individual's own academic freedom is protected with a salary that may not be adequate for financial independence (AAUP 1996). The AAUP suggests using a basic science salary line as a guidepost for determining salary guarantees for clinical faculty members.

Of late, it appears that the flash point for future controversies over tenure may be faculty governance over questions that surround the development of faculty compensation plans. Often at issue is the degree to which faculty has had input into or been involved in the decision-making process for instituting new salary structures. The AAUP has noted the importance of involving the faculty in arriving at a specific recommendation. In recognizing the difficulties of dealing with financial issues in the complex academic health center environment, AAUP notes that creative approaches not overtly at odds with existing association policy seem possible.

Gerald Bodner (1997), legal counsel to the Albert Einstein College of Medicine and Yeshiva University, recently argued that regardless of motivation, the reduction in salaries of tenured faculty is legally achievable. He notes that there is no requirement that tenure exist or, if it does exist, that it is to have any implication for salaries. Nevertheless, his analysis points to the paradox between what the institutional tenure rules state (they would appear to support the legal right to impose a salary reduction) and historical practice, which generally has shown no previous instances of salary reduction for tenured faculty, often even where grants were lost or private practice income not realized.

*Probationary Period.* In terms of AAUP guidelines, medical schools have historically evidenced a broader interpretation of issues than other schools of higher education, including longer probationary periods to fit particular circumstances of their faculty. Although the guidelines have been altered, they have not been stretched as far as many would believe. Seventy-three percent of the surveyed schools in 1994 maintained probationary periods of seven years or less for basic science faculty, the prescribed AAUP period. For clinical science faculty, the percentage was slightly less. Eleven percent of the schools had no fixed maximum period by which basic science or clinical science faculty had to present themselves for tenure review. The remaining schools had maximum probationary periods of from eight to eleven years, little changed since 1983. Of those medical schools that required faculty to be reviewed for tenure after a fixed maximum probationary period, 57 percent maintained strict "up-or-out" systems; the remainder permitted some faculty to be continued on a renewable appointment basis (Jones and Sanderson 1994).

In 1997, Jones and Gold (1998) found that 34 percent of the medical schools allowed basic science faculty eight years or more before they were required to be reviewed for tenure, with 42 percent of schools permitting the longer probationary period for clinical faculty. These figures also included schools for which the probationary periods were indefinite.

Although such modifications are still subject to debate, they have been seen as beneficial and necessary, particularly in light of the academic health center's unique environment, which requires, for example, a great deal of time for grant writing, clinical service, or preparation for subspecialty boards. The debate will likely continue over the extension of probationary periods, which the AAUP says weakens the system.

*Promotion and Tenure.* Linking faculty promotion to tenure in the classic sense (i.e., whereby it is automatically awarded with promotion to the rank of associate professor) occurred in only 35 percent of medical schools in 1994. Fifty-four percent of schools reported that the minimum rank at which faculty could be tenured was associate professor; 34 percent allowed an assistant professor to be tenured; and only three schools reserved tenure for faculty with the full professor title (Jones and Sanderson 1994).

In 1997, the AAMC found that 76 percent required a faculty member to achieve the rank of associate professor in order to be tenured; in 4 percent of schools faculty must achieve the rank of full professor. Forty-six percent of schools link tenure to promotion to a specific rank, most often associate professor (Jones and Gold 1998).

The termination of tenured faculty for cause was reported by 13 medical schools. Cause included misconduct in science, sexual harassment, disregard for the university code of conduct, interference with departmental functioning, and total lack of effort. There is probably considerable underreporting here, given that some schools may have negotiated settlements that permitted faculty to resign rather than face review (Jones and Sanderson 1994).

Eighty-two percent of schools limited neither the number of tenure eligible positions nor the number of faculty who could be awarded tenure (Jones 1994). Jones and Sanderson (1994) reported that limitations on the number of tenured positions or faculty, or both, usually occurred in public medical schools as a result of limitations set by state authorities.

*Post-tenure Review.* Post-tenure reviews are another area where aggressive change is underway. Bickel (1991) reported that, in 1989, schools had not moved aggressively in instituting post-tenure evaluations. Some schools conducted reviews annually; others, every five years. The reviews, ranging from casual to strict in form and consequence, are variously viewed as ways to enhance productivity, permit faculty flexibility in career interests and priorities, and get rid of deadwood. By 1997, post-tenure review was the focus of much attention, with mandated reviews for public institutions implemented or discussed in twenty-eight states, including Colorado, Hawaii, Kentucky, and Wisconsin (Beasley et al. 1997).

Some academics hold to an AAUP statement of 1983 that viewed post-tenure reviews as offering scant benefit and threatening academic freedom. Such reviews, they say, compromise or defeat the meaning of tenure. It is also understandable that post-tenure reviews are interpreted as an end to the tenure system. A variety of forms, functions, and outcomes is evident in these reviews. Some reviews, as at the University of California, are linked to salary and step increases; others are intended to enhance faculty growth and development, as at Northeastern Ohio Universities and the University of Cincinnati (Jones and Gold 1998). The University of New Mexico has annual reviews, and an outcome can trigger a more extensive review with consequences. Wake Forest University School of Medicine has reviews of tenured faculty on a five-year cycle. Department chairpersons report to the dean on the performance of each tenured faculty member. If performance is found to be lacking, the faculty member is notified and given a two-year probationary period in which to correct the deficiencies or resign (Bickel 1991).

The attitudes and reactions of medical school faculty to post-tenure review are not entirely clear. Recent news articles draw attention to other university faculty, many of whom have reacted quite strongly. They say that their work is judged all the time: they jump through hoops to win tenure, and again when they seek promotion to full professor. Many are evaluated annually when raises are awarded and again every time they write a book or teach a course (Magner 1995). Many professors question the need for more evaluations and view them as time-consuming activities that generate more paperwork and do little more than help administrators satisfy their critics.

The effectiveness and costs of post-tenure review are still open questions. At the University of Colorado where reviews were instituted in 1982, a survey found that professors found post-tenure review to be fair but of little value with no follow-up even after a review identified areas where a professor needed to improve (Magner 1995).

Faculty development initiatives are also on the rise, with faculty receiving more guidance on faculty tracks and the promotion process. Some administrators and faculty members have raised questions about the application of traditional faculty development models that only reward the triple threat—that is, faculty expertise in research, education, and patient care, in the current health care environment (Evans 1995). New models of health care delivery and changed environments for teaching require different reward systems, they say. Faculty reward and compensation plans are also under examination to define more clearly what scholarship means and to consider new strategies to reward performance.

Faculty performance has often been perceived as a function of age. Interestingly, a recent report by Drs. William Bergquist and Carole Bland reveals that productivity does not decline among senior faculty members, but that the ways in which they are productive do undergo change (Shaw 1997). This finding contrasts with a commonly held view expressed over a decade ago by Petersdorf (1984) that aging tenured faculty were expensive and unproductive.

*Contract vs Tenure.* Academic health centers have paid substantial attention to contracts as an alternative to tenure. In 1977, Spellman and Meiklejohn found interest in shifting to a system of renewable contracts of five or six years duration, but respondents expressed doubts about the ability of contracts to influence the rate of retention of faculty members positively. For those institutions using contracts, including Wake Forest University School of Medicine and Stanford University, contracts do not appear to be a deterrent to recruitment.

Jones found that nearly 50 percent of medical schools now provide multiyear contracts for some faculty in non-tenure clinical tracks. Multiyear contracts vary in length, ranging from two to six years. At Wake Forest University School of Medicine, untenured faculty are offered one- to three-year contracts; tenured faculty are offered a five-year contract. Although all positions are tenure eligible, the finances of a department must be able to support all of its tenured positions, a situation that may pose a problem for the future. Contract renewal tends to be at the discretion of the dean in consultation with the chair of the department in question.

## THE FUTURE: EVOLUTION OR REVOLUTION?

The literature on academic health centers speaks in terms of adaptation, that is, fashioning a system that works well for both the clinical service and traditional university education and research. Not yet clear is the extent to which (if any) adaptations and modifications to the tenure system undertaken so far have resolved academic health center problems created by the changing health care environment. Researchers must learn whether modifications to tenure are creating or increasing the institutional flexibility, competitiveness, efficiency, or other institutional capabilities which academic health centers say are needed to successfully respond to the market.

Moreover, we still don't know whether academic health center reforms of ownership, governance, organizational, or leadership policies and practices are indeed accomplishing their intended ends.

Thus, academic health centers stand at a crossroads, one in which their ties to the university may be at issue. As economic and societal pressures increase, along with America's preoccupation with transposing the corporate model of organizations to all enterprises, many academic health center leaders caution that it will become even more difficult to adapt and still maintain the delicate balance between the academic and corporate worlds.

## CONCLUSION

Adopting a corporate model for organizational change is a call that resounds throughout the academic health center community as these institutions are increasingly pressured by economic forces, including changing reimbursement systems and competition in the health care marketplace. Academic responsibilities are held high in the academic health center tradition and have been fulfilled successfully over the years. They are impelled in part by a regard for an unwritten contract with society and the synergy of the centers' tripartite mission, which presumes service to the public not only through direct care, but also through education and research.

The same interrelatedness that holds true for the tripartite mission of the academic health center holds true for tenure; its value has come from the interplay of its various components, and the risks and benefits of separating the parts from the whole must be weighed carefully.

If academic tenure is to play a diminishing role in the employment relationship for future generations of faculty, what price will be paid relative to the quality of education? Will modification of the system weaken the academic health center-university relationship? Will the evolutionary changes with regard to tenure result in the emergence of an organizational form less compatible with the university environment? Will the academic health center experience, with its growing categorization of the faculty, eventually lead to the bifurcation of the medical profession to a point at which some teach and some practice? The relationship between universities and academic health centers in this century has resulted in enhancing the quality of education, expanding the frontiers of biomedical research, and improving patient care. There is reason to believe that the next fifty years holds the same or even greater promise. It would appear that society would suffer a great loss if academics and their institutions could not push through the ideological rhetoric on tenure and together focus on knowledge and the role of the university in discovering and expanding the frontiers of knowledge through education and research for the future.

## REFERENCES

AACP (American Association of Colleges of Pharmacy). 1997. *Profile of Pharmacy Faculty 1996-1997.* Washington: AACP.

AADS (American Association of Dental Schools). 1997. *Survey of Dental Educators: 1996-97.* Washington: AADS.

AAHE (American Association for Higher Education). 1995. *New Pathways: Faculty Careers and Employment in the 21st Century.* Washington: AAHC.

AAUP (American Association of University Professors). 1995a. On full-time non-tenure track appointments (1986). In *Policy Documents and Reports.* Washington: AAUP.

____. 1995b. On periodic evaluation of tenured faculty (1983). In *Policy Documents and Reports.* Washington: AAUP.

____. 1995c. On the relationship of faculty governance to academic freedom (1994). In *Policy Documents and Reports.* Washington: AAUP.

____. 1995d. The status of non-tenure track faculty (1993). In *Policy Documents and Reports.* Washington: AAUP.

____. 1995e. 1940 Statement of principles on academic freedom and tenure with 1970 interpretive comments. In *Policy Documents and Reports.* Washington: AAUP.

____. 1997. *On Post-Tenure Review.* Washington: AAUP.

____, Committee on Academic Freedom and Tenure. 1915. The 1915 Declaration of principles: Academic freedom and tenure. *Bulletin* 1:41–42

____, Subcommittee of Committee A on Academic Freedom and Tenure. 1996. Tenure in the medical school. *Academe* (January-February): 40–45.

Adler, S. 1996. *Draft Policy on Faculty Compensation.* Pittsburgh: University of Pittsburgh.

AMA (American Medical Association). 1975. Undergraduate medical education in the U.S. (Section II) *Journal of the American Medical Association* 234:1333-1351.

—Arden, E. 1995. Is tenure obsolete? *Academe* (January-February):28–39.

Beasley, B.W.; S. Wright; J. Cofrancesco, Jr.; S. Babbott; P. Thomas; and E. Bass. 1997. Promotion criteria for clinician-educators in the United States and Canada: A survey of promotion committee chairpersons. *Journal of the American Medical Association* 278:723–728.

Benjamin, E. 1995. Five misconceptions about tenure. *AGB Trusteeship* 3(1).

Bennett, A. 1994. Tenure: Many will decry it, few deny it. *Wall Street Journal,* 10 October.

Berlin, L.E., G.D. Bednash, and D.R. Scott. 1998. *1997-1998 Salaries of Instructional and Administrative Nursing Faculty in Baccalaureate and Graduate Programs in Nursing.* Washington: American Association of Colleges of Nursing.

Bickel, J. 1991. The changing faces of promotion and tenure at U.S. medical schools. *Academic Medicine* 66, 249–256.

Bland, C.J., and R.L. Holloway. 1995. A crisis of mission: Faculty roles and rewards in an era of health care reform. *Change* (September-October):30–35.

Bodner, G. 1997. Does tenure protect the salaries of medical school faculty? *Academic Medicine* 72:966–971.

Bowen, H.R., and J.H. Schuster. 1986. *American Professors: A National Resource Imperiled.* New York: Oxford University, 235–244.

Brewster, Kingsman Jr. 1972. *Report of the President.* August 28. New Haven: Yale.

Brown, R.S., and J.E. Kurland. 1990. Academic tenure and academic freedom. *Law and Contemporary Problems* 53 (Summer).

Chait, R. 1997. Thawing the cold war over tenure: Why academe needs more employment options. *Chronicle of Higher Education,* 7 February.

*Chronicle of Higher Education.* 1996. New concerns over the meaning and value of faculty tenure. (Letters) December 16.

_____. 1997. Tenure is still a key ingredient of academic freedom. (Letters) March 21.

_____. The first amendment is no substitute for tenure. 1997. (Letters) April 11.

_____. Should colleges and universities adopt corporate practices? (Letters) November 28.

_____. The pros and cons of tenure in an era of financial adversity. (Letters) May 16.

_____. 1998. Does moving with the times mean an end to shared governance? (Letters) March 13.

Cohen, J. 1995. Academic medicine's tenuous hold on tenure. *Academic Medicine* 70:294.

Commission on Academic Tenure in Higher Education. 1973. *Faculty Tenure.* San Francisco: Jossey Bass.

Cotter, W.R. 1996. Why tenure works. *Academe* (January- February):26-29.

DePasquale, S.; M. Hendricks; and D. Keiger. 1997. Tenure under Scrutiny. *Johns Hopkins Magazine* (September):16-22.

Evans, C. 1995. Faculty development in a changing academic environment. *Academic Medicine* 70:14–20.

Finkin, M.W. 1997. The assault on faculty independence. *Academe* (July-August):21-23.

Franke, A. 1995. Tenure and the faculty pocketbook. *Academe* (March-April):108.

───── 1997. *Tenure and The First Amendment.* Washington: American Association of University Professors.

Froom, J.D., and J. Bickel. 1996. Medical school policies for part-time faculty committed to full professional effort. *Academic Medicine* 7:91-96.

Gray, M. 1997. The great tenure debate: Colleges need it. *Washington Post* (Educational Review), 27 July.

Hamilton, Neil. 1996. Buttressing the neglected traditions of academic freedom. *William Mitchell Law Review* 22(2): 549–572.

Hamilton, N. 1997. Peer review: The linchpin of academic freedom and tenure. *Academe* (May-June):333–355.

Happel, S. 1996. In defense of tenure. *Wall Street Journal* (Manager's Journal), 28 October.

Helfand, D. 1995. Tenure: Thanks but no thanks. *Chronicle of Higher Education*, 15 December.

Hofstadter, R., and W.P. Metzger. 1955. *The Development of Academic Freedom in the U.S.* New York: Columbia University.

Holden, C. 1997. Tenure turmoil sparks reforms. *Science* 276 (April 4):24-26.

Jolly, P., and D. Hudley, eds. 1997. *AAMC Data Book. Statistical Information Related to Medical School Financing.* Washington: Association of American Medical Colleges.

Jonas, H., S. Etzel, and B. Barzansky. 1994. Educational programs in U.S. medical schools, 1993–1994. *Journal of American Medical Association* 272:694–701.

Jones, R.F. 1993. Three views on faculty tenure in medical schools. *Academic Medicine* 68:588–593.

Jones R.F., and J.S. Gold. 1998. Faculty appointment and tenure policies in medical schools: A 1997 status report. *Academic Medicine* (73):212–219.

Jones, R.F., and S.S. Sanderson. 1994. Tenure policies in U.S. and Canadian medical schools. *Academic Medicine* 69:772–777.

Keyes J.A., M.P. Wilson, and J. Becker. 1975. The future of medical education: Forecast of the Council of Deans. *Journal of Medical Education* 5:319-327.

Kolodny, Annette. 1996. The dismantling of tenure. *Chronicle of Higher Education*, March 22.

Kurland, J.E. 1996. Commentary on buttressing the defense of academic freedom. *William Mitchell Law Review* 22(2):545–548.

Leatherman, C. 1998a. Faculty unions move to organize growing ranks of part-time professors. *Chronicle of Higher Education*, February 27.

———. 1998b. Shared governance under siege: Is it time to revive it or get rid of it? *Chronicle of Higher Education*, January 30.

Leatherman, C., and D.K. Magner. 1996. Faculty and graduate-student strife over job issues flares on many campuses. *Chronicle of Higher Education*, November 29.

*Lovejoy Papers*, American Association of University Professors.

Machlup, F. 1964. In defense of academic tenure. *AAUP Bulletin* (June):112–124.

Magner, D.K. 1995a. Beyond tenure: Colleges seek periodic reviews of professors who have already passed muster. *Chronicle of Higher Education*, July 21.

———. 1995b. A scholar provides an intellectual framework for plans to end or revamp tenure systems. *Chronicle of Higher Education*, February 14.

———. 1995c. Tenure re-examined. *Chronicle of Higher Education*, March 31.

————. 1997. An aging faculty poses a challenge for colleges. *Chronicle of Higher Education,* August 8.

Magrath, C.P. 1997. Eliminating tenure without destroying academic freedom. *Chronicle of Higher Education,* February 28.

Mandel, H.G. 1997. Downsizing of basic science departments in U.S. medical schools: Perceptions of their chairs. *Academic Medicine* 72:894-900.

Mangan, K. 1994. Hahnemann U. Angers faculty with threat to fire those who don't attract grant money. *Chronicle of Higher Education,* October 5.

McHugh, W.F. 1973. Faculty unionism and tenure. In *Faculty Tenure: A Report and Recommendations by the Commission on Academic Tenure in Higher Education.* San Francisco: Jossey-Bass.

McHugh, P.R. 1994. A letter of experience about faculty promotion in medical schools. *Academic Medicine* 69:877-881.

Metzger, W.P. 1973. Academic tenure in America: A historical essay. In *Faculty Tenure: A Report and Recommendations by the Commission on Academic Tenure in Higher Education.* San Francisco: Jossey-Bass.

NCES (National Center for Education Statistics). 1993. *Digest of Education Statistics* 173. Washington: U.S. Department of Education.

Nelson, C. 1997. The real problem with tenure is incompetent faculty hiring. *Chronicle of Higher Education.* November 14.

Nuchims, P. 1995. Will tenure end with this century? A pastiche of quotes and ideas leading to a challenge. *Academe* (January- February)

O'Toole, J. 1994. Tenure: A conscientious objection. *Change* (May- June): 78-86.

Parini, J. 1995. Tenure and the loss of faculty talent. *Chronicle of Higher Education,* July 14.

Perley, J.E. 1995. Tenure, academic freedom, and governance. *Academe* (January- February), 43–47.

————. 1997. Tenure remains vital to academic freedom. *Chronicle of Higher Education,* April 4.

Petersdorf, R.G. 1984. The case against tenure in medical schools. *Journal of the American Medical Association* 251:920-924.

————. 1997. Deans and deaning in a changing world. *Academic Medicine.* 72:953-958.

Power, B.M. 1997. The danger inherent in abusing academic freedom. *Chronicle of Higher Education,* June 20.

Quincy, J. 1840. *History of Harvard University.* (Vol. 1). Cambridge, MA: Harvard University, p. 281.

Rabkin, M.T. 1998. A paradigm shift in academic medicine? *Academic Medicine.* 73:127–131.

Robson, B. 1997. Destroying the university to save the university. *Minneapolis City Pages,* 18:853.

Shaw, G. 1997. *Career Status, Post-tenure Review Challenge Faculty Affairs Professionals.* Association of American Medical Colleges Reporter 7:1.

Smythe, C. McC., A.B. Jones, and M.P. Wilson. 1982. Tenure in medical schools in the

1980s. *Journal of Medical Education* 57:349-360.

Spellman, M.W., and G. Meiklejohn. 1977. Faculty tenure in American medical schools. *Journal of Medical Education* 52:623- 632.

Tallman, I. and D. Ward. 1997. The great tenure debate: No they don't. *Washington Post* (Education Review), July 27.

Trachtenberg, S.J. 1996. What strategy should we now adopt to protect academic freedom? *Academe* (January-February):23-25.

Trani, E. Tenure: Has its time passed? 1995. In *Academic Health Centers and Universities: Shaping a Common Agenda,* E. Rubin, T. Larson, and J. Griffith, eds. Washington: Association of Academic Health Centers.

Uhlman, M. 1994. Tenure runs afoul of bottom line. Some Hahnemann U. tenured faculty face an ultimatum; produce or resign. *Philadelphia Inquirer,* August 28.

Van Alstyne, W.W. 1994. Tenure: A conscientious objective. *Change* (May-June):88.

Volume is turning up on tenure question. 1994. *American Assembly of Collegiate Schools of Business (Newsline).* 24 (Winter):1 6.

Wilson, R. 1995. Scheduling motherhood: Women on the tenure track have trouble fitting children into career timetables. *Chronicle of Higher Education*, March 10.

# ASSESSING RESOURCE REQUIREMENTS AND FINANCING FOR HEALTH PROFESSIONS EDUCATION

*Meredith A. Gonyea, PhD*

O VER THE PAST FIVE YEARS, THE CENTER FOR Studies in Health Policy (CSHP) and the Association of Academic Health Centers (AHC) have been working to identify the resource requirements for the education programs associated with an academic health center, along with their costs and related sources of support (Gonyea 1997). Because initial reviews indicated that the main resource requirements and costs were associated with undergraduate and graduate medical education (UME and GME), the focus of the Gonyea study became that of medical education.

The study examined several questions, including:

- What does it cost to educate a medical student?
- How many educators are needed to run a UME program?
- What is the impact of shifting the educational setting from the hospital to the community?
- How do educators spend their time, and how is their productivity affected by teaching?
- How much UME teaching should residents do?

*Dr. Gonyea is president of The Center for Studies in Health Policy, Inc., in Washington, D.C.*

- Who supports the cost of the education programs in an academic health center?

This paper reviews some of the lessons we learned from an examination of data for U.S. medical schools for the 1995–96 academic year.

## LESSON 1.

It is possible to construct the resource requirements and identify the costs of health professions education.

A methodology that has been developed, tested, and refined over the past twenty-five years—the Program Cost Analysis/Construction Methodology (PCACM)—proved useful to our study. PCACM can be used to analyze an existing program by examining the values of key variables that affect costs. Once the analysis is complete, future alternatives can be developed. The concept of identifying all the resources required to provide an education program and then assigning a dollar value to each of them to calculate the cost of running a medical school was introduced in the classic Institute of Medicine (1974) study of the costs of health professions education. PCACM can be applied to any education program, but it is especially useful in analyzing health professions education programs that contain large clinical experience components.

Several key variables affect the resource requirements of a UME program and in turn the cost. The entering student class size, attrition, repetition, transfer, and graduates affect the magnitude of the resources required to provide a program. The major demand factor is the program curriculum structure, including the program length, the number of student contact hours, the mode of instruction, and the group size per teacher. This demand is usually expressed as educator contact hours per student output. The term *educator* includes full- and part-time faculty, preceptors, volunteers, and graduate trainees (for example, GME residents).

Once the *demand* has been quantified, the next step is to determine who will supply the resources. The type of educator assigned to teach is the main *supply* factor. The educator's activity profile, including hours available to teach, related research, and service activities, must be identified, and the related salary and fringe benefits then must be calculated. Other resource costs that must also be considered include support staff, supplies, facilities, and other administrative costs. The two types of costs are then added, and an average cost per student output is calculated.

We used PCACM to construct the average cost of educating a medical student in 1995–96 (table 1). In 1995–96, the average UME program was a total of 157 weeks spread over four calendar years, including 85 weeks of clerkship in groups that averaged four students per educator. The entering class size averaged 132 students, and the total number of student contact hours averaged about 4,700.

Table 1.
**COST TO EDUCATE A MEDICAL STUDENT, 1995–96**

| Key variables | Value |
|---|---|
| Student class size | 132 |
| | |
| Program length (weeks) | 157 |
| Total student contact hours | 4,702 |
| Clerkship weeks | 85 |
| Clerk-educator contact hours per week | 36 |
| | |
| Educator contact hours per student output | hours/student |
| Basic sciences | 86 |
| Clinical sciences | 794 |
| Total | 880 |
| | |
| Assignment of educators | % |
| Full-time basic sciences faculty | 100 |
| Clinical sciences faculty | 50 |
| Trainees | 50 |
| | |
| Educator salaries | $ |
| Basic sciences | 75,000 |
| Clinical sciences faculty | 126,160 |
| Trainees | 29,880 |
| | |
| Breakdown of essential education cost | % |
| Educator salaries | 41 |
| Other costs | 59 |
| | |
| Total Essential Education Cost | $ |
| Program | 56.2 million |
| Per student output | 425,559 |
| Average annual cost per student | 106,390 |
| Annual instructional cost | 34,517 |
| Total resource costs (inflation adjusted) | 106,390 |

Source: CSHP. US Average Analysis for 125 Medical Schools, 1995–1996 (i.e., 74 public and 51 private schools).

Because the two main types of educators involved in teaching undergraduate medicine are basic and clinical sciences educators, the educator contact hours are defined by basic and clinical science demand requirements. The total number of educator contact hours per student output (ECH/SO) averaged 880, of which 10 percent (86 ECH/SO) was spent by basic sciences educators and 90 percent (794 ECH/SO) by clinical sciences educators. The basic science demand is provided by full-time faculty from mutually exclusive discipline areas, which require critical masses to function effectively. By contrast, the clinical science demand can be assigned either to full- or part-time faculty or to trainees (residents). Of course, the greater the reliance on full-time faculty, the higher the cost will be. In 1995–96, the clinical sciences demand was assigned equally to full-time faculty and trainees.

In 1995–96, essential education salaries averaged $75,000 for basic scientists, $126,160 for clinical scientists, and $29,880 for residents. Educator salaries averaged 41 percent of the total essential education cost, and other costs accounted for the balance.

Essential education cost includes the instruction, research, and service costs related to the educational activities of educators. The data for 1995–96 that we analyzed revealed that the essential education cost of a UME program with 132 graduates is about $56.2 million. The total cost per student output is about $425,600, or about $106,400 per year.

From this analysis, we learned:

- The more weeks students spend in clerkships in small groups, the higher is the demand for resources.
- The size of the resident pool greatly affects the percentage of the full-time faculty that teaches in UME.
- What is included in "other costs" can significantly affect the total cost of a UME program.
- Many people do not like these numbers. (They are either too high or too low for their purposes.)

## LESSON 2.

PCACM can be used to determine why studies of the cost of educating a medical student produce different estimates.

In addition to our own study, we selected for our analysis five recent studies that looked at the cost of educating a medical student (Ginzberg et al. 1993; Valberg et al.1994; Goodwin et al. 1997; Rein et al. 1997; and Franzini et al. 1997). Table 2 presents the values of the key variables for each of these studies. These values can be compared both across the five studies and with the values shown in table 1.

As table 2 shows, the planned class size varies considerably, from ninety-six to two hundred. The total program length in weeks, by contrast, is quite similar, ranging from eighty to eighty-six. The two studies that clearly defined the total student contact hours in the program have higher values than the ones we calculated using 1995–96 data (table 1). The number of weeks in clerkship ranges from eighty to eighty-six. The number of weeks in clerkship has a direct bearing on resources required.

Educator contact hours per student output provides insight into assump-

Table 2.
COMPARISON OF FIVE STUDIES OF THE COST OF EDUCATING A MEDICAL STUDENT

| Key variables | 125 USMC '95-96 Avg | Ginzberg et al. '93 | Valberg et al. '96 | Goodwin et al. '94-'95 | Rein et al. '95 | Franzini et al. '95 |
|---|---|---|---|---|---|---|
| **Student program** | | | | | | |
| Class size | 132 | 150 | 96 | 169 | 139 | 200 |
| Length (weeks) | 157 | 158 | 152 | 155 | 152 | 154 |
| Total student contact hours | 4,702 | — | — | — | 5,070 | 5,989 |
| Clerkship weeks | 85 | 86 | 80 | 83 | 80 | 84 |
| Clerk-educator contact hours per week | 36 | 18 | 36 | 39 | 39-47 | 53 |
| Educator contact hours per student output | DEMAND | | | | | |
| Basic sciences | 86 | 43 | 50 | 28 | 19 | 20 |
| Clinical sciences | 794 | 311 | 800 | 968 | 868 | 1,624 |
| Total | 880 | 354 | 850 | 996 | 887 | 1,644 |
| **Assignment of educators (%)** | SUPPLY | | | | | |
| Basic sciences faculty | 100 | 100 | 100 | 100 | 100 | 100 |
| Clinical sciences | | | | | | |
| Faculty | 50 | 100 | 65 | 52 | 75 | 55 |
| Trainees | 50 | 0 | 35 | 48 | 25 | 45 |

## Table 2 (continued)

| Key variables | 125 USMC '95-96 Avg | Ginzberg et al. '93 | Valberg et al. '96 | Goodwin et al. '94-'95 | Rein et al. '95 | Franzini et al. '95 |
|---|---|---|---|---|---|---|
| **Educator availability to teach (hours/year)** | SUPPLY | | | | | |
| Basic sciences | 360 | 140-250 | 360 | 360 | 360 | 376 |
| Clinical sciences | | | | | | |
| Faculty | 450 | 1,920 | 450 | 450 | 450 | 940 |
| Trainees | 270 | 0 | 747 | 401 | 270 | 564 |
| **Educator salaries ($)** | | | | | | |
| Basic sciences | 75,000 | 81,000 | 69,176 | 54,242 | 62,500 | 76,200 |
| Clinical sciences | | | | | | |
| Faculty | 126,160 | 143,500 | 114,832 | 116,575 | 114,100 | 11,500 |
| Trainees | 29,880 | 0 | 32,426 | 30,000 | 33,298 | 32,580 |
| **Breakdown of total essential education cost (%)** | | | | | | |
| Educator salaries | 41 | 83 | 39 | 55 | 41 | 38 |
| Other costs | 59 | 17 | 61 | 45 | 59 | 62 |
| **Total essential education cost ($)** | | | | | | |
| Per student output | 425,559 | 44,700 | 351,530 | 279,967 | 349,394 | 413,295 |
| Average program annual cost per student | 106,390 | 11,175 | 87,883 | 69,992 | 87,349 | 103,324 |
| Annual instructional cost | 34,517 | 13,059 | 40,319 | — | — | 45,515 |
| Total resource costs adjusted for inflation | 106,390 | | 111,004 | 71,672 | 91,401 | 92,836 |

Source: Four articles on the cost of educating a medical student in *Academic Medicine* 72, 3 March 1997.

tions about the demand for resources. The basic sciences ECH/SO values for the six studies, when calculated as a percentage of total hours, fall in a narrow range (from 2 percent to 10 percent). Shifting over time from lectures and laboratory instruction to small groups and clinical integration causes the number to rise. The clinical sciences ECH/SO values for the six studies range from 311 to 1,624.

Although the study by Ginzberg et al. has the highest number of clerkship weeks (86), that study's assumption of only 18 hours per week of direct contact yields only 1,548 total hours of contact, about half as many total hours as we used (36 hours per week for eighty-five weeks, totaling 3,060 hours).

All six studies show 100 percent use of full-time basic sciences educators. The assignment of clinical sciences educators, by contrast, ranges from 50 percent to 100 percent use of full-time faculty. The recognition of residents as required teachers therefore ranges from 0 percent to 50 percent.

As for educators' availability to teach, the consensus of five of the six studies is 360 hours per year for basic sciences faculty. The Ginzberg study, by contrast, assumes 140 to 250 hours per year. The five studies we reviewed make significantly different assumptions regarding the availability of clinical sciences faculty to teach. Educator salaries, adjusted for inflation, are fairly similar across the six studies.

The values for other costs range from 17 percent to 62 percent of the total cost; in four studies, other costs account for about 60 percent of the total cost.

The estimate of the study by Ginzberg et al.—$44,700 to educate a medical student—stands out as the lowest estimate. It is the lowest because of the assumptions the authors made about student direct contact hours in clerkship, the size of clerkship groups, nonuse of trainees as educators, the teaching time profiles for clinical faculty, and the low value for other costs. The estimate of the study by Goodwin et al. is the second lowest among the five studies, mainly because the estimates of other costs and the salary of basic sciences faculty are the lowest of the six studies.

At the other end of the spectrum, the estimate by Franzini et al.—$413,295—is the highest of the six studies, mainly because the total number of clinical educator demand contact hours is quite high (1,644). The estimate is high because of the authors' assumption about the time students spend in patient care relative to direct contact teaching.

As this example shows, in comparing cost studies, it is important to look beyond the magnitude of the differences in total cost and determine what variables contribute to the differences. From this review of cost studies, we learned that assumptions that drive the demand or supply requirements up often can be negated by other assumptions that drive them down.

## LESSON 3.

PCACM can be used to assess how a shift from a traditional UME program to a more community-based program would affect resource requirements and cost.

In a traditional program, UME students spend an average of sixty hours per week in a hospital setting, thirty-six hours of which is spent in direct contact with a clinician educator or a trainee in a group of about four. In a community-based environment, students spend an average of thirty-eight to forty hours per week in a community setting. In addition, they spend about eighteen hours in direct contact activities, of which about ten hours are spent consulting one-on-one with an educator-clinician. Moving clinical training from a hospital to an ambulatory or a community-based setting therefore requires a change in the educator mix being used to supply the demand.

Table 3 shows the effect on resources and costs of a shift to a more community-based program. The shift that is illustrated assumes a class size of ninety-six students. It involves a two-week decrease (1 percent) in the program length; a ten-week decrease in clerkship time in the hospital and an eight-week increase in clerkship time in the ambulatory or community setting, effectively doubling the time; and a six-week shift in the second-year clinical experience from the hospital to the ambulatory care setting. Such a shift would necessitate a decrease in the number of educator-clinicians and lower-cost trainees in the hospital setting along with an increase in the number of educator-clinicians in the ambulatory and clinical settings. Although the net effect is only a 2 percent increase in the number of educators required, the requirement for community-based clinician educators doubles. The shift increases the essential education cost per student output by 5 percent. From this example, we leafned that shifting from a hospital setting to a community base requires significant changes in educator staffing and cost.

## LESSON 4.

The interaction of instruction, research, and patient care in UME, GME, and graduate biomedical education can be examined using PCACM, as can the implications for resource utilization, costs, and sources of support.

The typical academic health center provides an undergraduate medical education program; graduate medical education programs for generalists, specialists, subspecialists, and fellows; and graduate biomedical education programs for masters, doctoral, and postdoctoral students. Table 4 provides detail information for the program cost and sources of support for the average academic health center for 1995–96.

## Table 3
### EXAMPLE OF THE EFFECT ON RESOURCES AND COSTS OF A SHIFT FROM A TRADITIONAL PROGRAM TO A COMMUNITY-BASED PROGRAM

| | Value | |
|---|---|---|
| Key variables | Traditional | Community-Based |
| | Weeks | |
| **STUDENT PROGRAM** | | |
| Class size | 96 | 96 |
| Program weeks | | |
| Period 1: Academic | 36 | 36 |
| Period 2 | | |
| Hospital | 18 | 12 |
| Ambulatory | 18 | 24 |
| Total | 36 | 36 |
| Periods 3 and 4 | | |
| Hospital | 58 | 48 |
| Ambulatory | 16 | 16 |
| Community | 8 | 16 |
| Total | 82 | 80 |
| Total | 154 | 152 |
| | | |
| Educator requirement in full-time equivalents | | |
| Period 1: Academic | 12.2 | 12.2 |
| Period 2 | | |
| Hospital | 8.5 | 5.7 |
| Ambulatory | 8.6 | 11.5 |
| Total | 17.1 | 17.1 |
| Periods 3 and 4 | | |
| Hospital | 177.2 | 146.6 |
| Ambulatory | 50.6 | 50.6 |
| Community | 35.8 | 71.7 |
| Total | 263.7 | 269.0 |
| Total | 293.0 | 298.3 |
| | Dollars | |
| Essential education cost per student output | | |
| Period 1: Academic | 35,775 | 35,775 |
| Period 2 | | |
| Hospital | 18,218 | 12,145 |
| Ambulatory | 15,260 | 20,346 |
| Total | 33,478 | 32,492 |
| Periods 3 and 4 | | |
| Hospital | 182,612 | 151,127 |
| Ambulatory | 102,614 | 102,614 |
| Community | 51,157 | 102,314 |
| Total | 336,383 | 356,055 |
| Total | 405,637 | 424,323 |

Source: CSHP. "Activity Profiles and Total Program Constructions for Undergraduate and Graduate Medical Education."

## Table 4
## AVERAGE PROGRAM COST AND SOURCES OF SUPPORT OF AN ACADEMIC HEALTH CENTER, 1995–96

| Key variables | | Value | |
|---|---|---|---|
| **PROGRAM CLASS SIZE** | **Total (n = 125)** | **Public (n = 74)** | **Private (n = 51)** |
| Undergraduate medical (MD) | 132 | 132 | 132 |
| Graduate medical (GME) | | | |
|   Generalist/Specialist | 136 | 119 | 150 |
|   Subspecialist | 65 | 56 | 70 |
|   Fellow | 23 | 21 | 24 |
|   Total | 626 | 546 | 684 |
| Total GME slots/MD slots | 4.74 | 4.14 | 5.34 |
| Graduate biomedical | | | |
|   Masters | 15 | 14 | 11 |
|   Doctoral | 37 | 36 | 28 |
|   Postdoctoral | 55 | 52 | 41 |
| **AVERAGE COST PER STUDENT PER YEAR** | **Dollars** | | |
| Undergraduate medical (MD) | 106,390 | 104,379 | 108,144 |
| Graduate medical (GME) | | | |
|   Generalist/Specialist | 224,085 | 224,268 | 223,728 |
|   Subspecialist | 289,698 | 289,632 | 292,777 |
|   Fellow | 98,104 | 86,801 | 97,423 |
| Graduate biomedical | | | |
|   Masters | 71,500 | 75,586 | 79,040 |
|   Doctoral | 105,985 | 104,412 | 107,856 |
|   Postdoctoral | 58,500 | 56,980 | 58,316 |
| **ALL PROGRAM COSTS** | **Millions of Dollars** | | |
| Essential education cost | 228.4 | 206.8 | 237.1 |
| Complementary research and service cost | 56.4 | 47.2 | 79.6 |
|   Total | 284.8 | 254 | 316.7 |
| **SOURCES OF SUPPORT** | **Percent of Total** | | |
| Patient care | | | |
|   Faculty and clinic | 29.9 | 29.4 | 31.7 |
|   Student and hospital | 13.4 | 11.8 | 15.7 |
|   Other | 11.6 | 13.0 | 7.6 |
|   Total | 54.9 | 54.2 | 55.0 |
| Nonpatient care | | | |
|   Research grants and contracts | 25.7 | 22.4 | 30.9 |
|   State | 8.3 | 15.0 | 0.8 |
|   Gifts and endowments | 3.5 | 2.3 | 5.1 |
|   Student tuition and fees | 3.4 | 2.3 | 5.1 |
|   Federal | 0.3 | 0.5 | 0.1 |
|   Other | 3.9 | 3.4 | 4.2 |
|   Total | 45.1 | 45.8 | 45.0 |

Source: Construction by CSHP based on AAMC Data Book and *Journal of American Medical Association*, 1995–96.

Whether the academic health center is public or private, it costs the center approximately the same amount of money ($106,000) to train a PhD as it does an MD, even though a PhD requires 650 ECH/SO and an MD 880 ECH/SO. The costs are comparable because full-time basic science faculty provide 100 percent of the requirements for a PhD, whereas clinician educator faculty and trainees share training responsibility for an MD, thus lowering the supply cost.

As table 4 shows, the total program cost for the average academic health center is $284.8 million, $228.4 million (80 percent) for essential education and $56.4 million (20 percent) for complementary research and service. Tuition and fees support less than 4 percent of the total cost. We have learned that PCACM provides a means of decribing and evaluating all the key variables related to all the educational programs in an academic health center.

**LESSON 5.**

PCACM can be used to assign educator hours and costs to the missions of an academic health center.

The activities of educators in an academic health center can be assigned to the principal missions of the academic health center—teaching, research, and patient care—through an arbitrary process. The process is arbitrary because some activities can support more than one mission, for example, teaching students when research is being carried out during the provision of patient care. Once the time of all educators has been allocated to the various missions, preferably by a consensus of the involved decision makers, the costs related to each mission can be determined.

Based on faculty activity analyses, profiles of a dozen types of educators for the clinical sciences and a half-dozen for basic sciences have been developed. A profile of a clinical sciences educator-clinician, developed from a series of studies of faculty activities at U.S. medical schools, is provided in table 5.

As the table shows, an educator-clinician engages in two types of professional activities: activities that are essential to education and activities that are complementary to education. Essential education activities include direct contact teaching, research and patient care with students present, course preparation, research or scholarship without students present, professional improvement, and administration. Patient care without students is considered a complementary

## Table 5.
## CLINICAL SCIENCES EDUCATOR-CLINICIAN PROFILE AND COST ASSIGNMENT

| Activity Analysis | Total Hours/Week | Teaching Percent of Total | Teaching Hours /Week | Research Percent of Total | Research Hours /Week | Patient Care Percent of Total | Patient Care Hours/ Week |
|---|---|---|---|---|---|---|---|
| **ESSENTIAL EDUCATION** | | | | | | | |
| Direct contact teaching | 6 | 100 | 6 | | | | |
| Patient care with students | 18 | 20 | 4 | | | 80 | 14 |
| *Teaching total* | 24 | 42 | 10 | | | | 14 |
| Preparation for teaching | 4 | 100 | 4 | | | | |
| *Instruction total* | 28 | 50 | 14 | | | | |
| Research | | | | | | | |
| Scholarship | 14 | 5 | 1 | 85 | 12 | 10 | 1 |
| Professional improvement | 4 | 5 | | 80 | 3 | 15 | 1 |
| Administration | 4 | 15 | 1 | | | 85 | 3 |
| **COMPLEMENTARY** Patient care without students | 10 | | | | | 100 | 10 |
| TOTAL ACTIVITY | 60 | | 16 | | 15 | | 29 |

| EDUCATOR COST ASSIGNMENT | Total | Teaching | Research | Patient Care |
|---|---|---|---|---|
| **Total Educational Cost** | | | Dollars | |
| Educator salary | 152,000 | 38,000 | 38,000 | 76,000 |
| Other | 239,400 | 88,540 | 88,540 | 62,320 |
| Total | 391,400 | 126,540 | 126,540 | 138,320 |
| **Essential Education Cost** | | | | |
| Educator salary | 126,160 | 38,000 | 38,000 | 50,160 |
| Other | 218,211 | 88,540 | 88,540 | 41,131 |
| Total | 344,371 | 126,540 | 126,540 | 91,291 |
| **Complementary Cost** | | | | |
| Educator salary | 25,840 | 0 | 0 | 25,840 |
| Other | 21,189 | 0 | 0 | 21,189 |
| Total | 47,029 | 0 | 0 | 47,029 |

Source: CSHP (Center for Studies in Health Policy). Basic and Clinical Services Activity Profiles and Income Analyses.

activity. Adding the number of hours an educator spends in activities with students present (often defined as teaching activities) to the number of hours spent preparing for teaching gives the total number of hours spent in instruction.

Of the sixty hours per week this educator-clinician spends in professional activities, fifty hours (83 percent) are assigned to essential education activities and ten hours (17 percent) to complementary patient care activities. Ten essential education hours are assigned to the teaching mission, six hours from direct contact teaching and four hours from patient care with students. This is a key variable because it indicates the amount of educator time (supply) available to meet an educational program (demand) requirement for teaching. Approximately 25 percent of the total professional time of this educator-clinician is assigned to teaching, 25 percent to research, and 50 percent to patient care.

On the basis of these assignments, an allocation of education costs can be made. With a salary of $152,000 and other costs of $239,400, the educator-clinician's total education cost is $391,400. Of the essential education cost of $344,371, $126,540 (32 percent) is assigned to the teaching mission, $126,540 (32 percent) to research, and $91,291 (23 percent) to patient care. The complementary cost assigned to the patient care mission is $47,029 (12 percent). The percentages shown in the income analysis do not correspond to those in the activity profile because the other cost factors for the teaching, research, and patient care activities vary.

Armed with the kind of information shown in table 5, an academic health center can then begin to address the question, Who should pay for what?

Also, when productivity is mentioned in relation to clinician-educators who are major patient-care providers, answers can be developed to deal with the question, How many patients can the provider service? This question is best answered by constructing "what ifs" based on assumptions about existing activities and the productivity of students and educators. Productivity depends in large measure on the program structure and an educator's style of practice. The analysis of educator activities has helped us to better understand the relationships among activities, direct contact teaching, mission assignment, and, most importantly, allocation of cost to missions.

## LESSON 6.

PCACM can be used to compare the resource requirements and cost of educating various workforce members.

PCACM can shed light on the debate about which health professionals can best provide primary health care at the least cost to the health care delivery system. The methodology can help answer the question, How many primary care providers can I get for the cost of one allopathic physician? As shown in table 6, it costs about $1,650,000 to educate an allopathic physician specialist during eleven calendar years of postsecondary education, a little more than the cost of educating an osteopathic physician for eleven years. The same amount of money could educate twenty-five doctors of chiropractic for six years; fourteen advanced nurse practitioners for six years or twenty-eight for two years beyond the bachelor's degree; twelve physician assistants for four years; thirty-three physical therapists for six years; or thirty occupational therapists for six years.

The lesson learned here is that the key variables identified in PCACM not only help describe the elements and assumptions behind these costs; they also

Table 6.

**COMPARISON OF THE RESOURCE AND COST REQUIREMENTS OF EDUCATING SELECTED PRIMARY HEALTH CARE PROVIDERS**

| Providers | Program calendar years | Average educator contact hrs/output | Cost/output SMD/$PCP | PCP/ MD |
|---|---|---|---|---|
| Doctor of allopathic medicine | | | | |
|    Specialist | 11 | 1,840 | 1,647,000 | 1 |
|    Generalist | 9 | 1,795 | 1,635,000 | 1 MD |
| Doctor of osteopathic medicine | 11 | 1,830 | 1,464,000 | 1 |
| Doctor of chiropractic medicine | 6 | 265 | 67,000 | 25 DC |
| Advanced nurse practitioner (ANP) | 6 | 343 | 114,000 | 14 ANP |
| ANP (BSN + 2 years) | 2 | 171 | 58,000 | 28 ANP |
| Physician assistant | 4 | 315 | 133,000 | 12 PA |
| Physical therapist | 6 | 200 | 51,000 | 33 PT |
| Occupational therapist | 4 | 280 | 55,000 | 30 OT |

Source: Center for Studies in Health Policy. September 15, 1997. In "Primary Care Professionals Comparison."

help identify where effective changes can be made, particularly in program structure and educator staffing, in a cost-beneficial manner.

## LESSON 7.

PCACM can provide a basis for the solicitation of funding.

Table 7 illustrates an allocation of annual essential education cost per student to the instruction, research, and patient care missions. If, for example, an academic health center wanted to solicit a large donation for the endowment fund, the total essential education cost—about $110,000 per year, or $450,000 for the four-year program—would be a good gift. The center could request a state appropriation of $35,000—the essential instruction cost—for each enrolled student, or about $18.5 million.

Service mission costs represent 39 percent of the total essential education cost, so the center might request $41,000 for each enrolled student from the practice plan fund, or about $22 million. Finally, research mission costs are about $31,000 per student per year. The research grants and contracts would be

---

Table 7.

**THE AVERAGE ALLOCATION OF ESSENTIAL EDUCATION COST PER STUDENT TO THE THREE MISSIONS OF AN ACADEMIC HEALTH CENTER**

| Key variables | Value ($) | % of total |
|---|---|---|
| Instruction | | |
| Basic sciences | 6,500 | 6 |
| Clinical sciences | 28,017 | 26 |
| Total | 34,517 | 32 |
| Research | | |
| Basic sciences | 6,500 | 6 |
| Clinical sciences | 24,306 | 23 |
| Total | 30,806 | 29 |
| Service | | |
| Basic sciences | 0 | 0 |
| Clinical sciences | 41,067 | 39 |
| Total | 41,067 | 39 |
| Essential education total | | |
| Basic sciences | 13,000 | 12 |
| Clinical sciences | 93,390 | 88 |
| Total | 106,390 | 100 |

Source: CSHP. US Average Analysis for 125 Medical Schools, 1995–1996.

expected to generate about $16.4 million per year.

It should be noted that in this average program, 100 clinician-educators are volunteering their teaching time. The time of each clinician-educator can be valued at about $127,000 per year, for a total "savings" or "noncost" for the program of about $1.3 million.

## SUMMARY

By providing a means for identifying all the education elements; their resource requirements; particular educator staffing; and their costs and sources of revenues, the program cost- construction method provides an approach to calculating the costs to educate a physician from undergraduate through graduate medical education, and also obviates the need for a major new cost accounting study. Thus, the method is a powerful tool for shaping responsible planning strategies for institutional and public policies at all levels of decision making.

Among the conclusions we can draw from our study are the following:

- We can construct answers to all the resource requirement and cost questions we posed and thereby develop information that can be used to examine present activities and explore alternatives.

- In comparing cost studies, determining the magnitude of differences is not as valuable as determining why the differences occur.

- Planning alternative futures and discussing their impacts on resource requirements, costs, and potential sources of support before implementation can be very cost effective.

- Not all sources of support are recorded in medical school accounts, but cost construction allows the determination of total costs and their potential sources of support by the type of cost.

- Productivity can go up or down depending on the design of the program structure and the educator's style of practice.

- Cost construction works to describe all types of health professions education and allow for consistent comparison.

# WORK CITED

Franzini, L., M.D. Low, and M.A. Proll. 1997. Using a cost-construction model to assess the cost of educating undergraduate medical students at the University of Texas-Houston Medical School. *Academic Medicine* 72(3).

Ginzberg, E., M. Ostow, and A.B. Dutka. 1993. *The Economics of Medical Education.* New York: Josiah Macy, Jr. Foundation.

Gonyea, M.A. 1997. Unpublished. The constructed cost of physician and graduate biomedical science education: An analysis of educational resource requirements in various medical schools. Washington: Center for Studies in Health Policy.

Goodwin, M.C., W.M. Gleason, and H.A. Kontos. 1997. A pilot study of the cost of educating undergraduate medical students at Virginia Commonwealth University. *Academic Medicine* 72(3).

Institute of Medicine. 1974. Report of a Study: Costs of Education in the Health Professions (parts 1–3). Washington: National Academy of Sciences.

Rein, M.F., W.J. Randolph, J.G. Short, K.G. Coolidge, M.L. Coates, R.M. Carey. 1997. Defining the cost of educating undergraduate medical students at the University of Virginia. *Academic Medicine* 72(3).

Valberg, L.S., M.A. Gonyea, D.G. Sinclair, and J. Wade. 1994. Planning the *Future Academic Medical Centre: Conceptual Framework and Financial Design.* Ontario Canadian Medical Association.

# THE RESEARCH MISSION
# OF ACADEMIC HEALTH
# CENTERS

*David Blumenthal, MD, MPP*

S
TIMULATED BY THREATS TO THEIR FINANCIAL
viability, much of today's discussion on the future of academic
health centers (Iglehart 1994, 1995; Blumenthal and Meyer 1996;
Blake 1996; Gold 1996; Commonwealth Fund 1997) has, predictably enough, concentrated on the changes in public policy and academic
health center behavior required to enable academic health centers to attract
patients in the increasingly price-competitive health care market.

Considerably less attention has been devoted to several important related
questions. They include, first, the potential effects—positive and negative—of the
survival strategies that academic health centers are adopting to protect their academic missions. The second set of questions concerns whether academic health
centers are exploiting available opportunities to improve the efficiency with
which they conduct their academic missions. Such improvements could help academic health centers do more with less as market forces restrict discretionary
funds that have helped support these missions in the past.

Failure to address these issues early and explicitly could prove unfortunate
for academic health centers. Academic health centers could adopt strategies that

*Dr. Blumenthal is executive director of The Commonwealth Fund Task Force on
Academic Health Centers, and Chief, Health Policy Research and Development
Unit, Massachusetts General Hospital, Partners HealthCare System, Boston, and
assiociate professor of medicine and health care policy at Harvard Medical School.*

preserve their financial viability and assure their survival as institutions, only to find that they have fundamentally undermined their raison d'etre in the process.

Even if academic health centers avoid this pitfall, it seems that resources to support mission-related activities will be scarcer in the future than in the past. This suggests the need for academic health centers to make whatever resources they have stretch further—to be smarter and more efficient in their conduct of research, education, and clinical innovation, just as they are struggling to do in patient care. Recognizing these dangers and opportunities, this paper addresses the problems and options facing academic health centers in the conduct of one of their core missions: health care research.

## THE RESEARCH MISSION

Academic health centers (including both medical schools and their affiliated clinical facilities) conduct about $12.5 billion of health care research each year (Causino et al. 1995). These funds derive from several sources: Federal and state government, private industry, private philanthropy, endowment, and net revenues from clinical operations. This last has been by far the fastest growing funding mechanism.

Using these funds, academic health centers pursue a variety of types of research, ranging from quite fundamental molecular biology to quite applied clinical research. Unfortunately, though it is possible to identify qualitatively the types of biomedical research that academic health centers conduct and the types of support they receive, the data do not permit us to quantify how much of each type of research they do or how dependent each type is on particular external or internal sources. This makes it difficult to identify with precision the future vulnerability of alternative varieties of research to changes in public policy or private markets.

### Fundamental Investigation

Fundamental, or basic, investigation is classically thought to concentrate on identifying the basic mechanisms that underlie normal and abnormal biologic processes. Research of this type generally takes place in medical school and university laboratories, although some hospital-based laboratories also conduct such investigation. The National Institutes of Health (NIH) is the predominant supporter of this type of work in academic health centers (NIH 1997).

Because fundamental research is funded predominantly by the NIH, the fortunes in academic health centers are likely to track the funding patterns of this agency. In recent years, NIH has fared reasonably well in the Federal budget process. Even in the face of cutbacks in other domestic discretionary programs, NIH's budgets have increased faster than inflation: about 6.1 percent annually since 1990 (NIH 1997). Thus, for academic health centers that participate to a significant extent in fundamental research, the NIH type of mission-related activity would seem to have fairly bright prospects.

Adding to this optimistic picture is the growth of academic-industry relationships (AIRs). AIRs supply only about 13 percent of all research funding at academic health centers, and most do not support fundamental investigation. However, a number of long-term strategic alliances between large pharmaceutical companies and academic health centers have, in fact, included important commitments to quite basic research. This is because academic health centers have a comparative advantage in the conduct of such investigation; by using the centers, large companies can gain access to highly talented investigators without incurring the fixed costs associated with creating their own basic research labs (Blumenthal et al. 1996a). In a sense, AIR support of fundamental biology can be seen as another version of the outsourcing that is so prevalent among major companies in the United States currently.

Nevertheless, fundamental investigation in academic health centers is not completely insulated from market forces in the health care system. Though the precise sum is unknown, a significant proportion of the revenues transferred from academic health center clinical operations to medical schools and universities goes to support fundamental investigation.

Clinical funds assist research leaders at academic health centers to accomplish several tasks related to basic research.

First, these cross-subsidies make up for research expenses that NIH does not support. One such expense is the cost of capital. The Federal government makes no explicit payments for major core facilities or new buildings, although interest and depreciation can be included in indirect costs. Another expense for academic health centers results from the tendency of the Federal government to displace operating costs onto grantees. The NIH caps the salaries of investigators at artificially low limits and refuses to pay for certain routine expenses, such as secretaries. The result is that parent institutions must complement Federal funds with additional money or risk losing premier investigators to other institutions.

Second, institutions rely on clinical revenues to support young investigators who have not yet acquired the track record they need to compete for their first investigator-initiated (so-called RO1) NIH grant. Many of the nation's most prominent senior basic investigators began their careers supported by discretionary funds that clinical department chairpersons and other mentors sequestered from clinical revenues.

## Clinical Investigation

Some of the basic investigation conducted at academic health centers could probably be handled just as well in universities without clinical connections. This situation is definitely not true, however, of clinical research, which requires both access to patients and involvement by trained investigators. Clinical investigation and its associated transfer of technology from bench to bedside are functions that academic health centers are uniquely suited to perform. They may also be the functions that are most dependent on cross-subsidies from clinical operations.

There are three types of clinical research occurring at academic health centers (Crowley and Thier 1996), as follows:

1. Translational clinical research—Closest to fundamental investigation, involves exploration of basic biological questions using humans as research subjects. It is often a necessary step to moving basic insights into application, but may not lead directly to new medical technologies. Typical of translational investigation is the work that goes on in inpatient general clinical research centers (GCRCs) funded by the NIH. These centers explore such questions as how sleep is regulated or how the calcium content of bone is hormonally controlled in normal humans. Some research of this type is funded by NIH, but many observers believe that translational investigation is particularly dependent on clinical cross-subsidies.

2. Clinical trials—A step closer to application than translational investigation, generally involves defined diagnostic or therapeutic technologies that are under evaluation for their safety or efficacy. The most advanced form is the so-called phase III clinical trials, which are funded by drug companies to provide

data required for approval by the Food and Drug Administration (FDA). Clinical trials are regarded as much less dependent on internal academic health center funding because of industry's strong interest in supporting them. The exception may be studies of drugs and devices that are not protected through existing intellectual property statutes or are inherently unprofitable because their markets are small. Examples include studies of the costs and efficacy of off-patent medications or of surgical innovations that cannot be patented.

3. Clinical investigation, or so-called outcomes/health services research— Includes a wide variety of studies that examine the natural history of illness, develop better ways to measure the effects of treatment, and study methods to improve the efficiency or quality of health services through organizational or financial interventions. Outcomes/health services research is a relatively new field in biomedical investigation, and it has depended largely on funding from a small Federal agency, the Agency for Health Care Policy and Research (AHCPR) and on private philanthropy. Recently, however, market pressures may actually be working in favor of this area of investigation, since private health care providers increasingly view it as important to improving their competitive positions.

A widespread perception exists that clinical investigation is more dependent than fundamental investigation on cross-subsidies from clinical revenues. This perception is based on anecdotal and modest empirical evidence. First, leaders of clinical units in academic health centers report that they have commonly used clinical revenues to support research by their faculty. Much of this support does not show up on academic health center budgets. It occurs as part of the routine administration of an academic health center unit. Department chairs may use the funding for such expenses to gain protected time for a young investigator, hire a research assistant for a laboratory, and rent space for an expanding unit. For example, the General Medicine Unit at the Massachusetts General Hospital (MGH) at one time used revenues from its practice to subsidize the unit's research. Individual faculty may actually divert some of their personal clinical revenue to fund their own research efforts. The author of this article did precisely this during critical startup years of MGH's Health Policy Research and Development Unit (HPRDU).

Second, studies of publication patterns in clinical disciplines suggest that a considerable amount of scholarly work is not supported by external sources. At least 23 percent of studies published in major medical journals result from research with no explicit extramural sponsorship of any type (Stein et al. 1993). Unsponsored research accounts for 84 percent of studies published in the field of pathology, 62 percent in internal medicine, and 74 percent in surgery (Berman et al. 1993, 1995). Apparent dependence of clinical research on patient care revenues suggests that this type of investigation may be more vulnerable to changes in market forces than basic research. However, this vulnerability is likely to vary among the three types of clinical investigation.

Because clinical trials are funded by industry and respond to regulatory mandates, these, too, may be somewhat buffered from changes in patient care markets, although, as we shall see, they are unlikely to be completely protected. In contrast, translational research may have the least secure extramural support, and thus, may be most vulnerable to declines in academic health center net income from patient services.

## DEALING WITH THREATS TO SURVIVAL

A variety of developments pose potential problems for the research missions of academic health centers. For purposes of discussion, I have divided these developments into those that are either external or internal to these institutions.

### External Threats

External threats to the research missions of academic health centers originate in two sectors: public and private. Private sector developments have received the most publicity, but those in the public sector are equally important to the future of research at academic health centers.

The advent of competition in private health care markets is the first and newest factor affecting the research missions of academic health centers. Brought about by purchasers' interest in reducing their health care premiums, price competition among providers for managed care contracts threatens to reduce the net clinical revenues of academic health centers. Declining clinical surpluses jeopardize academic health centers' ability to cross-subsidize their research missions.

Documentation of the effect of competitive pressures on the research missions of the centers is scarce, so the extent of the threat is difficult to quantify. As noted previously, our qualitative understanding of the funding sources for academic health center research suggests that clinical research would be more affected by declining clinical income than would basic research, but that basic research may not be completely unaffected by trends in health care markets. In addition, because young researchers often compete less successfully for extramural funds, they may be more vulnerable to reduced clinical subsidies than are the more established investigators.

Besides affecting the funding for academic health center research, price competition in local markets may also affect the availability of patients for clinical experiments. This situation would occur if managed care organizations (MCOs) tended to steer patients away from academic health centers, thus reducing the supply of patients who can participate in clinical investigation.

Anecdotal evidence supports the impression that resources available to subsidize research are declining in clinical departments. Together with Dr. Paul Griner at the Association of American Medical Colleges, we conducted fifteen case studies of academic health centers over the last year (Moy et al. 1997). Especially in competitive markets such as Boston and Oregon, department chairs in areas such as medicine and surgery reported that clinical surpluses were reduced or had completely disappeared. Equally interesting was the finding that the intellectual energy of senior academic leaders is now consumed by day-to-day management problems aimed at improving the competitive position of their institutions in local markets. One major department chairman commented that instead of devoting 50 percent of his own energy to research and teaching as he did a decade ago, he now devotes only 3 to 5 percent of his time to this purpose. The same was true, he said, of the regular meetings of department chairs at his academic health center.

Recently, more systematic empirical evidence has emerged to support the hypothesis that markets adversely affect research missions. The recent study by Moy and colleagues found that academic health centers in markets with a high managed care enrollment tend to compete less successfully for NIH funds than sister institutions in less competitive areas. As the researchers predicted, the effects were most marked in clinical departments. A complementary study by Campbell and colleagues (1997) found that clinical investigators in competitive markets tend to be less academically productive (as measured by publication rates in peer-reviewed journals) than clinical investigators in noncompetitive areas. This effect was not found for basic researchers, suggesting that NIH-funded work may be comparatively protected in competitive environments. Campbell and colleagues also found that in competitive markets, there seemed to be greater pressures on young investigators to participate in clinical care, which is consistent with the hypothesis that young clinical investigators are most vulnerable to market pressures.

As yet, there have been no empirical studies of the availability of patients for clinical studies in competitive as opposed to noncompetitive areas. Therefore, the potential adverse effects of competition on the supply of patients for clinical investigation cannot be assessed.

Another private sector development with important potential implications for the research missions of academic health centers is the advent of so-called contract research organizations (CROs), for-profit entities that conduct clinical research for large pharmaceutical clients. In 1995, more than 200 CROs were located in North America, representing about 25 percent of all CROs worldwide (Hughes 1996). A study of the impact of CROs on academic research found that in 1993 more than half (57 percent) of all clinical trials were performed by investigators not affiliated with academic institutions (Center Watch 1995).

Among the leading reasons pharmaceutical companies give for turning to CROs is the greater time and costs associated with clinical research in academic health centers. A 1994 study by Pharmco LTD (Center Watch 1996) a large pharmaceutical firm, of its sponsored clinical studies found the average time from IRB submission to contract approval was 60 to 150 days for university hospitals, 30 to 60 days for private hospitals, and 7 to 28 days in private practices. Not only have CROs demonstrated they can initiate trials faster than academic health centers, but their costs per patient are also 15 percent lower than academic institutions (Center Watch 1995). More recently, CROs themselves have encountered competition from groups of physicians who are forming so-called site management organizations (SMOs). Using their physicians' access to and control over patients, SMOs negotiate profitable fees with CROs or pharmaceutical companies to participate in the conduct of (or directly undertake) clinical trials.

Though the actions of the public sector have attracted somewhat less attention than private sector developments in recent years, changes in public policy may also affect the research missions of academic health centers. Efforts by Federal and state governments to encourage enrollment of Medicare and Medicaid patients in managed care organizations are likely to increase the intensity of price competition in local markets as managed care organizations seek the same savings in caring for public sector clients as they do for private sector enrollees. Among Medicare beneficiaries, predicts the Congressional Budget Office, the proportion enrolled in managed care organizations will grow from its current figure of 10 percent to 22 percent by 2002 (Commonwealth Fund 1997). If managed care organizations direct Medicare patients away from expensive academic health center hospitals, it could also affect the availability of patients for clinical research on the problems of the elderly.

Equally important are recent provisions of the Balanced Budget Act of 1997 (BBA), which reduce a variety of Federal Medicare payments to academic health centers. According to the Prospective Payment Advisory Commission (ProPAC 1997), hospitals have been making handsome margins from Medicare business in recent years, on the order of 9 percent. Major teaching hospitals have done even better, earning Medicare margins of 18 to 19 percent. Not surprisingly, these figures have encouraged Congress to curtail inpatient Medicare payments to hospitals, in general, and to academic health centers, in particular. Under the BBA, Medicare reimbursement for hospital care is expected to be reduced by $44 billion over the next five years compared to the reimbursement under current law. Two changes will particularly affect academic health centers: the reduction of indirect medical education adjustment (IME) from 7.7 to 5.5 percent over four years, and the reduction of disproportionate share payments by 5 percent over five years.

Although seemingly justified by high Medicare margins, these changes in Medicare payment policy may have a disproportionate effect on the research missions of academic health centers. Whether rightly or wrongly, academic health centers have grown increasingly dependent on generous public sector payments to maintain the clinical surpluses that cross-subsidize their research missions. Though Medicare margins are generous at major teaching hospitals, total margins at these facilities are only 3.8 percent (ProPAC 1997). The inescapable conclusion is that earnings from other payers are minimal or negative. Reduced Medicare payments, added to fierce price pressures from private payers, may thus cause a number of academic health centers to experience operating deficits and force reductions in clinical cross-subsidies.

## Internal Threats

Changes in private markets and public policies have prompted responses from academic health centers that are designed to protect the centers' research and other academic missions. Of the many options available to the centers for this purpose, two seem most commonly employed. The first is to develop integrated health care delivery systems that compete more effectively with local community-based health care institutions and thereby preserve market share, revenue, and clinical income. Clinical income can then be used to continue research subsidies.

A second, nearly ubiquitous strategy is to seek increased industrial support for research, or to commercialize academic health center research results more aggressively, thereby developing funding streams that can compensate for losses of clinical revenue.

Just as potentially beneficial treatments may have unintended adverse side effects, so too may the regimens that academic health centers have adopted to cope with environmental pressures. Some of these potential problems may be simply unavoidable consequences of the changed rules of the markets in which the centers now exist. Still, if center leaders are to minimize the risks of their actions, it is essential that they be familiar with the disadvantages as well as the benefits of the strategies they are implementing.

In addition to the external forces that will reduce resources available to academic health centers to support research are the potential, equally important, effects of coping strategies on the constrained resources that remain at the disposal of the centers.

Those resources come in two primary forms: human capital and financial capital. Faced with increased clinical competition, academic health centers are likely to divert both types of capital away from traditional uses in support of research and other academic missions.

Academic health centers are now devoting large amounts of financial and human capital to building integrated delivery systems that can compete for managed care business. These monies are used to develop primary care and specialty networks, create management systems to run those networks, develop marketing campaigns to attract patients, establish information systems to demonstrate and improve quality and efficiency, and acquire complementary health care services. Numbers on the amounts of money that academic health centers are expending on these activities are not available, but it is not unusual for a single, major academic health center to budget tens or hundreds of millions of dollars for these purposes.

The need for such new initiatives seems indisputable, at least for academic health centers that want to stay in the patient-care business. However, the associated opportunity costs are also sizable. If the same monies and creativity were devoted to developing the research and teaching missions of the centers, the result would be new research buildings, more modern equipment, more talented young people who have been trained, and possibly, greater progress in biomedical research. Some of the nation's most powerful and wealthy academic health centers—usually venerable private institutions with large endowments and substantial capital reserves—may be able to forge ahead both with major new clinical projects and with research expansions. However, only a small minority of centers are this fortunate.

The development of integrated delivery systems by academic health centers is likely to have unforeseen effects on the research activities of these organizations that extend well beyond the opportunity costs of capital. Even successful, wealthy centers that create thriving integrated systems will find that, as a result, they are fundamentally changed as organizations. They will be much bigger and more diverse. They will incorporate large, community-based networks of providers who account for a substantial portion of the organizational revenues and contain hundreds or thousands of employees, including clinicians, with less understanding of and commitment to the traditional academic missions of academic health centers.

The diversity and complexity of the new academic health center will be reflected in its governance. Department chairs and the faculty they represent will be one constituency among many with seats on governing councils. The power of chairs and faculty will inevitably be reduced compared with their current status. Their influence will not be enhanced by the fact that they will often appear in governing bodies as supplicants, requesting support from the integrated system to fund faculty research.

Even if representatives of community-based clinical units have a deep sympathy for the research missions of academic health centers, this new arrangement will create tensions between the academicians and clinicians. The latter, it seems likely, will demand, at a minimum, some influence over how their contributions to research missions are expended. In other cases, their sympathy for department chairs and academic faculty may erode over time because of differing perspectives and values. Faculty may come to resent the intrusions of academically unsophisticated community physicians. Community clinicians—pushed ever harder to be efficient—will come to resent the arrogance of faculty and their apparent insulation from the exigencies of day-to-day practice.

Such economic and cultural divisions will be played out in the governance and management of integrated academic health care systems. Department chairs and faculty leaders will find themselves more involved than ever in internal politics and further diverted from their roles as research leaders. Because of their complexity and resulting internal tensions, academic systems may be more difficult to manage than their community-based competition, leading to decreased agility in responding to market developments. Eventually, leaders may be forced to reduce internal strife and simplify their management by separating their research and clinical operations both financially and administratively. The result could be to deprive research activities of the subsidies for which the integrated system was created, and to separate the investigative side of the organization from the clinical side. If this situation occurs, the capital that academic health centers will have diverted to integrated health will have been used primarily to create clinical organizations that differ little from the nonacademic organizations with which they must compete.

One additional internal threat to the research missions of academic health centers may arise from the effects of coping strategies on the values of the academic enterprise. This issue is raised most visibly by the growth of academic-industry relationships and by the efforts of academic health centers to commercialize their research.

AIRs have documented benefits for both companies and academic health centers, and have been actively promoted by Federal and state policy (Blumenthal 1992). Nevertheless, industrial research relationships among academic health centers also carry risks. It is now well-documented that AIRs are associated with secrecy among faculty and delay in dissemination of research results (Blumenthal et al. 1997). Research supported by industry also tends to be more applied in nature than research supported by governmental (especially NIH) sources. These findings raise questions about whether commercially oriented strategies to preserve the research missions of academic health centers may change the values and attitudes of enough faculty to change the nature and direction of the missions themselves. Many observers are also concerned that over the long-term, efforts by universities to forge stronger links to companies and to commercialize their own research will reduce public confidence in the quality and objectivity of the academic biomedical research enterprise.

## STRATEGIES FOR SURVIVAL

The above review of threats to the research missions of academic health centers has dwelled on the negative forces and effects created by the current health care environment. There is, however, another perspective on the situation.

Academic health centers are resourceful institutions, populated by very talented individuals. A select few institutions are actually well positioned to adapt to the rigors of competitive markets and, in the process, to preserve their research missions. Even those academic health centers not among these favored few can act to reduce the risks to their research missions posed by the current environment. In pursuing those opportunities, some academic health centers may actually emerge as stronger, more diverse research enterprises. The optimal set of strategies for any particular institution is likely to vary from center to center and market to market. This section reviews a generic set of approaches that particular institutions may wish to consider as they design their individual approaches.

It should also be noted that public policy also has an essential role in preserving the research capabilities of academic health centers. One public policy option is the creation of an Academic Health Services Trust Fund that would protect the academic missions of academic health centers from market forces (Commonwealth Fund 1997). (Because of insufficient space, we do not deal with public policy options explicitly in this paper.)

## MANAGING EXTERNAL THREATS

As previously noted, academic health centers' research missions face three types of external threats in the current competitive environment: reduced revenues to finance those missions; reduced access to patients to conduct clinical research; and competition from for-profit CROs and SMOs. Here we discuss options for countering each of these problems.

### Financing the Research Mission

To finance their research in competitive markets, academic health centers have two basic choices. They can develop new sources of revenues, or they can find ways to do more with less by increasing the efficiency with which they conduct research.

A variety of strategies offer opportunities to increase the funds available to academic health centers for their research mission. These can be roughly categorized as clinical and nonclinical revenues.

*Increasing clinical revenues.* The most straightforward approach to preserving academic health center ability to cross-subsidize research activities is the one that many centers have adopted, namely, to compete successfully on the basis of price and quality for clinical business, while controlling clinical costs well enough to generate the margins necessary to support their research (Blumenthal and Meyer 1996). The potential costs of this approach in financial and human capital have been discussed above. The potential benefits remain unclear at this point.

There is a widespread impression based on anecdotal evidence that primary care networks have not fulfilled their promise: that many are losing money and failing to generate tertiary and quarternary referrals. Some academic health centers seem to be concluding that they underestimated the costs of building primary care systems and overestimated their ability to capture referrals from affiliated primary care physicians, who often continue to rely on community-based specialists. In response, academic health centers seem to be embarking on another potentially costly wave of network development, this time aimed at creating systems of affiliated specialists. The shortcomings of primary care networks to date are also likely to spur increased efforts to manage these networks to make them more efficient, and also spur an increased interest in creating an insurance function within academic health-center networks. The latter, it is hoped, will enable centers to capture and retain the profits that MCOs have enjoyed on the managed care business.

Despite early problems, the strategy of competing for clinical business has a reasonable chance of paying off for centers that enjoy certain advantages. These advantages include ample reserves of capital, deep management benches (or the working cash to acquire the necessary talent), a sterling reputation in local markets, and modest local competition from other providers (especially aggressive for-profit hospital and HMO chains). Examples of institutions that may fit this description include Partners HealthCare System (PHCS) in Boston, University of Pennsylvania Health System in Philadelphia, University of Alabama Health Science Center in Birmingham, Emory Health System in Atlanta, and Washington University/BJC Health Systems, Inc., in St. Louis. It should be noted that many of these institutions are in stage I and II markets by University HealthSystem Consortium (UHC) standards, and that the Boston market is often considered atypical because, despite its high managed care penetration, its MCOs are predominantly nonprofit (Bourne and Malcom 1996).

Many academic health centers, however, do not enjoy the advantages that these few favored institutions possess. A number of the less well-endowed centers are taking a radically different approach to enhancing clinical revenues for the support of research and other missions. These centers have decided to cash in on their long-term investment in clinical infrastructure by selling their teaching hospitals and putting the money in the bank—in effect, capitalizing a clinical asset and using the resulting funds to endow their research and other academic enterprises. At a minimum, this approach protects an academic mission against the threat of debilitating clinical deficits in the future. Examples include Tulane University, which sold its primary teaching hospital to Columbia/HCA, and University of Minnesota, which sold its teaching hospital to the nonprofit Fairview chain.

Getting out of the business of owning hospitals has a number of advantages. At the right price, the sale can generate a comfortable nest egg. With stock markets booming, return on invested capital may exceed return on assets tied up in the hospital business. Only time will tell whether academic health centers are actually selling for the right price. Some observers fear they are not (Anderson

1997). Also, this strategy frees up human capital to concentrate on enhancing academic missions. One academic health center leader commented during a recent interview with this writer that, ever since the sale of his teaching hospital, he wakes up every morning feeling liberated from the burden of managing a vulnerable teaching hospital.

*Increasing nonclinical revenues.* A number of nonclinical strategies for enhancing revenues to support research missions are also available. The first is the tried-and-true approach of increasing philanthropic donations. Because gifts have come to constitute about 2 percent of medical school revenues (and are assuming a similar figure for hospitals), philanthropy has received less emphasis in academic health centers recently (Krakower et al. 1996). However, some institutions are taking a new look at this option. The new wealth created by the high-tech and biotechnology revolutions and by the stock market offers new fundraising opportunities. Many state institutions, in particular, have never aggressively exploited their philanthropic options, in part because they feared they would not be able to retain control of the funds they raised. Now, some state-owned academic health centers, such as the Oregon Health Sciences University, have arranged to be freed from direct state control, a situation that may make philanthropy more appealing as a funding source.

Here again, not all academic health centers face equally interesting prospects. Those with long histories of fund-raising and major national and local reputations are likely to do better than newcomers. The Massachusetts General Hospital has recently embarked on a $160 million capital campaign that, for the first time in the institution's history, will be devoted exclusively to endowing its research program. The $160 million goal was met 1.5 years early and, as a result, the campaign was doubled to $320 million and extended until the year 2000. At present, MGH has collected more than $200 million and expects to reach the $320 million goal ahead of schedule. Not many centers, however, have the development resources of this venerable hospital.

Another potential source of nonclinical revenues for academic health center research missions may be enhanced contributions from state governments. States have long supported publicly owned academic health centers through annual appropriations for educational and, to much lesser extent, research activities. These contributions have become less and less important to public academic health centers over time as clinical revenues have increased and as states have reduced their contributions. However, two factors may alter this situation now.

The first is that the financial fortunes of the states are improving because of booming local economies, with resulting increases in state revenues and declines in welfare and Medicaid rolls. The second factor is that some states may soon enjoy unexpected windfalls in the form of settlements on suits against tobacco companies. Florida, for example, just agreed to accept $11.3 billion over five years from tobacco companies to settle such a suit. It will receive a $1 billion down payment in the first year of the agreement (Blumenthal and Meyer 1996). Multiplied across the forty states that are now suing the tobacco companies, such agreements could bring major new revenues into state coffers. The theory behind the suits has been that tobacco use increased state health expenditures for Medicaid beneficiaries. Finding better ways to prevent and treat tobacco-related illness would seem a compelling use of these new monies, and investing in research at local academic health centers might, therefore, be a justifiable and appealing use of new state funds.

A third possible source of new nonclinical revenues to support academic health center research is industrial support of this research. As previously noted, this strategy has both benefits and risks. Methods of managing the risks are discussed below. Here we merely note that the opportunities remain substantial, especially in the area of fundamental investigation. In a 1994–1995 survey of a representative sample of companies that support biomedical research, we found that 60 percent intended to maintain or expand their current investment in academic research (Blumenthal et al. 1996b).

Very aware of the opportunities for industrial support, many academic health centers are actively pursuing such funds. In general, however, these efforts seem focused on attracting clinical research dollars. Academic health centers, especially those with strong basic research infrastructures, should make certain they do not lose sight of opportunities to secure such funding to enable the institution to pursue fundamental investigation.

*Instituting peer review of internally supported research.* A widespread impression exists among academic health center research leaders that some of the work supported by internally generated resources is not highly meritorious. Whether or not this is true, it is clear that very little of the research supported predominantly by internal center resources is subjected to the kind of rigorous peer review that occurs with most extramurally funded research.

The initiation of formal peer review of internally supported research could potentially free up funds for the most meritorious academic health center projects. It would also create a fair and impartial process for allocating increasingly scarce research funds. This might help reduce the conflict that will inevitably arise as research support decreases (Campbell et al. 1997).

*Improving research efficiency.* A final potential source of revenues for support of academic health center research missions is found in opportunities for savings in the conduct of research. Such savings would constitute found money that could be used to support work threatened by falling clinical revenues.

In a series of case studies of academic health centers, we have observed that their leaders have rarely devoted much thought to reducing research-related expenses as a way of augmenting available funding for their research enterprises. The first reaction of some research managers and academic health center leaders to the suggestion that research efficiency may be improved is a blank stare, followed by an expression of skepticism that meaningful cost savings can be realized. This relative inattention to research costs stands in stark contrast to their widespread and growing concern with clinical expenses. The one exception is in the area of industrially supported clinical trials, where competition from for-profit CROs and SMOs is forcing such attention to improving research productivity. This potential response of academic health centers to CROs and SMOs is discussed later in this paper.

The skepticism of academic health center leaders about prospects for reducing research costs is understandable. Biomedical research is an inherently decentralized and spontaneous activity. Suggestions that it can be managed to improve its efficiency raise concerns about efforts to control the research in ways that will reduce its quality and provoke legitimate opposition from faculty. Furthermore, the processes underlying research are diverse, variable, and constantly changing. This makes it difficult to undertake the kind of process reengineering that lies at the heart of efforts to reduce expenses in the clinical and administrative arenas.

On the other hand, the proposition that significant cost reduction is feasible in the clinical work of academic health centers was also greeted with skepticism ten years ago. If funds available to support research become scarce, research leaders may become more receptive to restructuring research management for the purpose of increasing efficiency. If so, it is worth considering some of the available options. We mention a number of possible approaches here, though space limitations prevent us from considering each in full detail.

Lacking serious external pressure to improve the efficiency of their research, academic health centers have not always made the best use of scarce research resources. Space has often been allocated based on historical arrangements—deals cut between powerful faculty or department chairs and deans or CEOs—rather than on the quality and promise of the work. Leaders have lacked the incentive or political strength to force laboratories to consolidate or co-locate, even when this approach might have been in the best interests of the institution or of the work of individual investigators.

Opportunities also exist for the creative use of core resources, that is, capital-intensive facilities that can service the needs of multiple labs. Classic examples include animal facilities, X-ray crystallography, and electron microscopy units. More recently, core resources to produce useful cell lines or clones of animals with special genetic compositions offer additional opportunities. The widespread impression from our unpublished case-study results and interviews, although hard to document, is that academic health centers are moving more slowly than might be expected to take advantage of core facilities, in part because of difficulty in building internal consensus on how the resources should be used and controlled.

Another opportunity for improving the efficiency of research is in the developing multidisciplinary research centers that cross departmental boundaries. Most academic health centers are developing multidisciplinary centers of some kind. Typical are the neuroscience center at Duke University Medical Center and the cancer center at Mt. Sinai. Multidisciplinary research is increasingly recognized as central to future research productivity and competitiveness. However, cross-departmental units create potential conflicts with traditional departmental structures that conform to clinical disciplines. Such conflicts may somewhat impede the ability of academic health centers to take advantage of opportunities to reengineer their research programs for maximal efficiency. One persistent issue is power to promote faculty. At Mt. Sinai, the cancer center has such power to promote faculty, but this is rare. It is not clear whether multidisciplinary programs will reach their full potential in research until the respective roles of clinical departments and research centers are clarified.

Improved use of space, core facilities, and multidisciplinary research are three of the most obvious ways to increase the efficiency with which research resources are used. They are easily described because at least some academic health centers have identified their potential and begun to implement them. There may be other opportunities that will not become apparent until academic health center managers devote the same energy to reducing research expenses and improving research productivity that they have already begun applying to reengineering clinical processes. Some of the necessary changes may even require cooperation among centers. For example, it may be possible for centers to pool their resources for training fellows in basic laboratory skills and to consolidate their purchasing power and thereby gain better prices for large research-related capital acquisitions (the way they currently do for drug and supply purchases on the clinical side).

How much money could be saved through these types of efforts to improve research efficiency? Let's assume the amount was 10 percent on average. In an academic health center with a $50 million research budget, it would come to $5 million annually. This may not seem like much, but if expendable income on endowment is 5 percent annually, savings of this amount would yield the same benefits as a $100 million capital campaign.

## Enhancing Access to Patients for Clinical Research

Another external threat to the research enterprise of academic health centers is the potential loss of patients to MCOs that do not use academic health center clinical facilities because of the higher costs. Without patients, clinical research of all types—translational, trials, and outcomes/health services research—is threatened.

Two general strategies seem to be appropriate responses to this threat. The first is to increase the competitiveness of clinical services. However, since the research missions of academic health centers are partly responsible for their higher costs, it is unlikely that the centers will ever have prices as low as their community competition (Gold 1996). The second strategy, therefore, would be to depend to some degree on the willingness of customers to pay higher prices in order to contribute to the research enterprise.

The potential success of the second strategy—to have customers willing to pay higher prices in order to contribute to the research enterprise—is far from assured. However, the existence of the following situations will increase the probability of success.

• A well-organized business community with a history of commitment to civic causes—Pride in local institutions can be a very strong motivating factor in some markets. Business leaders, especially those already participating as board members and fund-raisers for academic health centers, may be willing to pay somewhat higher prices for health care (especially in good economic times) in order to sustain premier local health care institutions. Cities in which business communities may display this type of civic-mindedness include St. Louis, Rochester, Chicago, and Atlanta.

• A strategy of approaching health care purchasers directly for their support—Academic health centers have tended to focus their political energy and their wrath on managed care organizations, assuming that MCOs are controlling the flow of patients and dollars that affect the centers' vital activities. In fact, however, MCOs themselves are often merely doing the bidding of price-conscious purchasers—e.g., major employers, unions, and purchasing coalitions—seeking to control their premiums. Academic health centers are unlikely to convince MCOs to pay the higher prices at teaching facilities unless MCO clients are willing to do so as well. In making the necessary case to purchasers, academic health centers would do well to identify the contributions of biomedical research to the local economy. Extensive empirical studies have demonstrated the range of such contributions to the creation of new companies and jobs in the markets where the research occurs (Jaffe 1989; Zuker et al. 1994).

• Development of academic health center research consortia—Even if academic health centers are able to maintain local market share (and especially if they fail to do so), they should explore opportunities to work with other academic health centers locally and nationally to acquire the patient populations necessary to conduct clinical research. This strategy will require improved communication across locations, but it could also enhance the quality and reduce the costs of large-scale clinical trials.

## Managing Internal Threats

For each of the potential internal threats to the research missions of academic health centers—diversion of resources, changes in governance and management, and changes in values and attitudes—the centers can adopt specific policies or programs to minimize those risks. As always, the available and optimal strategies will vary from center to center and market to market.

For academic health centers that have the human and financial capital and the market opportunity to develop price-competitive integrated health care systems, setting aside the money and management resources necessary to secure this option may be the preferred course of action. If nothing else, the academic health systems formed through such efforts may provide valuable assets that can be sold to nonacademic health systems in the future. The proceeds of such sales may then constitute substantial endowments to support the research and academic missions.

Those academic health centers that choose to stay fully engaged in clinical competition would nevertheless be wise to minimize the potential risks to their research missions by consciously investing in the leadership and infrastructure of their research enterprise. This stance requires, at a minimum, a careful strategic review of the current status of that enterprise: its areas of weakness and strength and priorities for future development. An essential ingredient in this process is the identification and cultivation of research leadership. Also essential is the commitment of financial resources to the growth of the research enterprise.

An example of one approach to this challenge is the PHCS in Boston. While building a major primary care and hospital network, PHCS has also appointed a director of research for its organization, Dr. Eugene Braunwald, former chief of medicine at Brigham and Women's Hospital (BWH) and an eminent figure in U.S. biomedical research. The Massachusetts General Hospital, one of Partners' subsidiaries, has appointed its own research director, Dr. John Potts, former chief of Medicine at MGH and also a very distinguished researcher. PHCS is conducting a strategic review of its huge investigative program, which currently brings in nearly $400 million annually in extramural funding. As noted above, MGH, in anticipation of hard times to come, is undertaking a $320 million capital campaign to provide discretionary funding for its priority research areas. Both BWH and MGH have already set aside modest revenues from operations—on the order of several million dollars annually—to be used by their research leadership for start-up ventures.

One of the most important consequences of such investments in human and financial capital is to bolster advocates of research within academic health systems. As these organizations become more and more consumed with maintaining far-flung clinical enterprises, it is essential that respected individuals and groups with a stake in research missions continue to have regular access to senior management and continue to sit at the table when major strategic decisions are made for the entire organization.

However, once granted such access, research leadership must also find ways to keep the interest and support of the clinical enterprises on which they will depend for financial and political sustenance. A number of approaches are worth exploring in this regard.

One is improving communication with the clinical side of academic health systems. Researchers are not accustomed to having to justify their value within academic health centers. They assume that their work speaks for itself through its contribution to the peer-reviewed literature and to the knowledge in their field. Unfortunately, what is self-evident to biomedical investigators may not be evident to community-based clinicians who are being asked to contribute some portion of their hard-earned and sometimes shrinking clinical income to support a research endeavor that they may not understand. Academic health centers must find ways to inform all members of their communities about the value and contribution of the daily work that goes on within their laboratories. This will require a new emphasis on internal public relations that is foreign to many academic institutions and to biomedical investigators. The latter must be educated to the importance of such activities.

Another way to maintain the interest and support of members of academic health center clinical enterprises is to increase investment in research and development that is relevant to the needs of that enterprise. For the most part, this will consist of clinical research and particularly clinical trials and outcomes/health services research. The former can be used to involve community-based clinicians—especially specialists—in a form of research that they may find relevant and personally gratifying. Even if few are interested, they may welcome being asked. The Duke Health Sciences Center is developing a clinical genetics research initiative with the specific purpose of enlisting specialists in work that seeks to relate the varying phenotypes of presenting illnesses to the varying genotypes identified by laboratory geneticists. Outcomes/health services research can be used to address operational problems that are essential to improving the efficiency and quality of care, and thus the competitive position of community-based clinicians.

Another set of reforms in governance and management that may benefit research missions of academic health centers is the development of a research management infrastructure. Most centers have grants management units that are responsible for processing applications and tracking funds. However, few have the management capability to enhance the efficiency of research through the methods discussed above: improved space planning, process reengineering, the evaluation of business plans for core facilities and multidisciplinary research centers, and peer review of internally funded projects. Again, there are undoubtedly many ways to build these capabilities, and it will be essential to draw heavily on the expertise of faculty in the process.

A number of policies and management approaches can help academic health centers minimize the risks to academic values that may accompany increasing reliance on industrially funded research.

• Promulgation of clear policies regarding openness in research—To combat the secrecy that seems to accompany some industrial research arrangements, academic health centers need to make clear to faculty and research managers, including technology transfer officers, that academic health centers will not accept agreements or behaviors that interfere with sharing research results. The exception is modest delays required to file patents prior to publication. The latter should not exceed the sixty to ninety days allowed by most academic centers at the current time.

• Limits on the proportion of research funds derived from industrial sources—Evidence suggests that there is an inverse relationship between the proportion of funds that individual investigators derive from industrial sources and the productivity and quality of their work. Specifically, investigators who receive more than two-thirds of their extramural research support from industry tend to publish less and to publish in less highly cited journals than colleagues who receive smaller proportions of their funds from outside companies (Blumenthal et al. 1996b) Although a causal relationship between magnitude of industrial funding and research productivity has not been definitively established, it would seem prudent for academic health centers to avoid excessive reliance on such support and to encourage faculty and research groups to derive the bulk of their funds from nonprofit sources.

• Institution of formal conflict-of-interest management procedures—In addition to clear policies regarding conflict of interest, academic health centers would be wise to create formal conflict-of-interest review procedures that are independent of their technology transfer offices. The latter will have a natural bias toward promoting AIRs and the commercialization of research.

## CONCLUSION

Academic health centers face an uncertain world in which many will have to struggle to survive as institutions. From a societal standpoint, however, their survival per se is less important than the assurance that they will continue to perform the essential social functions that they are uniquely suited to accomplish. As academic health center leaders manage the crises that increasingly consume their daily lives, they will find it tempting to put off the decisions that are necessary to maintain the health of those missions. Doing so will ultimately undermine the rationale for the existence of academic health centers. Many of the approaches suggested in this paper are not extraordinarily costly in financial terms but will require that leaders invest a certain amount of time and political capital. There is every reason to expect that this investment will pay off handsomely.

## WORK CITED

Anderson, G. 1997. The role of investment bankers in nonprofit conversions. *Health Affairs* (Millwood) 16(2).

Berman, J., A. Borkowski, and W. Moore. 1993. Letter to the Editor. *Journal of the American Medical Association* 270(1)

Berman, J., A. Borkowski, H. Rachocka, and W. Moore. 1995. Impact of unfunded research in medicine, pathology, and surgery. *Southern Medical Journal* 88(3).

Blake, D.A. 1996. Whither academic values during the transition from academic medical centers to integrated health delivery systems? *Academic Medicine* 71.

Blumenthal, D. 1992. Academic-industry relationships in the life sciences: Extent, consequences, and management. *Journal of the American Medical Association* 268(23).

Blumenthal, D., E.G. Campbell, N.A. Causino, and K.S. Louis. 1996a. Participation of life-science faculty in research relationships with industry. *New England Journal of*

*Medicine* 335(23).

Blumenthal, D., N.A. Causino, E.G. Campbell, and K.S. Louis. 1996b. Relationships between academic institutions and industry in the life sciences—an industry survey. *New England Journal of Medicine* 334(6).

Blumenthal, D., E.G. Campbell, N.A. Causino, and K.S. Louis. 1997. Withholding research results in academic life science: Evidence from a national survey of faculty. *Journal of the American Medical Association* 277(15).

Blumenthal, D., and G.S. Meyer. 1996. Academic health centers in a changing environment. *Health Affairs* (Millwood) 15.

Bourne, S., and C. Malcom. 1996. *Market Classification and Revisions and Review.* Chicago: University HealthSystem Consortium.

Campbell, E.G., D. Blumenthal, and J.S. Weissman. 1997. Relationship between market competition and the activities and attitudes of medical school faculty. *Journal of the American Medical Association* 278(3).

Causino, N.A., D. Saglam, and D. Blumenthal. 1995. Analysis of research related funding of academic health centers from Federal and non-Federal sources. Unpublished.

Center Watch. 1995. Can academic centers remake themselves? *Center Watch* 2(3).

Center Watch. 1996. The academic center as CRO. *Center Watch* 3(3).

Commonwealth Fund Task Force on Academic Health Centers. 1997 *Leveling the Playing Field: Financing the Missions of Academic Health Centers.* New York: Commonwealth Fund.

Crowley, W.F., Jr., and S.O. Thier. 1996. The continuing dilemma in clinical investigation and the future of American health care: A system-wide problem requiring collaborative solutions. *Academic Medicine* 71(11).

Gold, M.R. 1996. Effects of managed care on academic medical centers and graduate medical education. *Academic Medicine* 71.

Hughes, G. 1996. CROs under the microscope. *Pharmaceutical Visions* 5(1).

Iglehart, J.K. 1994. Rapid changes for academic medical centers, 1. *New England Journal of Medicine* 331:1391–1394.

Iglehart, J.K. 1995. Rapid changes for academic medical centers, 2. *New England Journal of Medicine* 332:332–401.

Jaffe, A. 1989. Real effects of academic research. *American Economic Review* 79(5).

Jaffe, A., M. Trajtenberg, and R. Henderson. 1993. Geographic localization of knowledge spillovers as evidenced by patent citations. *Quarterly Journal of Economics* 108(3).

Krakower, J.Y., J.L. Ganem, and P. Jolly. 1996. Review of medical school finances, 1994–1995. *Journal of the American Medical Association* 276(9).

Moy, E., A.J. Mazzaschi, R.J. Levin, D.A. Blake, and P.F. Griner. 1997. Relationship between National Institutes of Health awards to medical schools and managed care market penetration. *Journal of the American Medical Association* 278(3).

NIH (National Institutes of Health). 1997. Analysis of NIH data available at: http://www.nih.gov/news/budget98/IMG00001.GIF. Accessed September 5.

ProPAC (Prospective Payment Advisory Commission). 1997. *Medicare and the American Health Care System: Report to Congress.* Washington: ProPAC.

Stein, M., L. Rubenstein, and T.J. Wachtell. 1993. Who pays for unfunded research? *Journal of the American Medical Association* 269(6).

Zuker, L., M.R. Darby, and J. Armstrong. 1994. Intellectual capital and the firm: The technology of geographically localized knowledge spillovers. Working paper no. 4946. Cambridge, MA: National Bureau of Economic Research.

# RESTRUCTURING THE
# RESEARCH ENTERPRISE
# FOR THE FUTURE

*Ralph Snyderman, MD*

O NCE CONSIDERED A PROFESSION, HEALTH CARE is today increasingly viewed as an industry—indeed, representing approximately one-seventh of the nation's gross national product, it is one of the largest. American business has been quick to recognize the tremendous financial opportunities in the area of health, and is devoting substantial energy to exploiting them. As a result, American health care has now shifted to a largely for-profit, market-driven model of managed care. Seeking to control costs, this new managed care system emphasizes primary care, limits specialty care, and is reticent to invest in new therapies or technologies. Although these developments have forced the entire health care system to cut costs and become more efficient, they have had a uniquely unsettling impact on the nation's academic health centers (Iglehart 1997)—the institutions that have historically been the drivers of new therapies, technologies, and specialty medicine. Until recently, cost-consciousness was not the hallmark of the academic health center.

Today, academic health centers find themselves competing with commercial providers for increasingly discounted health care contracts. This situation has created threats to the clinical margins of the academic health center. Contract

---

*Dr. Snyderman is chancellor for health affairs and dean of the School of Medicine, Duke University Medical Center, and CEO, Duke University Health System.*

revenues now account for 48.4 percent of revenues for U.S. medical schools (Ganem and Krakower 1997). These revenues represented only 10 percent and 3 percent in 1970 and 1960, respectively. Margins from clinical practice that had been used to support the research and educational missions are increasingly in danger of disappearing.

## THE TRIPARTITE MISSION

To ensure survival, academic health centers must undergo a rapid transformation that enables them to maintain their academic responsibilities while securing revenues more effectively in the free market. As a result, many academic health centers have been aggressively developing restructuring strategies for survival in the current market-driven health care environment.

Most of the focus has been on restructuring the clinical area by developing comprehensive physician and hospital provider networks, acquiring the ability to deliver managed care, and lowering clinical delivery costs (Rogers and Snyderman 1994; Shortell and Gillies 1996). In my view, such approaches are essential and appropriate to the times. However, to be able to preserve their true strengths, academic health centers also need to restructure their educational and research missions. Such restructuring will allow them not only to support their academic programs more effectively, but also to deliver higher quality clinical programs (Snyderman 1997).

How do leaders of academic health centers do this? An important first step is to view each of the center's core missions—education, research, and clinical programs—as business operations, that is, to analyze them in terms of their size, revenues, expenses, and value to the institution and society. Each of these businesses must be operated as efficiently as possible without compromising its unique attributes. Clearly, as currently constituted, the education and research missions will be deficit operations. These needless deficits must be minimized through efficiency efforts, appropriate sizing, and the identification, from within, of new sources of revenue. Ultimately, through reorganization, components of the educational and research missions (particularly research) can be structured to enhance the value of the clinical operations and to generate substantial new sources of revenue (Snyderman 1996).

## RESEARCH

We need to think of biomedical research as made up of a number of different components, each with its own values and loci for integration with the health system, as follows:

Basic discovery
    Nondisease oriented
    Disease oriented
Clinical research
    Translational research
    Clinical trials
    Outcomes research
    Classic epidemiology
Health policy

## BASIC DISCOVERY

Pure discovery RO1 research is valuable in its own right for its contributions to our understanding of biology. Beyond serving this function, RO1 research will every once in a while spin off discoveries with practical and commercial applications. Academic health centers must, therefore, support investigator-oriented basic research while at the same time providing the continual surveillance that recognizes when findings of commercial application occur and then ensure that the full value of such discoveries accrue to the benefit of the investigator, the institution, industry, and the public.

## CLINICAL RESEARCH

### Translational Research

Leaders of academic health centers need to understand the nature and value of translational research; phase I, II, III, and IV clinical trials; postmarket surveillance, outcomes research, and classic epidemiology—the components of clinical research. This research pipeline ultimately transforms an innovation into improved medical care; each type of research contributes to the understanding and treatment of disease and requires different resources and sources of funding. To varying degrees, all are appropriate for the academic health center setting.

Translational research is usually investigator-initiated and funded by the

National Institutes of Health (NIH), often through RO1 funding mechanisms, but increasingly through requests initiated by NIH institutes.

## Clinical Trials

Academic health centers are expanding their primary care activities and their community-based infrastructure. They will, therefore, be able to determine the value of new clinical strategies as well as determine cost-effectiveness and benefit. The development of disease-management strategies and standards of care can and should be coupled to an outcomes research apparatus. The best information can then be used to develop strategies for treating disease, thereby creating a high standard of care throughout an academic health center's health system and measure its efficacy.

## Outcomes Research

In this context, academic health systems can use their strengths to develop the most cost-effective new models for evidence-based quality care. This emerging model for health care delivery is based on the congruence of research

Figure 1.
**HOW FEEDBACK LOOPS CONTINUOUSLY IMPROVE STANDARDS OF CARE**

### Disease Management

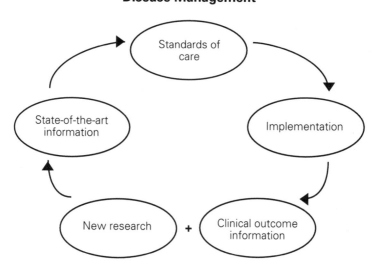

advances, integrated delivery systems, information systems, and methods of outcomes analysis (figure 1). Working this strategy into the clinical infrastructure can become one of the real strengths of the academic health center.

## Classic Epidemiology

As organized health care increasingly focuses on preventive care of captured lives within managed care types of practices, the methodology and findings of classic epidemiology have become more publicized and relied on to drive medical practice. Findings from two classic community- or hospital-based epidemiologic studies, for example, undergird two of the most frequent and least controversial behavioral interventions: (1) the findings from the British case-control studies of smoking and carcinoma of the lungs during the early 1950s (Doll and Hill 1950); and (2) the findings on the increased risk for cardiovascular disease from elevated cholesterol from the Framingham Heart Study (Dawber and Kannel 1966).

Epidemiologic methods and the long-standing association of epidemiologic studies and biostatistics support the methods of statistical analysis of virtually all clinical research studies, from clinical trials to etiologic studies. They help physicians and health care organizations weigh the relative risks to health of behavior and other factors that are subject to intervention, and thereby enable health caregivers to determine the relative value of instituting a prevention program. In addition, the experience gained from classic epidemiology (and companion disciplines such as biostatistics) facilitate the design, implementation, and analysis of virtually all clinical research efforts. Academic health centers should, therefore, maintain their emphasis on a range of investigative endeavors, from molecular biology to classic, community-based epidemiology.

## FUNDING SOURCES

Currently, the Federal government is spending about $14 billion per year for biomedical research, and industry is funding well over $15 billion per year nationally for research and development. Although the Federal government and industry are making considerable investments in biomedical research and development, some important differences between the two sources of funding should be noted.

---

Figure 2.
**RECIPIENTS OF PUBLIC AND PRIVATE INVESTMENTS IN BIOMEDICAL R&D**

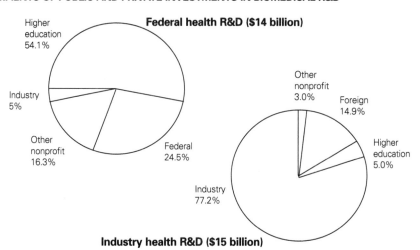

The Federal government invests more than 50 percent of its research budget in discovery research performed in academic institutions. Industry funds only 5 percent of its R&D at academic institutions; most of their funding is internal and devoted to development and clinical research. Internal funding may make sense for industry, given proprietary issues and the need for secrecy and control. However, as competition grows and the complexity of biomedical research and clinical trials increases, it is likely that more opportunities will arise for academic health centers to increase their share of industry R&D funding. On the other hand, it is less likely that the academic health center's percentage share of Federal health R&D funding will increase substantially (figure 2).

It is important to view the academic research enterprise as being in partnership with industry. These enterprises have complementary missions and capabilities. The focus of the academic health center is on discovery and types of clinical research; the focus of industry is on the development of marketable products to the health care provider. There is good reason for industry to want to partner with academia and for academia to partner with industry. A partnership can be achieved without sacrificing the academic health center's academic mission, if leadership in both sectors fully understands the inviolate principles on which an academic health center is based.

## THE NATIONAL RESEARCH
## INFRASTRUCTURE

It is important that the public appreciate the value of research operations at academic health centers. Clearly, discovery research is valuable for its contribution to understanding life and human biology. Follow-your-nose research sometimes leads to unexpected observations that, in turn, open the way to practical application. For example, work on bacterial DNA repair enzymes recently led the way to understanding susceptibility to colon cancer (Parsons and Li 1993). Indeed, most of our significant clinical advances stem from discovery research.

But research has advantages to the academic health system that go far beyond successes. For example, the kind of infrastructure that results in improved quality care is heavily dependent on research conducted in the academic health center. What is not well understood by the public and our politicians is that the quality of the American health care system and the ability of the commercial health care provider to provide good health care at a reasonable price is dependent on the progress made by the research infrastructure. True, many advances occur within the pharmaceutical, biotechnology, and medical device industries. But research within the academic health center system provides a vital base for therapeutic interventions. Moreover, academic health centers perform clinical trials, enhance the fields of biostatistics and epidemiology, and perform outcomes research. Through the development of integrated clinical delivery systems, linked by clinical information systems, an entirely new field of outcomes research will inevitably develop. The research infrastructure needed to support evidence-based medical practice (through developing and implementing standards of care, analyzing outcomes, and refining practice standards) will require academic health centers.

## STRATEGIES FOR SURVIVAL

As currently structured, the research endeavors of the academic health center require institutional subsidization. Even when fully funded by the Federal government, laboratory research at academic health centers does not support all of an institution's research costs. Even with robust external research funding at Duke University, internal subsidization is approximately 15 cents on the externally funded dollar. Because we are currently performing about $225 million a year worth of sponsored research, this university subsidy represents a significant amount of money to the center.

With appropriate restructuring, however, the research missions of the academic health center could become self-sustaining. In some institutions, research could even provide margins for funding other activities. More important, the research components of an academic health center can be designed to enhance the quality of the institution's health care system, thus providing a competitive edge in terms of the quality of its health care delivery.

The strategies needed to restructure the research enterprise in the academic health center are multifactorial, and they vary according to type of research. In the aggregate, the institution must maximize opportunities for funding, decrease needless inefficiencies, provide value-added core technologies, and create an environment that fosters and nurtures good research, provides leadership, and, when appropriate, provides direction and integration.

I believe that the first task of the academic health center in this regard should be to focus on the more effective use of current resources. It is helpful for department chairs as well as faculty to understand the true costs of their research operations and the degree to which they are being subsidized institutionally. The importance of institutionally subsidized research should not be underestimated, but we need to know when and where it occurs and make sure we are deploying our resources appropriately.

## DUKE'S RESPONSE TO CHANGING TIMES

At Duke University Medical Center, we have provided our department chairs with data (in dollars per square foot) on how much research space they occupy, the cost to the institution, and the recovery rate of their investigators. The data allow the department chair as well as our medical center to deploy its resources and subsidization more efficiently.

### The Research Infrastructure

Recognizing that it is important to provide the very best infrastructure to help faculty carry out their research, secure grants, and identify additional opportunities for funding, the medical center has taken a proactive role in restructuring the research mission through the creation of administrative initiatives and new resources for research.

## Core Technologies

The availability of important core technologies institutionally can make investigator research more effective as well as more cost effective. At Duke, our investigators identify for us those core technologies that they feel will most greatly enhance their research. We have devoted considerable resources (approximately six million institutional dollars per year) for the following shared core technologies.

| | |
|---|---|
| Cell culture scale-up | Microscopy |
| Crystallography | Molecular biology databases |
| DNA sequencing | Nuclear magnetic resonance (NMR) |
| Fermentation | Phosphoimaging |
| Flow cytometry | Protein microsequencing |
| Macromolecular graphics | Transgenic and knock-out mice |
| Mass spectrometry | |

The allocation of resources is largely faculty driven through representative committees advising the vice chancellor for academic affairs and the director of the Comprehensive Cancer Center. A description of institutional resources for biomedical research at Duke follows.

*Office of Grants and Contracts.* It is very important to have an outstanding office of grants and contracts with a commitment to excellent communication with faculty and aggressive strategies for informing investigators about funding opportunities. A goal of the office at Duke is to be as responsive as possible to investigators' needs and to be proactive in providing them information and opportunities so that we can help them enhance their success in securing grants. This task is accomplished through a service-oriented mind-set on the part of staff, use of electronic communication, frequent grant-writing seminars and workshops, and a regular review of departmental performance of grantsmanship.

*Office of Science & Technology.* We believe there is a benefit to having a separate office responsible for medical center-industrial relationships. We therefore created an Office of Science & Technology (OST) responsible for commercializing medical center and university intellectual property and developing various forms of interaction with industry. The office is also responsible for managing new ventures based on businesses that can evolve out of medical center intellectual properties and technologies.

Duke's OST is also responsible for determining how our intellectual properties can best serve our own clinical mission. For example, the office looks at how investments in clinical information systems and disease management programs can be used to manage our own health care system to make it more competitively advantaged in the commercial marketplace. This approach is leading to diverse projects, including the development of disease-management programs and CD-ROMs for physicians and patients. Such programs are used internally but may also be sold or licensed to others.

OST also makes recommendations for internal investments in research initiatives that could further raise the cost-effectiveness of our clinical enterprise. It also plays an important role in securing funds for ongoing research, faculty recruitment, research facilities, and the development of partnerships, joint ventures, and new businesses. The number of commercially supported research projects for clinical and nonclinical faculty has grown by 25 percent in each of the last two years. The key to the success of such an office is for everyone involved to understand its importance to the missions of the academic health center. Thus, administrators must make certain that the office reports to the head of the medical center, that it has the appropriate internal leadership, and that it has the resources necessary for success.

The leader of the office should be a person who understands both the value of academic research and the world of business. Obvious attributes include academic experience and credibility; small-business experience; large-business experience; and experience in dealing with intellectual property.

Another important role for this office is to find practical ways to apply the benefits of our research toward generating additional revenues and bringing discoveries to clinical practice for the benefit of our medical center and our partners (table 1). It would be wrong to value OST solely on its ability to secure licensing revenues or revenues from patents. Such incomes are not insignificant, but they will not be able to float the research enterprise. Unless the institution is extremely fortunate in having a big hit—for example, the discovery of warfarin,

Table 1
**DUKE UNIVERSITY MEDICAL CENTER'S OFFICE OF SCIENCE & TECHNOLOGY**

| Methods | 1990 | 1992 | 1994 | 1996 |
|---|---|---|---|---|
| Invention disclosures | 57 | 89 | 98 | 108 |
| Patent applications | 25 | 51 | 74 | 31 |
| Patents issued | 7 | 8 | 28 | 37 |
| License agreements | 19 | 31 | 23 | 27 |
| **Revenue (dollars)** | | | | |
| Royalty income | $304,092 | $616,938 | $1,457,453 | $1,667,948 |
| Other income | — | ~3,000,000 | ~5,000,000 | ~7,200,000 |
| OST budget | (450,000) | (1,000,000) | (1,100,000) | (1,400,000) |
| Net income | — | 2,616,938 | 5,357,453 | 7,467,948 |

Gatorade, Cis platinum, or the Cohen-Boyer patent, it is unlikely that licensing revenue will bring in more than several millions of dollars per year.

An effective OST is also capable of fostering interactions with industry that support basic research. It can identify opportunities for fostering clinical trials and corporate gifts as well as interesting start-ups and new ventures. It is important that OST be intimately familiar with the research going on within the institution and also have excellent relationships with venture capitalists and the biotechnology, pharmaceutical, and device industries.

Duke's OST has taken the lead in developing such creative partnerships. In two cases—an information technology joint venture and a production facility for gene therapy vectors and cell therapy scale-up—the resources of an industrial partner fully complement the academic research perspective. In the latter case, the corporate expertise in good manufacturing practice (GMP) allowed us to have a facility unique to academic medicine.

*Office of Development.* Another on-campus focus for additional revenues for research is the Development Office. This office should understand the work of the investigators along with the intentions of foundations and potential donors. Our institution is now embarking on a capital campaign for the medical center. Much of the fund-raising effort will be directed at gaining support for our research investigators and the institution's research infrastructure. Our goal is to raise $150 million from philanthropy for research over the next five years. Another role for the Development Office is working with the vice chancellor for academic affairs to enhance foundation funding for research.

## Conducting Translational Research

Each of the many types of clinical research in the academic health center has an important role to play. Each also requires a substantial infrastructure and resources. Ultimately, however, they can bring value not only to clinical research but also to the development of appropriate clinical information systems and databases that benefit the practice of medicine throughout the academic health center.

The availability of an NIH-funded General Clinical Research Center (GCRC) at Duke is invaluable for supporting much translational research at the medical center. Today's increasing interest and opportunity in clinical genetics, gene therapy, and cellular therapies has led to the development of some institutional programs in these areas. Duke is fortunate to have an active GCRC, and this center receives substantial institutional support and subsidization. The chancellor for health affairs and dean of the school of medicine is the principal investigator on the university's GCRC grant and he plays an active role in facilitating its operations.

*Clinical Research Institute.* Duke's Clinical Research Institute (DCRI), established in 1994, is a large academic clinical research organization that conducts large multiinstitutional and multinational clinical trials, usually Phase III or IV research. One of the largest clinical research organizations worldwide, this institute is a strong proponent for evidence-based medicine locally and nationally (Snyderman 1995). It has an outstanding clinical database, particularly in cardiovascular disease.

Currently, DCRI has 57 active clinical trials, 1,500 participating sites worldwide, a $140 million budget, $40 million in 1966 revenues, and 500 employees. It receives funding that can be used to support the clinical research enterprise as well as salaries of clinical faculty involved in clinical trials. This funding helps offset salary costs. We believe that the institute is important not only to Duke but also to academic medicine in general. Its functions include serving as source for new trials; providing statistical, data management, and accrual support; and performing financial management, site monitoring, and the pharmacy function.

At Duke, just as in health care delivery elsewhere, commercialized clinical research organizations have emerged because of the high profitability margins.

Industry is already spending well over $7 billion nationally per year for clinical trials. It is therefore increasingly important for academic health centers to play a major role in conducting clinical trials and assure that the data are published regardless of the trial's outcome. Quality assurance and objectivity can only be ensured in appropriately organized trials under the scrutiny of academicians with no vested financial interest in the outcome.

Given the magnitude of the DCRI, as well as its potential for additional growth, we envision that the DCRI will interact with faculty in every clinical department and, indeed, with most divisions in the clinical departments. The DCRI provides our clinical faculty with opportunities to participate in clinical trials in their area of interest once they have had sufficient instruction to become competent clinical investigators. (It is important for medical center leaders to recognize that not all clinicians, particularly those without specific training in clinical research, are capable of participating in the types of clinical trials performed by the DCRI.) In addition to the support that the DCRI provides to a large number of clinical faculty, it also provides the educational infrastructure for teaching clinical research to faculty, fellows, and medical students.

*Center for Human Genetics.* The understanding of human genetics will have a profound an impact on the future of medicine. Understanding the genetic basis of common diseases plus the ability to predict susceptibility will alter the practice of medicine in ways that can barely be grasped at this time. The new information will also lead the way to untold therapeutic targets.

Duke has invested in an infrastructure that allows for the identification of genes responsible for both common and rare diseases. A primary objective of this Center for Human Genetics (CHG) is to act as a catalyst, fostering research collaborations across the entire medical center. For nascent projects, the CHG provides the expertise for generating preliminary design and data collection so that outside funding (public, private, and corporate) can be obtained. For established projects, it is used to efficiently map and identify genes causing or influencing human disease. The genetic epidemiology and family ascertainment component of the CHG provides the necessary expertise for development of the overall study design, data collection and storage, and analysis of the clinical and molecular data. Its molecular component provides the technical expertise for sample collection and storage, DNA extraction, tissue culture, and high throughput genotyping. It also houses resources critical to positional cloning and candidate gene analysis.

As genetic information plays an increasingly central role in the practice of medicine, molecular diagnostics will become increasingly important. However, attendant to these exciting developments will be the responsibility to ensure that the technologies are utilized properly, ethically, and legally. The institution that can handle the above functions and also address the social questions they pose in an integrated manner will be a leader in the field.

*Center for Genetic and Cellular Therapeutics.* Gene therapy is in its infancy, and cellular therapy is a newly developing clinical strategy. Both will play increasingly important roles in clinical medicine. At Duke, therefore, we have developed a Center for Genetic and Cellular Therapeutics (CGCT) to enable us to support research in these emerging areas and provide our patients with the latest opportunities for conquering or controlling severe diseases that may be often life-threatening.

Duke's CGCT is also a bridge between clinical programs and six basic science departments (genetics, cell biology, microbiology, immunology, biochemistry, and pathology). Serving as a locus for staff engaged in gene therapies and translational research, the mission of the center is (1) to develop gene transfer technologies, methods, and protocols for ex-vivo cell processing and clinical programs for cell and gene therapy, and (2) to establish institutional cores for gene technologies, cellular processing, and regulatory oversight and reporting. We believe that this center will not only undergird Duke's position at the forefront of treating important and serious diseases, but also increase the value of our health system to others. It will also allow us to put these scientific accomplishments into practice most cost-effectively and, we hope, to receive Federal and industry funding to support these activities.

## Training Clinical Investigators

Duke has a long tradition of training clinical investigators, and opportunities in clinical research are available at both the undergraduate and graduate levels. Duke medical students who spend their third year in independent study can choose among the following options: laboratory experience at Duke, NIH clinical research training, NIH Cloister program, or Howard Hughes Medical

Institute research training fellowships. The most recent offering is a twelve-month course of study at the University of North Carolina at Chapel Hill that culminates in a master of public health; students pursuing this option receive both the MD and MPH degrees in four years.

Duke's Department of Medicine has had a long record of success in training physician-scientists. The department encourages both basic and clinical research and has designed its house-staff program in a way that facilitates individualized training for those interested in academic medicine. In addition to its traditional subspecialty fellowship training, the department offers a clinical investigator pathway and a physician-scientist program. The Clinical Investigator Pathway is designed to encourage house-staff to consider careers in basic or clinical investigation. One year of internship and one year of residency are followed by two years of research training within a subspecialty division. The Physician-Scientist Program is a faculty development program designed for house-staff who wish to make a longer-term commitment to basic science training. The objective is to train young physicians to become physician-scientists proficient in the fundamental techniques of modern biomedical research with performance levels comparable to those with PhD research training.

At the postgraduate level, Duke offers both degree and nondegree programs in biometry and clinical research. The biometry program, established in 1986, is primarily designed for clinical fellows and physicians training for academic careers. The program offers formal courses in research design, statistical analysis, decision analysis, research ethics, and research management. The degree option leads to the masters of health sciences offered by the School of Medicine. This program allows the student to integrate the program's academic training with his or her clinical training. Course work, taken during two 16-week semesters, can be completed in one academic year. The nondegree option is available to those who want to acquire specific skills but who do not want to pursue the master's degree. Clinical fellows, faculty members, postdoctoral fellows, graduate students in the basic medical sciences, and other health professionals are the most frequently enrolled.

Because of the changing nature of clinical research from its predominant emphasis on clinical trials to increased concerns with outcomes research in cost-effective medicine, genetic epidemiology, and preventative medicine, Duke decided to modify and expand the biometry program. Thus, a new program at the medical center will offer the master of health science in clinical research with an emphasis on outcomes research, cost-effective medicine, genetic epidemiology, and preventive medicine.

## Organizational Structure for Funding Research

Each academic health center should develop an appropriate organizational structure for funding its own research infrastructure. Research must be a valued component of the academic health system and the appropriate resources should be dedicated to it. The health system at Duke is currently close to becoming a $1.2-billion enterprise. It is justifiable for a vibrant, growing health system to support research and development internally as well as externally. By industry standards, a 4-percent figure for internal investment in R&D is not outlandish. Interestingly, Duke allocates approximately $40 million to support all unfunded research, including faculty salaries and infrastructure costs. Simply

Figure 3.
**RESOURCES FOR BIOMEDICAL RESEARCH,
DUKE UNIVERSITY MEDICAL CENTER**

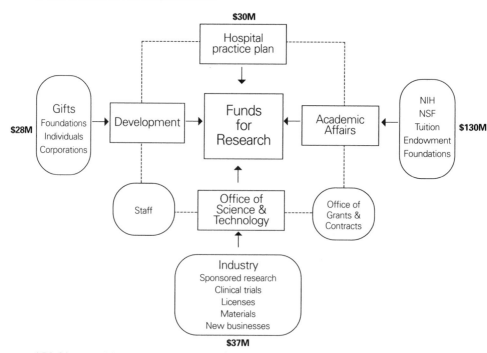

put, our goal is to maximize the value of this investment through the strategies described above. It would be fortunate for (and fair to) America's health if the commercial providers of health care also assume responsibility for funding this research infrastructure.

One way to view the sources of funds for research appears in figure 3. At Duke, we believe that each source of funding needs its own leader and strategy. There may need to be ongoing subsidization from clinical revenues for unfunded research within clinical departments and the hospital. But because the availability of these dollars will shrink, the center will have to aggressively pursue funds from the Federal government, foundations, and philanthropy in support of investigator-initiated research.

Moreover, at Duke, we intend to use margins from our health system enterprises to support research and development efforts that can enhance the value of our clinical enterprise. This strategy is clearly a social good and also a sound way to improve the health care we deliver. In addition, the value of the research output, to the extent possible, should be directed at acquiring new revenues or improving the value and, hence, competitive position of our health system.

## CONCLUSION

Restructuring the academic health center must be based on the understanding that research is a mission that is not only worthy of subsidization for its own intrinsic value, but is also a mission that can represent a competitive strength for the integrated academic health system. Academic health centers must continue to support biomedical research and advocate its societal benefits to the public and the government. The academic health center must, however, restructure its research enterprise to be compatible with the realities of the health care marketplace. In doing so, the institution need not compromise the quality or integrity of its research; however, it may need to readjust its size and efficiency. Where possible, research with commercial application should be positioned to generate new revenues to support unfunded components. The research mission can be deployed over time to enhance the quality of care. In this way, the integrated academic health system can utilize its research functions to improve health care. By doing so, it will provide social good and position itself as a formidable market force.

## ACKNOWLEDGMENTS

The author acknowledges the conceptual and technical contributions of Vicki Saito who contributed greatly to the development of this manuscript.

## WORK CITED

Dawber, T.R., and W.B. Kannel. 1966. The Framingham study: An epidemiological approach to coronary heart disease. *Circulation* 34.

Doll, R., and A.B. Hill. 1950. Smoking and carcinoma of the lung: A preliminary report. *British Medical Journal* 2.

Ganem, J.L., and J. Krakower. 1997. Review of U.S. medical school finances, 1995–1996. *Journal of the American Medical Association* 278.

Iglehart, J.K. 1997. Listening in on the Duke University Private Sector Conference. *New England Journal of Medicine* 336.

Parsons, R., and G.M. Li. 1993. Hypermutability and mismatch repair deficiency in RER+ tumor cells. *Cell* 75.

Rogers, M.C., and R. Snyderman. 1994. Cultural and organizational implications of academic managed-care networks. *New England Journal of Medicine* 331.

Shortell, S.M., and R.R. Gillies. 1996. Clinical integration; maximizing patient value. In *Remaking Health Care in America*. San Francisco: Jossey-Bass.

Snyderman, R. 1995. Model for a 21st century academic health system. In *The Academic Health Center in the 21st Century*, R. Snyderman and V. Saito, eds. Durham, NC: Duke University Medical Center.

———. 1996. Development of academic health systems. In *The AHC Responds to Health Care Reform*, R. Snyderman and V. Saito, eds. Durham, NC: Duke University Medical Center.

———. 1997. The HMO hazard: How the quest for short-term profits may undermine our whole health care system. *Washington Post*, January 6.

# RESEARCH ADMINISTRATION FOR THE 21ST CENTURY: THE UCSF RESEARCH ADMINISTRATION PROJECT

*Karl J. Hittelman, PhD, and Mary Beth O'Connor, MBA*

THE UNIVERSITY OF CALIFORNIA, SAN FRANCISCO (UCSF), is a research-intensive, public, health sciences university striving to maintain its preeminence into the 21st century. This serious task is occurring in an environment shaped by permanent decreases in state funding, erosion of indirect cost recovery, and ferocious competition for all sources of research support—Federal, foundation, and corporate. To remain competitive, the UCSF faculty must be able to depend upon the campus for research administration services of every kind that are timely, efficient, and effective and that can also adapt swiftly and nimbly to a rapidly changing environment. This job will be difficult using the existing research administration procedures: Except for the significant new responsibilities added over the years, research administration is carried out in 1997 largely as it was in 1967.

In these days of intense competition for funding, faculty report that good science is not enough of a goal anymore. Funding proposals must now be essentially bulletproof and, for Federal awards (from the National Institutes of Health, in particular), it is no longer safe to assume that grant renewals will be

*Dr. Hittelman is associate vice chancellor for academic affairs, University of California, San Francisco; Ms. O'Connor is a partner in the Higher Education Consulting Practice, Coopers & Lybrand, LLP.*

easily forthcoming. As a result, to maintain the scope and vigor of their research programs, more faculty than ever before are turning to private—often corporate—sources for funding.

Although public funding sources continue to account for the largest proportion of awards at UCSF, the number of awards from private sources grew by 54 percent in the past few years (figure 1). During the same period, awards from public sources decreased by 9 percent. Stated another way, between FY 1990 and FY 1997, the annual number of awards from private sponsors rose from 27 percent to 38 percent of all annual campus awards. The increased volume and

Figure 1
**NUMBER AND PERCENT OF RESEARCH AWARDS, UCSF, FY 1990 AND 1997**

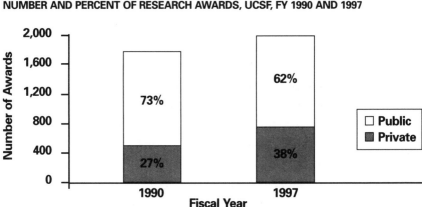

increased complexity of awards, combined with constraints on both the number of administrative staff and their functions, are having dramatic effects on research administration at UCSF. For example:

- The number of UCSF extramural proposals and awards increased substantially between FY 1980 and FY 1997 (figure 2). This dynamic growth was not accompanied by commensurate increases in research administration staff, particularly at the campus level. At the same time, newly imposed restrictions on indirect cost recovery make UCSF's resources for research administration problematic.

- As faculty submit more proposals to an increasingly diverse range of sponsors, both public and private, the administrative workload on department, school, and campus-level staff increases. In particular,

Figure 2
**NUMBER OF PROPOSALS SUBMITTED AND AWARDS
RECEIVED, UCSF, FY 1980, 1989, AND 1997**

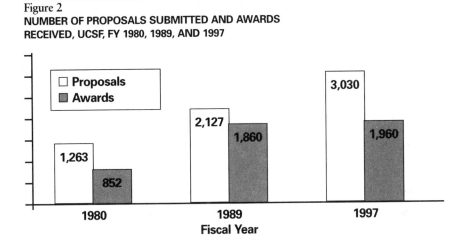

increasing administrative resources and effort must be directed toward administration of proposals to, and awards from, private sponsors. Both the pre- and postaward administrative requirements of these privately sponsored proposals and awards are much more complex than for relatively simple Federal awards, and thus much more labor intensive.

- The increased complexity of both proposals and awards requires increased levels of coordination among research administration staff who have interrelated functional responsibilities. For example, contract negotiators must be in communication with administrators of conflict-of-interest policies. Institutional review board staff must coordinate activities with contracts and grants staff and, often, with intellectual property administrators. These functions are not all located conveniently to one another, a situation that would not be a problem if truly effective and efficient computer links and data sharing existed between these units. They do not.

- The number and complexity of Federal regulations continues to increase, driving up the cost of regulatory compliance even as the administrative component of the indirect cost rate is capped.

## CURRENT 'SYSTEM'

To establish a context for discussing the UCSF Research Administration Project, it is helpful to look at a thumbnail sketch of the current research administration "system." Briefly, it is one in which authority is highly centralized and, quite appropriately, requires extensive financial accountability.

### Authorities

At the University of California, grant, contract, and gift policies emanate from the Board of Regents and, typically, procedures for implementing them are extensively transaction based with numerous control points at which signed approvals are required. It is a system of "checkers checking checkers," as one university administrator characterizes it. Indeed, research administration procedures in universities seem to have originated in a primordial administrative soup where meticulous financial control procedures for the management of extramural funds (virtually all that were needed at the time) conferred a distinct survival advantage. Accountants were the first nonfaculty research administrators, and most institutional research administration procedures still reflect a heavily transaction-based approach strongly indicative of their accounting origins.

Academic units at UCSF have no approval authority for preaward activities except for such internal matters as space allocations, salaries, and appropriateness of research. University authority (i.e., legally delegated signature authority) to make commitments on behalf of the Regents (e.g., to submit grant proposals; negotiate and sign contracts, including clinical trials; accept awards; and execute other approvals) resides solely with central units.* Gifts up to a certain amount may be solicited by faculty or their representatives but must be accepted centrally. To prevent inadvertent, simultaneous solicitation of large gifts from the same sponsor, central approval is required for soliciting gifts above the threshold.

Authority for postaward activities is slightly more evenly distributed between the local and central levels. However, although academic units have wide latitude to make hiring and spending decisions within university policies,

---

* The terms "academic" and "local" refer to schools, departments, divisions, organized research units, and other academic jurisdictions. The term "central" refers to units with campuswide jurisdiction that report to UCSF's chancellor.

the ultimate approvals and control points still remain at the central level. All official financial records are kept centrally, with typical, periodic feedback (usually monthly) to academic units for such activities as ledger reconciliation. The need for more current data has driven many units to create their own shadow systems to monitor research expenditures in real time.

## Procedures

Procedurally, pre- and postaward activities are largely, but not absolutely, separated. Central units, such as the Division of Contracts and Grants (pre-award) and the Accounting Office (postaward), are responsible for large amounts of transaction processing. The pre- and postaward functions report to two different vice chancellors. In general, the academic vice chancellor is responsible for most pre-award activities, and the administrative vice chancellor handles most postaward activities. The development function (pre-award) reports to yet a third vice chancellor.

Nonfinancial regulatory matters (e.g., governance of the use of human and animal subjects) are under central authority, but because of the nature of these activities, centralization is the preferred mode. From the perspective of staffing, it offers economies of scale, easing the burden that service on regulatory committees places on faculty and fostering consistency in the application of UCSF policies, practices, and standards.

As is described in more detail below, current procedures are transaction based and paper driven, lack a faculty focus, and fail to make sound use of new technologies. This system can no longer adequately support either current levels of proposal and award activity or the increasing complexity and intensity of effort demanded by diverse funding sources—at least for a price we can afford into the foreseeable future.

In response, the UCSF administration endorsed a proposal to undertake a comprehensive review of research administration at UCSF with the specific goal of creating a faculty-oriented system that would be an adjunct, not an impediment, to the competitiveness of the faculty. The project soon became known as the Research Administration Project (RAP). From the time it was launched it has had—and continues to enjoy—unequivocal support from the highest levels of campus administration, a fact essential to its success.

## DESIGN FOR A NEW SYSTEM

RAP is being conducted in three phases. Phase 1 was a discovery phase in which the eight major research administration activities were analyzed. Phase 2, based on the findings from phase 1, was a redesign phase in which a model for research administration at UCSF was conceived. Phase 3, where we are now, is an implementation phase that has two parts: a pilot phase for testing and refining features of the model (including its computer technology component), and a final, campuswide implementation phase.

Figure 3 shows the project organization. The work has largely been carried out by the RAP Work Group made up of middle-level research administra-

Figure 3
**RESEARCH ADMINISTRATION PROJECT, UCSF**

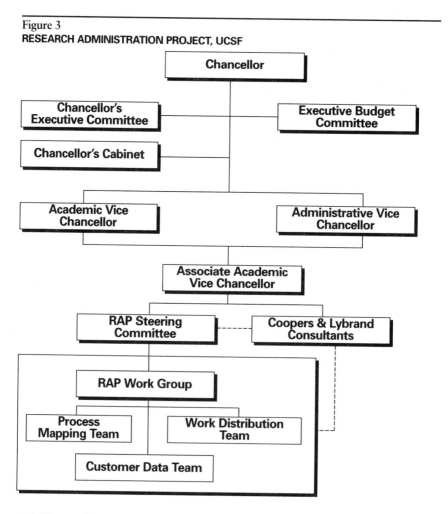

tion staff from both the central and the academic units. Department managers, unit directors from central administration, and other key staff actively engaged in pre- and postaward research administration, internal audit, budget, and human resources have joined forces to (1) collect and analyze data illuminating in detail how research administration is currently conducted at UCSF, and (2) conceive a new research administration model for the campus.

The Work Group has made recommendations to a Steering Committee of senior faculty and upper-level campus and school management (associate and assistant vice chancellors and associate deans) chaired by a member representing the academic side of the campus. The Steering Committee determined the overall direction of the project and approved for action the recommendations of the Work Group. Through its chair, the Steering Committee reported regularly to the chancellor's Cabinet and the chancellor's Executive Committee.

The Higher Education Consulting Practice of Coopers & Lybrand, LLP, was retained as consultant to this project, with mutual agreement that control of the project would reside firmly with UCSF. Coopers & Lybrand's role was to provide support and expertise to UCSF in a variety of ways. They included helping develop data-collection tools, training campus personnel to use a variety of such tools necessary to conduct the project, carrying out data analyses, and providing guidance for the evaluation of work-flow processes, management structures, and other aspects of UCSF's research administration system. Coopers & Lybrand acted as facilitators at meetings, kept records of proceedings, and occasionally collected data where it was felt that data collection by a third party was needed. The consulting practice staff were expected to be actively involved in discussions at all levels of the project. Their participation and support made it possible for the very busy and heavily committed UCSF staff to focus efficiently on core project activities.

## PHASE 1: DISCOVERY

Phase 1 of RAP, completed in May 1996, provided us with a comprehensive, data-based understanding of how research administration is conducted at UCSF. Research administration can be viewed as a cyclic process, or a continuum, that can conveniently be analyzed by breaking it into the eight activities, from identification and development of funding opportunities to closing out the

---

Figure 4
**RESEARCH ADMINISTRATION PROCESS, UCSF**

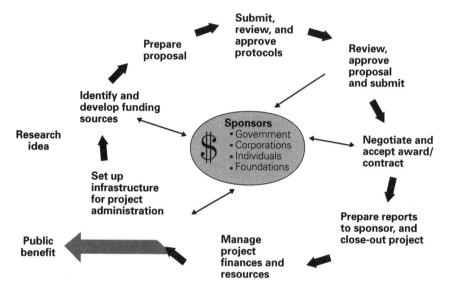

project. Each activity is a discrete segment of the continuum. This cyclic process, depicted in figure 4, is nearly universal at U.S. academic research institutions.

*Methods*

To develop a thorough understanding of existing research administration practices, five different methods were used to collect data from faculty and staff in all campus-level offices and a stratified sample of academic units. These data concerned user satisfaction, process flow, control points, governing policies, computing support, and organizational issues. The methods were:

1. Surveys of faculty and staff to determine their satisfaction with, and assessment of, the importance of current research administration services.

2. Work-flow mapping, combined with identification and assessment of control points, to illustrate the sequence of actions in both academic and central units.

3. Analysis of the distribution of effort allocated to research administration tasks and responsibilities (work distribution analysis) to estimate the cost of research administration and the degree to which work was

fragmented among individuals and units.

4. Assessment of computing and network support to identify the current level of technological support available for research administration activities.

5. Interviews with department chairs, members of key faculty and management committees, and senior management to illuminate institutional strategies, initiatives, and priorities.

## Findings

Detailed analyses of the data yielded conclusions in a number of areas of concern. None of the conclusions came as a great surprise. Every institution has its bureaucratic horror stories, and UCSF is no exception. Nevertheless, if a convincing case for change was to be made—particularly for very significant change in such an important functional area as research administration—it was clear that the argument would have to be data based; it could not stand merely on anecdotal accounts. Thus, the findings behind the conclusions were particularly interesting because they set before us the facts about the institution.

We had determined customer satisfaction through a survey of faculty and research administration staff. Relative costs were calculated from a work distribution study conducted during RAP. At the time these data were collected, UCSF was spending the smallest proportion of funds in what turned out to be the two areas of greatest dissatisfaction: identification of funding sources and negotiation of contracts (figure 5).

Faculty and staff were dissatisfied with many of the services provided to support research administration.* (Nevertheless, it was widely acknowledged by faculty that UCSF has a cadre of dedicated, diligent staff who strive to provide the best service possible under the existing constraints of the system.)

Efforts to identify and solicit funds for research, particularly from private (including industry) sponsors, were cited as inadequate to support faculty needs. Seventy-nine percent of faculty and their support staff felt this service is of high

---

* Survey instruments for assessing customer satisfaction were sent to a stratified sample of 1,166 faculty and 140 research administration staff representing all four schools. The overall return rate was 25% (328 responses)—faculty, 23%; staff, 36%. Response rates from the schools were very similar, ranging from 24% (medicine) to 30% (nursing).

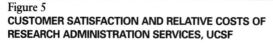

Figure 5
CUSTOMER SATISFACTION AND RELATIVE COSTS OF
RESEARCH ADMINISTRATION SERVICES, UCSF

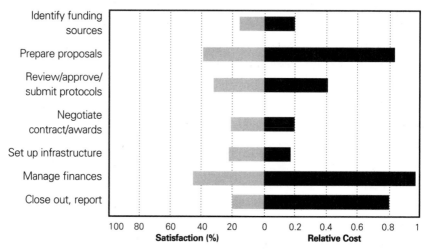

importance, yet only 16 percent expressed satisfaction with the existing services. Until very recently, only a minority of faculty supported the commitment of campus resources to this activity. Only 21 percent of faculty and staff were satisfied with the services to negotiate terms and conditions of contracts. They were least satisfied with services related to private contracts and clinical trial agreements.

Forty-three percent of faculty and staff expressed frustration and dissatisfaction with the services available for managing finances. Only 20 percent of faculty and staff were satisfied with the services provided to prepare reports to sponsors and to close out projects.

Summed across all levels of the campus departments and schools, UCSF spends approximately $11 million annually (about 3 percent of FY 1996 awards) on staff salaries and fringe benefits alone in support of research administration. (Campus-level services—accounting, development, environmental health and safety, contracts and grants, and regulatory affairs—account for about 15 percent of this amount.) Yet this investment has clearly not resulted in high levels of faculty and staff satisfaction.

If faculty effort at research administration is included in this estimate, the total expenditure almost doubles to $19 through $21 million annually (about 6 percent of the extramural awards total). Obviously, this situation stems from the high faculty salaries that drive up research administration costs significantly, even though faculty contribute a relatively small portion of the total effort.

There is no formal institutional investment in identifying funding opportunities for faculty. As a result, faculty spend significant amounts of their own time seeking funding sources. Several departments have created their own systems to track funding opportunities at the expense of considerable duplication of effort across the campus.

UCSF has a minimal complement of skilled and trained staff to conduct contract negotiations. This lack of staff contributes to long delays, faculty frustration, and, occasionally, unsatisfactory contracts.

Approximately 60 to 75 percent of research administration activities could be classified as nonvalue-added (figure 6), suggesting that there is ample room for improving the campus return on investment. To evaluate UCSF's return on investment in research administration, research administration activities were assessed (using work-flow diagrams) for nonvalue-added (NVA) activity.* The following five questions guided this assessment.

---

Figure 6
**ESTIMATES OF VALUE-ADDED, NONVALUE-ADDED, AND NONVALUE-ADDED BUT MANDATED ACTIVITIES IN RESEARCH ADMINISTRATION PROCESS, UCSF**

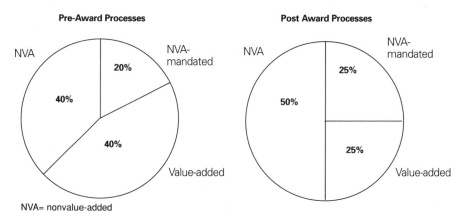

NVA= nonvalue-added

---

* Clearly, many activities in UCSF's overall process of acquiring funds and managing research are required, and so add value to the process. Such value-added activities are, for example, those that are essential to the functional continuity of the process, those that are mandated by external authorities, and those that assure responsible stewardship of resources.

1. Could the activity be eliminated if it were handled differently or correctly?
2. Could appropriate technology eliminate the activity?
3. Could the activity be eliminated without negative effect on the final outcome?
4. Is the activity required by an external party (e.g., sponsor, regulatory body)?
5. Would the faculty member pay for the activity?

The high estimate of NVA activity must be viewed with caution, of course, for some NVA activities are mandated by regulations. But others are self-inflicted by UCSF's own internal procedures. In addition, rework, error correction, and inadequate use and coordination of computing contribute significantly to NVA activities. NVA activities increase the time and cost required to complete the process and preclude staff from conducting other activities that would enhance service to faculty. A number of examples of nonvalue-added activities were discovered. Some examples follow.

- Ninety percent of new full-committee human- and animal-use protocols were returned to the investigator with a contingency letter, and required corrections or additional information before final approval could be granted, adding twelve to nineteen days to the process.
- Forty percent of cost transfers were returned to departments because the form used was incorrect or documentation was missing.
- Ninety percent of Federal grant proposals required some administrative modification prior to being submitted to the sponsoring agency, adding one to three days to the process.

To account for all private funds entering the institution, UCSF policy requires that private grants and contracts be processed and set up through the Development Office. This duplicates the effort of the Division of Contracts and Grants, which will usually have reviewed or negotiated the award, and the Accounting Office, which will formally have established the project account in the campus accounting system.

Of the estimated 60 to 75 percent of NVA activity, approximately 20 percent is mandated by UCSF or sponsor policies. For example, campus and School of Medicine policies require that the division chief, department chair or organized research unit director, dean, and contracts and grants officer each review and approve all funding proposals before they leave the campus.

The research administration process is very complex and requires extensive navigation by faculty and department staff to obtain service or find information. Seven to nine campus-level offices and each of the campus's academic units provide research administration services to faculty. Together, they are involved in approximately seventeen to twenty-four individual approvals. At least six campus offices and the sponsor are involved in the process. At some hand-off points between offices, redundant data entry may be required because of inadequate technological support of the process.

Figure 7 illustrates the complexity of the process for the submission of an NIH RO1 grant. Each unit provides a specific service, and in some cases these services overlap. Staff and faculty are frustrated with the difficulty of obtaining complete, accurate, and timely answers to questions without having to make telephone calls to several offices. Three to five units participate in the processing and management of a Federal grant award; three to eight are involved in a pri-

Figure 7
**PATHWAY OF AN NIH RO1 GRANT, UCSF**

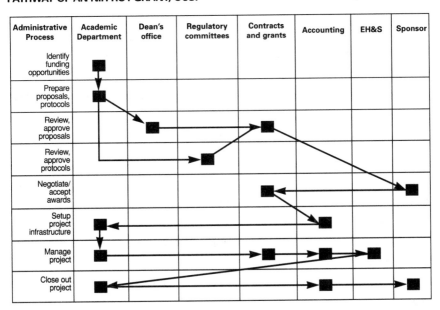

| Administrative Process | Academic Department | Dean's office | Regulatory committees | Contracts and grants | Accounting | EH&S | Sponsor |
|---|---|---|---|---|---|---|---|
| Identify funding opportunities | ■ | | | | | | |
| Prepare proposals, protocols | ■ | | | | | | |
| Review, approve proposals | | ■ | | ■ | | | |
| Review, approve protocols | | | ■ | | | | |
| Negotiate/ accept awards | | | | ■ | | | ■ |
| Setup project infrastructure | ■ | | | | ■ | | |
| Manage project | ■ | | | ■ | ■ | ■ | |
| Close out project | ■ | | | | ■ | | ■ |

EH&S= Environmental Health and Safety

## Table 1
### FRAGMENTATION OF RESEARCH ADMINISTRATION EFFORT, UCSF

| | Head count [a] | FTE [b] | Fragmentation ratio [c] | Average effort [d] (%) |
|---|---|---|---|---|
| Identify funding sources | 37 | 3.02 | 12.3 | 8.2 |
| Prepare proposals | 111 | 14.28 | 7.8 | 12.9 |
| Review, approve, and submit protocols and proposals | 68 | 8.15 | 8.3 | 12.0 |
| Negotiate and accept contract/award | 34 | 5.93 | 5.7 | 17.4 |
| Set up project infrastructure | 67 | 6.39 | 10.5 | 9.5 |
| Manage project finances and resources | 117 | 24.54 | 4.8 | 21.0 |
| Prepare reports; close out projects | 89 | 10.02 | 8.9 | 11.3 |
| ALL RESEARCH ADMINISTRATION | 523 | 72.33 | 7.2 | 13.8 |

[a] Head count: Number of people who contribute some level of effort to the proccess indicated.

[b] FTE (Full-time employee): Calculated from (a) average based on the percent effort each person reported contributing to the process indicated.

[c] Fragmentation ratio: Ratio (a)/(b) showing the degree to which effort on the process indicated is fragmented among staff. The higher the fragmentation ration, the more fragmented is the effort put into the process.

[d] Average effort. Ratio (b)/(a) showing the average percent effort any one person contributes to the process indicated.

vate award. For example, the Development Office and the Division of Contracts and Grants both process private grants. The Development and Accounting Offices both deposit checks and set up private grant accounts.

The duties of research administration staff are fragmented, especially in the academic departments; furthermore, staff assigned solely to research administration duties are the exception, not the rule. Our work distribution analysis revealed that, with rare exception, no one staff member spent more than about 20 percent of his or her time on any segment of the research administration process (table 1). The data were derived from a work distribution study conducted among staff with research administration duties. Note that in the head count column, people were counted more than once if they participate in more than one of the eight major research administration activities.

Because staff are spread over many administrative activities, from answering telephones to ledger reconciliation, numerous handoffs necessarily occur. The varying degrees of staff expertise in both proposal preparation and financial management, coupled with the lack of formal and ongoing training, contribute to a very high level of rework. The lack of development of staff expertise perpetuates inefficiency and unsatisfactory service and contributes to a high turnover rate of staff.

Responsibility for different aspects of the research administration process is dispersed across a number of vice chancellors and deans (figure 8). This approach diffuses authority and accountability for the process at all levels; it also means that policies are interpreted and communicated in numerous and sometimes inconsistent ways, leading to confusion and uncertainty about requirements and procedures. At the same time, these staff are held responsible for adhering rigidly to existing policies, with no authority to adapt them to the diverse and changing needs of investigators and the university. As a result, faculty work around the process and sometimes appeal to higher levels for exceptional treatment or waivers of policy. The result makes for inconsistent application of these policies, compromises the credibility of staff, erodes morale, and wastes faculty time.

There is a proliferation of computing systems used to support research administration. Because they are largely idiosyncratic and not integrated across functional lines, redundant data entry often occurs, and valuable data are not accessible to those who need the information.

Figure 8
OFFICES RESPONSIBLE FOR RESEARCH ADMINISTRATION SERVICES, UCSF

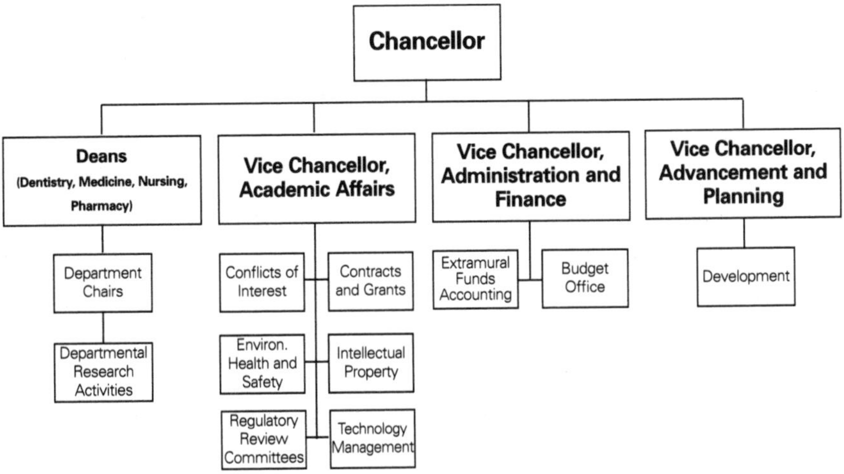

At the time this analysis was conducted, UCSF lacked integrated computing systems and on-line access to data, forms, templates, policies, guidelines, and procedures. Seven stand-alone systems had been developed for use by campus-level units to administer research, resulting in a staggering amount of redundant data entry. This lack of integrated technological support for research administration is a major contributor to a high degree of nonvalue-added activity. In addition, almost every department or other academic unit has developed its own system to track proposals and manage project finances.

At the time of this analysis, private grant proposal or award information was being entered into university systems eight times: thrice at the department, twice at the Division of Contracts and Grants, twice at the Accounting Office, and once at the Development Office. Standardized templates and on-line forms (e.g., for budgets, protocols, financial disclosure, proposals, reporting) were not provided to administrative staff, causing each department to find or develop its own. The profusion of stand-alone computer systems and databases results in redundant, and sometimes inconsistent, data collection and reporting, further adding unnecessary cost to the process.

## GOALS AND PRINCIPLES

The data from phase 1 pointed clearly to a number of problems that had to be addressed. But the Work Group was wary of the danger of creating a model that might address the problems only partially, especially if the simplistic approach of merely revising procedures was adopted. So, before proceeding directly to the complex task of fixing research administration, the Work Group undertook to derive a fundamental set of institutional goals and principles. Discussions in the Work Group, and subsequently between the Work Group and the Steering Committee, led to a statement of goals and principles. The intent was to provide a clear framework for a model that would address the problems that had been identified in phase 1 and position UCSF advantageously for the 21st century.

RAP established that its goals were to provide service to the faculty that would support research excellence and enhance competitiveness, and help the university fulfill its obligations to sponsors in an accurate and timely manner. Six principles were then identified as fundamental to delivering research administrative services in an accurate, efficient, effective, and ethical manner, as follows:

1.  *Leadership to guide and coordinate the system, ensure its consistency, and develop policies, procedures, and guidelines that secure the delivery of the highest quality services*—Both faculty and staff had commented upon the dispersed authority for research administration. The practical effect is that no one campus officer is held accountable for research administration policies and practices, let alone the quality of service, as a whole. This dispersed authority complicates coordination of pre- and postaward activities, which report to different vice chancellors, and sometimes makes it difficult to get unequivocal answers and definitive policy interpretations. Undertaking large-scale policy and procedural changes is also difficult, as exemplified last year by the complex logistics that were necessary to implement the recent revisions to OMB Circular A-21.

2.  *Ethical standards that promote the highest level of integrity in professional conduct*—The need for carefully thought-out and consistently applied ethical standards for research administration was a topic that came up from both faculty and staff, at times with considerable passion. A broad range of integrity issues was cited during phase 1. For example, faculty and some staff raised questions about the relationships between the university and industry sponsors of research (principally related to intellectual property matters) and between faculty and their industry sponsors (principally conflict-of-interest issues). Staff, on the other hand, raised the problem of pressure applied by faculty—sometimes subtle, sometimes not—to do things they might judge to be unethical or to violate policy. (I don't care what you have to do or how, just get it done!) And from an external perspective, the university has an obligation to its sponsors to manage funds and activities in a manner that is beyond reproach.

3.  *Coherence as a system, characterized by accountability that is unambiguously defined and delegated; consistency in the interpretation and application of and compliance with policies; adaptability, ensuring responsiveness to changes in faculty needs and the external environment; delegation, minimizing administrative processing by faculty;*

*ongoing assessment, supporting continuous improvement of the system; comprehensive training for all, commensurate with roles, responsibilities and authorities; and indexing of the workforce to the workload*—Currently, the organizational separation of pre- and postaward activities, dispersed authority, lack of training, fragmentation of staff responsibilities, and intensively transaction-oriented procedures all converge to make the existing system seem anything but coherent.

4. *Team approach, characterized by mutual trust underlying a collaborative working environment among faculty and staff; a commitment to staff development to assure recruitment and retention of the most outstanding possible staff in the service of the faculty's research activities; availability of information and appropriate training for faculty to support them in their roles at the center of the campus's research enterprise; and relationship building, to achieve rapport among faculty, staff, and research sponsors*—Both faculty and staff had stressed the importance of developing a model in which teamwork prevails. For staff, it would mean assuming virtually all administrative responsibilities for faculty, something they are eager to do, and working closely with faculty to handle the administrative needs of the faculty. Faculty would welcome escape from the administrative treadmill that such service would afford them.

5. *Simplicity, characterized by a single point of service for faculty at any stage of the research administration continuum; and single entry of data, capturing information once, obviating redundant data entry*—During phase 1, research administration procedures at UCSF had been mapped in detail. The resulting metabolic chart was staggering in its complexity. For example, just to submit a simple NIH RO grant application, an investigator's proposal had to transit six different offices and get at least six different approvals.

6. *Technological power, characterized by rapid communication; accessibility to faculty and staff of funding opportunities, proposal and award information, and the current forms, templates, policies, procedures, and guidelines required for research activity; and integrated*

*capture, management, sharing, and use of information, limiting the amount of data entry necessary and the creation and flow of paperwork*—Faculty and staff had remarked about the need for a campuswide, integrated computing capability for managing research administration, from identifying potential funding opportunities to closing out projects, and especially for tracking and projecting their expenditures.

## PHASE 2: REDESIGN

To design a model suitable for the campus, the Work Group decided to start with a simple, high-level conceptualization of research administration and then, using the Goals and Principles statement, develop a fully operational and functional model.

All research administration activities, from the identification of potential funding sources to project closeout from the academic unit to the campus level were simplified. The three principal activities now are identifying a source for research funds, applying for and obtaining research funds, and managing the funded project from start to finish. Some of the major processes that go into these three principal activities begin to reveal themselves when we take a closer look

Figure 9
PROCESS FLOW: FIND MONEY

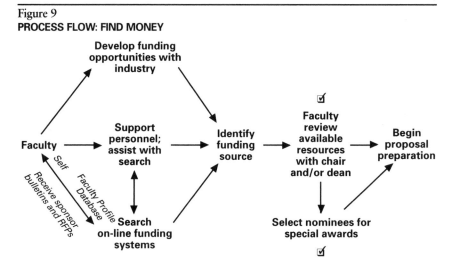

☑ Control point
RFP = request for proposal

Figure 10
PROCESS FLOW: GET MONEY

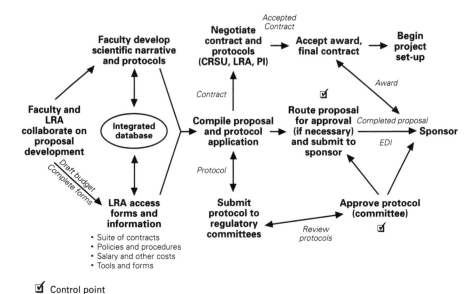

☑ Control point

at each activity. Figures 9, 10, and 11 are a simplistic depiction of the new world of research administration at UCSF.

In contrast to the current process, this model is designed with the faculty-client in mind. Data are maintained in a single, integrated database. Three essential pillars—computer technology, training, and integrity of data establish the foundation for developing the model.

Currently, the technology supporting UCSF's research administration process resides in seven stand-alone systems in central units and a multitude of department-based shadow systems. These systems seldom provide access to data by those who need it to manage their research portfolios.

Because the campus has relatively few people wholly dedicated to research administration, the model proposes establishment of a cadre of staff whose full-time responsibilities are to deliver administrative services in support of research to the faculty. This situation is very different from the current state of affairs, particularly at the school and department levels, where staff are fragmented across

Figure 11
PROCESS FLOW: MANAGE MONEY

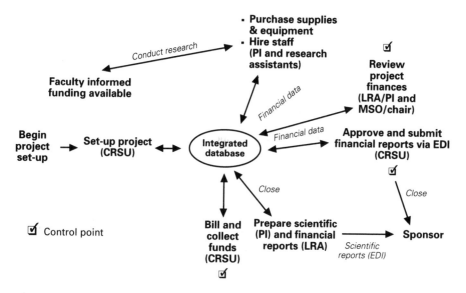

a multitude of activities. Implementation of the model will require the creation of new positions at UCSF and the modification of many existing ones.

The issue of the integrity of the research process that arose a number of times during phase 1 of this project from a number of levels—faculty, staff, and administrators—carried the same fundamental message: Develop a system that is internally consistent and fault intolerant.

## Technology

It is intended that the hallmarks of technology in the model be integration and accessibility. Computing technology, accessible at all UCSF academic sites, using a comprehensive research administration database and other campus systems, will provide the power to collect, maintain, manipulate, and distribute information easily and efficiently. For example, downloadable forms, applications, templates, policies, handbooks, and guidelines will all be readily available on-line. Data for budget development (e.g., salaries, fringe benefit and indirect cost rates, per diem costs for animal care) will be easily obtainable from on-line databases for accurate budget development. Similarly, access to project financial data will facilitate accounting, expenditure projections, cost transfers, and financial reporting. And, of course, such a system will facilitate rapid communication among staff involved in all aspects of managing extramural funds.

## Training

It will be imperative to develop training programs to support the personnel who will fill these newly created or modified positions.

Indeed, training will go further than just supporting the transition of staff into new positions. Intensive and comprehensive training will familiarize staff with all university research administration policies and procedures, including ethical ramifications. It will be tailored to the level of need and scope of responsibilities within the research administration process. For example, a typical, entry-level research administrator (called a local research advocate, or LRA) working in an academic unit will be fully trained in processing NIH RO1 grants but will not receive training on negotiating contracts until it becomes a required skill. Ongoing training programs will be available to assure that research administration staff at all levels have the most up-to-date knowledge and required skills to serve the faculty. Research administration will become a well developed and, we hope, attractive career track at UCSF.

## Integrity of System

The issue of integrity was recognized as very complex. Yet, because UCSF aspires to develop a research administration model based on the highest ethical standards, the issue is hardly controversial.

In practice this means that policies must be interpreted uniformly across the campus and that procedures must be uniformly applied.

To ensure that the integrity of UCSF, its employees, and its research is protected, special attention will be paid to developing a supporting organizational structure with appropriate accountability and reporting lines that will protect faculty, staff, sponsors, and the university.

## Primary Characteristics

The model does not simply create a different flow of activity supported by new policies and procedures. It goes further, establishing a new organizational model with clearly defined roles and responsibilities for participants. It will have a number of defining characteristics that clearly distinguish it from the current system and significantly simplify research administration at UCSF. Each characteristic is based on the computing technology-training-integrity function.

Each faculty member at UCSF will need to contact only one person to get the information, service, or needed contact with current and potential sponsors regardless of where in the research process a problem or question may lie. This does not mean that one person will be responsible for all tasks at any required level of detail or expertise associated with research administration. Nor should it suggest that every LRA will be responsible for a complete understanding of all regulations, policies, and procedures governing the process. Instead, one point of contact simply means that each faculty member will have a personal account manager who will make certain that all of the faculty member's needs are met and delivered in a timely way and at a high level of quality, whether personally or through referral. Research sponsors will also have the option of a single point of contact for any matter pertaining to an individual faculty member. Depending on the size of the unit's research portfolio, service units will be organized at the level of the school, department, division, or organized research unit to deliver service close to the source of need.

Much of the authority needed to conduct research administration in an efficient, client-oriented manner will be delegated to the level of academic units. Staff will receive appropriate training to certify them as qualified to exercise signature authority. Several levels of certification will permit assigning different levels of authority commensurate with a staff person's training and the complexity of funding instruments.

To ensure that the delivery of services occurs in a consistent manner across all units, the people responsible for delivering research administration at UCSF will be organized into two teams: Local Research Service Units (LRSUs) and a Central Research Support Unit (CRSU). LRSUs will consist of cadres of highly trained, full-time, certified research administration generalists. This new class of university employee will be trained to provide cradle-to-grave service (i.e., information or service across the entire continuum of research administration). The CRSU will consolidate the currently dispersed central research administration services reorganized into one coordinated unit reporting to a central officer. In addition to having advanced expertise, CRSU staff will provide training and technical support to LRAs.

## Technological Power

The research administration process and its organization will be supported by a new system of technology that will offer distributed access to the community and integrated information resources necessary to conduct both pre- and postaward activities.

Distributed access means that the model will have a data-management system that makes it possible to capture information only once and makes that information accessible to all those authorized to have access to it. Forms, applications, templates, policies, handbooks, guidelines, and other information sources and useful tools will all be readily available on-line, allowing staff to do it right the first time.

Integrated information resources means that the research administration data system will house all pre- and postaward information and be integrated with university financial, personnel, payroll, and purchasing systems. LRAs will be able to track all proposal and award information on-line and in real time.

## Organizational Structure

The two teams — the LRSUs and the CRSU — will be supported by a new system of human resource principles and practices that includes a professional career path, performance evaluations, and training programs.

An LRSU will be organized to facilitate the delivery of services to faculty directly at the local level. Depending on the number of faculty served, the LRSU may be attached to a school, department, division, or other academic subunit. Each LRA within the LRSU will be the equivalent of an account executive responsible for all aspects of research administration for a portfolio of faculty clients. The number of faculty clients an LRA serves will depend upon several factors, including the pace and intensity of research activity, the number and dollar amounts of grants and contracts, and the requirements of sponsoring agencies.

This organizational structure serves two important purposes: (1) It establishes the faculty orientation of the model by identifying an account manager who acts as the faculty member's single point of contact for any and all administrative questions about a research activity; and (2) it provides the opportunity to staff each LRSU with LRAs having the skills and expertise most appropriate for the academic unit. For example, the LRSU serving a clinical department would need one or more LRAs with capabilities to administer clinical investigation; a basic science department with no such clinical investigation need might emphasize support for National Institutes of Health and National Science Foundation funding.

A number of important features of the model can be determined only empirically. The number of faculty assigned to an LRA's portfolio, the number of LRAs constituting an LRSU, and the number of LRSUs the campus might require can only be approximated at this time. To whom the LRSU reports is a very important question. Solely for discussion purposes, it has been assumed that each LRA can manage about twenty faculty members and that an LRSU might comprise five to seven LRAs, with one of the LRAs serving as the team's leader. Efforts will be made to constitute LRSUs with staff with varying expertise (e.g., regulatory, financial, proposal development) to assure that, as a team, the LRSU staff can offer its faculty a breadth of experience and expertise. The reporting relationship of the LRSU will be some function of the academic unit served. For example, if the LRSU supports a school, the unit may report to the dean, whereas an LRSU supporting a cluster of small departments may report to one of the department chairs.

Taking into account these rough approximations plus the number of principal investigators at UCSF, we get an approximate distribution of one LRSU each for the Schools of Dentistry, Nursing, and Pharmacy, and about fifteen for the School of Medicine. It is anticipated that in the early stages of implementing the model, empirical studies in the form of pilot projects will refine these numbers. Some proposed pilot studies are discussed below.

Because it is intended that the LRAs be generalists in research administration (with particular strengths deriving from their backgrounds) capable of answering many, but not all, faculty questions, there will inevitably be problems for which an LRA will have to seek help. This level of support will be the responsibility of the CRSU staff. Made up of highly accomplished experts in the various aspects of research administration (e.g., contracts, human subjects regulations, accounting, intellectual property), each CRSU will be made up of a team of people with advanced knowledge and skills in research policies and procedures. When the model is mature, CRSU staff will no longer bear routine processing responsibilities. Rather, their responsibilities will be to provide high-level expertise for policy interpretation and communication, education and training, support for regulatory compliance, computer technology support, problem solving, and managing exceptional cases. One outstanding organizational element yet to be defined is how authority and responsibility should be consolidated to deal with the problem posed by the current dispersion of these functions.

The introduction of new organizational models into the current UCSF structures requires the development of new strategies to manage human resources. Because a clearly defined career path is proposed for LRAs and the experts in the CRSU, a new performance management system and training program must be designed to guide and encourage the development of a professional research administration career; in this way, UCSF can recruit and retain first-rate research administrators.

The new organizational model offers the possibility of a career track for research administrators, a feature of particular interest to the Work Group and to the campus. In the model, an individual may begin work as an assistant to an LRA, move on to become an LRA, advance through increasingly responsible levels of certification, become an LRA leader, and even eventually move into a position in the CRSU. No such career track currently exists at the University of California. Developing and managing individual careers to progress along such a track will provide distinct competitive advantages for recruiting, retaining, and advancing highly competent research administration staff.

To support the realization of a professional career for the LRAs and experts in the CRSU, a new performance management system will be developed to motivate staff to work productively, build core skills, and consistently provide excellent service. Such a system will serve as a tool in the professional development of staff and as an ongoing team-management and communication device, rather than as a source of documentation for personnel actions. It will emphasize both individual and group performance, incorporating the feedback of the team leader, peers, and faculty so that the quality of customer service can be measured. It is also intended to play a role in salary decisions—a radical departure from the existing system.

A four-level training and certification program will be developed to provide consistent levels of service to researchers across LRSUs and the CRSU. Coupled with training on the new process design, all research administrators will receive basic training to develop their technical, people, and computer skills.* However, as a person progresses in his or her career, other training courses will be required based on scope of responsibility. For example, a level 2 research administrator will be trained to draft and negotiate industry contracts while continuing to hold the authorities of level 1 (signature authority for grants and fellowships) and level 2 (signature authority for Federal government-sponsored contracts, subcontracts, and clinical trials). At the entry-level (tentatively identified as "intern"), prospects will receive the basic training and earn hours toward certification at level 1. At this writing, the Work Group is not aware of the availability, either commercially or from an academic institution, of a single package of integrated software that will support cradle-to-grave project management.

Many resources for finding potential research support are available on the Internet. These resources are being made widely available to faculty and staff at very modest cost to the campus. If UCSF chooses to increase its investment in this particular activity, it will probably do so by building a faculty expertise database and incorporating so-called expert systems for matching faculty interests to available funding opportunities.

*Getting money.* A handful of prototypes have been built to support the development of proposals, particularly the swift and accurate assembly of project budgets.

*Regulatory (financial and nonfinancial) compliance.* This module monitors compliance with both financial and nonfinancial regulations. Examples of financial regulations are Office of Management and Budget Circulars A-21 and A-110 and the recently imposed Cost Accounting Standards. Many institutions

---

* Technical training will include courses in on-line system searches, budget development, financial management, and regulatory requirements such as the preparation of animal and human subject protocols. People skills training will include course work on customer service, leadership, time and stress management, and communication. Computer skills training will include training in basic software such as Microsoft Word and Excel, and the university's On-Line Financial System, On-Line Payroll/Personnel System, and Ledger Link.

have developed databases for managing nonfinancial regulatory function (e.g., for the protection of human and animal subjects or the use of ionizing radiation or biohazardous substances). UCSF has long had such computerized capabilities. However, like most computerized functions at UCSF, they are isolated and idiosyncratic, and have not been developed with software or hardware that allows them to be used on a distributed basis.

These two regulatory elements—financial and nonfinancial—may be thought of as separable because they have distinctly different sets of regulatory, audit, and reporting requirements. In practice, however, they may not be separated so easily. In any event, each has some attributes, such as being table- and rules-driven, that provide highly desirable, time-saving features that ensure accuracy and compliance with policy. However, to the best of our knowledge, none of the systems in use is part of a larger system that will support all research administration activities.

*Managing money.* This module consists of the functions associated with extramural funds accounting commonly required by institutions and investigators to manage accounts. Such on-line financial systems are commercially available. UCSF has already acquired one such system, and it is anticipated that tools for using this financial system will be developed specifically to aid research administrators in managing research project finances.

Another feature of fully integrated software support for research administration (and the one that is perhaps most coveted by both faculty and department-level managers) is an analytical tool that uses current financial data to project expenditure rates. For faculty, such a tool allows a measure of precision in planning within the project budget. For department managers, the tool protects against (or, at worst, is an early warning system for) overdrafts of research funds. Of course, such an analytical module would serve many other management purposes. Suffice to say that it would provide a powerful management tool, useful from the individual to the institutional level.

Some of the pieces required for such computing support are already available, again, not as a single, integrated package.* The identification, testing, and

---

* This area is so active and evolving so rapidly that it is not possible for us to enumerate all the players. However, because there is so much interest, it might be useful for us to cite a few. Carnegie-Mellon, MIT, Minnesota, and Stanford are among a few institutions that have systems in use for some aspects of their research management. UCLA, in collabora-

implementation of a system to manage research administration is one of the biggest hurdles standing between UCSF and the success of this project.

The model is specifically designed to address the many problems of UCSF's research administration identified in phase 1 of this project. We anticipate that it will offer a host of benefits to all participants in the research administration process—faculty, staff, and sponsors—because it is designed explicitly with client needs in mind. By providing a consistently high level of service through LRAs and experts in the CRSU, the tools to help identify potential funding sources, the software to develop budgets and expenditure projections, and tools and training for large reductions in rework, the model should increase customer satisfaction dramatically.

Although the model is not expected to reduce UCSF's research administration costs, over the long term it will be an investment in the campus's research vitality. As faculty and staff avail themselves of training opportunities, tools, and technologies to reduce research administration burdens, faculty should be able to recapture time they can apply directly to their research activities.

The model seeks to reduce the level of nonvalue-added activities by having one point of contact for faculty, training staff in both pre- and postaward activities, integrating-technology systems, and by reducing the numbers of required approvals. By reducing staff time now lost to re-work, redundant data entry, or obtaining approvals, staff will be able to spend more time on value-added activities.

Instead of navigating through complex processes and dispersed central units to obtain service or find information, faculty will be able to obtain the full breadth of research administration services and avoid time-consuming and frustrating searching through one point of contact. CRSU staff will serve primarily as technical resources rather than transaction processors and approval authorities; redundancies across central units will be eliminated; and delegating authority for selected activities to the local level will minimize delays and internal

---

tion with IBM, is developing a system, called R/Net, that is intended to provide distributed processing capabilities for all of its research administration activities. A consortium of institutions is developing a system called GAMS, the Grants Administration Management System, that already partially meets the needs of the consortium's members. In the private sector, Oracle and PeopleSoft are developing research-management products that presumably will integrate with their current suites of financial and other management programs.

deadlines. Appropriate controls and training will be in place to ensure high-quality service and adherence to applicable policies and regulations.

As UCSF departs from the existing highly fragmented, transaction-based mode of support and, instead, provides service through the LRSUs, emphasis will be placed on providing comprehensive (cradle-to-grave) support to faculty. With full-time research administration staff supported by CRSU experts and a rigorous training and certification program, handoffs among staff will be minimized, with a concomitant increase in the consistency and quality of the work product. Even as LRSU staff build their individual skills, incentives will encourage teamwork so that LRAs can turn to each other as sources of expertise and knowledge in addition to turning to expertise of CRSU.

To coordinate and manage research administration effectively, the CRSU will report to one campus officer. In each of UCSF's smaller schools, the LRSUs will probably report to the associate dean, and, in the School of Medicine, to a chair or management-services officer of the department being served. This organizational structure eliminates the present functional management structure shown in figure 8 and facilitates a process-based structure. Moreover, authority and accountability for research administration will be aligned, facilitating the ease with which change can be managed, enabling consistent communication of policies and procedures, and representing a unified and consistent image to the external environment.

At both academic and central units, a new, integrated technology system for research administration will eliminate redundant data entry and maintenance of individual shadow systems. Moreover, staff will have access at any time to consistent, timely, and accurate information from a single source. Availability of on-line forms and templates will increase efficiency and timeliness, and routine and ad hoc reporting and analytical capabilities will enable individual staff to obtain required information quickly and manage the research portfolios of their respective principal investigators efficiently and effectively.

## SOME 'QUICK WINS'

During the course of this project, a number of examples of policies and procedures were identified that the Work Group, at first glance, believed could be changed immediately. However, close examination revealed that in many cases the proposed changes could have significant ramifications; thus, special attention had to be paid to limit quick changes to those that would not inadvertently wreak havoc. The Work Group therefore proposed, and the Steering Committee accepted, a set of criteria by which proposed changes could be assessed for feasibility. Proposals for such changes were reviewed carefully by the Work Group, then recommended to the Steering Committee, which had the authority to approve or disapprove them. Feasible changes became known as "Quick Wins." To be considered for Quick Win status, a proposed change had to (1) reduce the impact of a well-defined problem; (2) be part of a long-term solution (no Band-Aid); (3) produce a highly focused impact on research administration processes (with only negligible side effects that might inadvertently complicate other activities); (4) fall under the authority of no more than two departments; (5) require less than twelve weeks to implement; and (6) cost $20,000 or less.

The Work Group identified a number of candidate Quick Wins that met these criteria. To date, several have been implemented. For example:

- The campus has invested in several databases of funding opportunities and now offers access and instruction to faculty for using resources available on the Internet.
- Authorities were altered to simplify correction of certain accounting errors.
- Databases were modified to enhance tracking and reporting capabilities.
- Electronic linkages were established between some units with closely related responsibilities, facilitating data- and file-sharing.
- Web-based distribution mechanisms were established for some forms and templates that were lingering in diskette or paper format.

The Quick Wins served two purposes. First, they achieved rapid solutions to a number of simple and straightforward, but nagging, problems. Second, they emphasized that improvements could be made and, by being ascribed to RAP, they also enhanced project visibility and credibility.

## PHASE 3: IMPLEMENTATION
## OF THE MODEL

UCSF is now entering phase 3. It will take place in two stages. The first will be a pilot stage, anticipated to take about two years, in which a few pilot projects will test some of the assumptions of the model. An implementation team will be responsible for shepherding this stage, providing coordination, facilitation, expertise, and other needed support. Participation in pilot projects will be strictly voluntary; participants will be units with a desire to improve their research administration services and a commitment to see the model succeed. The second stage, which will occur once the model begins to prove itself, will be the expanded, long-term rollout to UCSF at large.

UCSF has had valuable experience with a client-oriented service model similar to the one described here; thus, an organizational model for research support services to the faculty is not novel. Some years ago, UCSF had an Environmental Health and Safety (EH&S) unit staffed by separate, specialized technologists for each of the required safety areas. Because each area had its own quasi-independent safety program, faculty were subjected to several different safety inspections, each from a different technologist; in addition, numerous contacts had to be made to get service for different problems. This way of doing business was, to be charitable, not very popular with the faculty.

In 1993, faculty discontent and other factors led to the decision to reorganize EH&S services along lines now echoed by the new research administration model. For example, once they are hired into the EH&S program, technologists (whatever their specialized backgrounds) receive training to make them into generalists who can deliver basic services in radiation, chemical, bio, or laboratory safety and also work collaboratively with laboratory personnel to comply with all laboratory safety requirements. Each UCSF laboratory has a single EH&S technologist assigned to it who conducts all inspections and handles the vast majority of its safety problems and questions. If necessary, complex problems or policy issues beyond the expertise of the technologist can be referred to specialists in the unit. Others conduct education and training programs.

There is no doubt that this single-contact, generalist model is strongly preferred by the faculty and offers better service than did its predecessor. UCSF has an exemplary laboratory safety record. The strength of the model, of course, is that service is delivered within the context of an established relationship between client and provider. In pioneering this model of service delivery, the UCSF Office of Environmental Health and Safety is a national model. The system also has unqualified administrative support: Since its inception, it has permitted the EH&S budget to be reduced by $2 million even as services and client satisfaction have been vastly improved.

## Pilot Stage

The pilot stage of the RAP will lay the foundation for the model. During this time, a few pilot studies will also be conducted to determine empirically the answers to some operational questions that cannot otherwise be adequately answered. The pilot stage is intended to achieve three principal goals. The first two will be pursued in parallel. However, pursuit of the third goal must await achievement of the first two goals. The goals are:

1. Install the technological (computing) foundation—Acquire and prepare to test the computer technology hardware and software necessary to support the new research administration model. This task is being referred to as the technology limb of the pilot phase.

At this stage of the project, we have conceptually redesigned research administration at UCSF but have not yet developed in detail how processes will flow through and among units for all types of grants, contracts, and other funding instruments. It is our intention to have our redesigned processes drive the technology, not the reverse. We must also develop methods for measuring progress and evaluating the effectiveness of the model.

2. Position the human resources and the organizational structures—In those academic units volunteering to participate, and among central support units, put in place the staffing and organizational components that the pilot projects required. This human resources limb will include:

- Development of job descriptions, training programs, and evaluation techniques for the new LRAs and CRSU staff.
- Recruitment of people to be trained as LRAs.
- Recruitment of academic units to participate in pilot projects.
- Organization of the LRSUs and the CRSU.
- Development of methodologies for data collection and analyses that

will permit evaluation of the pilot projects and of the new research administration model.

3. Test the new research administration model—Once the technology is available and the people and organizations are in place, the pilot projects will test the model in four different organizational units. Three will be academic units, the fourth will be the CRSU.

## Implementation Team

The six-member implementation team, reporting to the associate academic vice chancellor, will consist of one project manager, two computing experts to manage the technology limb, and three human resources experts to manage the HR limb (figure 12). The initial tasks of the team will be to work closely with personnel from both central and academic units to lay the foundation for the model. For example, the project manager, who must keep the project moving, will, among other tasks, coordinate, facilitate, monitor, and record the critical activity of redesigning work-flow to make it more efficient and effective. However, the highly detailed aspects of this redesign will rely heavily on personnel in academic and central units who are the day-to-day users—and current critics—of these processes. In a similar fashion, one of the HR experts will be skilled in the design and presentation of training programs, but program content (e.g., how to develop a project budget or properly prepare a protocol for the Committee on Human Research) must be supplied by existing campus experts.

Once pilot studies actually begin in central and local service units, the implementation team will shift some of its focus to work closely with these units to monitor, evaluate, troubleshoot, and facilitate logistical support.

## Evaluation

Evaluations during the pilot phase of RAP will address two basic questions. The first is: Does the new research administration model work? The answer requires obtaining the answers to four other questions:

1. Does the model result in higher levels of faculty and sponsor satisfaction than does the existing system?

2. Does the model satisfactorily meet the business requirements of the campus?

Figure 12
ORGANIZATION CHART, PROJECT IMPLEMENTATION PHASE, UCSF

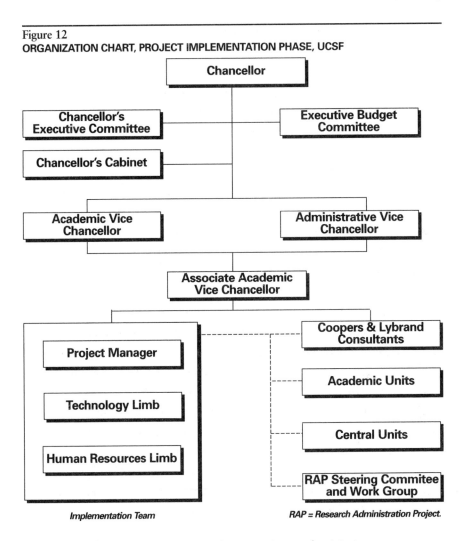

*Implementation Team*          *RAP = Research Administration Project.*

3.  Does the model increase administrative productivity?

4.  Do faculty served by the model spend less time at research administration than they did under the old system?

To get meaningful comparisons between the model and the current system, baseline data will be collected under current conditions; these benchmark data will be compared with data acquired under the model. For example, measures of customer satisfaction, error rates, and efficiency and productivity can all be made under both the current system and the model, allowing us to make comparative assessments of the old to the new.

The second basic question is: How can we make it work better? To answer this question, there are a great many other questions that should be asked. Among these are:

- Is training for staff appropriately designed? Are the certification levels for LRAs appropriate? Does the evaluation system for LRAs work?

- Is training for investigators appropriately designed? Is it reaching a sufficient number? Do they regard it as a service that adds value?

- Is compliance with university and sponsor requirements adequate? What improvements can be made to the technology?

- Do staff perceive that the model supports the six basic principles underlying its design: leadership, ethical standards, coherence as a system, a team approach, simplicity, and technological power? If not, what needs to be changed?

- What is the optimal number of faculty an LRA can serve effectively? What are the determinants of this decision: Number of grants? Number of contracts? A sum or ratio of these two? Total amount of funds managed? Amount of regulatory activity? Some combination of these that needs to be determined empirically?

- What is the optimal number of LRAs needed to create a fully functional LRSU? How does this vary by type of academic unit served? Are reporting lines acceptable and functional?

- Is communication among staff easy and effective? Do local staff get their questions answered by the central experts quickly, accurately, and with consistency?

As the pilot projects become better defined, mechanisms for collecting data to answer to such questions will also be developed. Evaluations will be an integral part of the project.

## Potential Pilot Projects

Discussions are currently under way with a few academic units that have indicated an interest in participating in the RAP. They will be chosen with care to achieve necessary diversity and permit us to answer a number of important questions. We seek the following types of academic units in which to conduct pilot studies.

The basic science departments in our School of Medicine are generally satisfied with their present research administration systems. However, we believe that offers of training, advanced technological capabilities, and delegation of some signature authorities may provide incentives for participation. In addition to providing data on the four principal evaluation questions (previously discussed), the inclusion of some basic science departments in this phase would enable us to make a direct comparison between the new research administration model and the current practices that appear to function at a high level of faculty satisfaction. Faculty satisfaction and adequacy of compliance would be specifically evaluated. In addition, because most of the funding in the basic sciences is via relatively simple instruments such as NIH grants, we would look carefully at questions related to the LRA composition and the training levels required to make up an optimal LRSU for the basic sciences. A pilot study conducted with an interdepartmental group in the basic sciences would also give us the opportunity to examine how well the model functions in a situation where there is only one LRA leader but more than one department chair.

We seek a cluster of units within one of our smaller schools as another test bed. In addition to providing data on the four principal evaluation questions, it is anticipated that a pilot project with some small schools would yield comparative data on how well the model functions compared to business-as-usual in other units in the school, as well as under conditions where, unlike the basic science departments in the School of Medicine, services may be limited and faculty satisfaction variable. Because the LRA might report to an associate dean, this pilot would also offer the opportunity to examine how well the model functions when it reports to someone other than the academic units it serves.

In our large clinical departments some faculty have high levels of research administration support and some who receive support with little continuity and inadequate skill levels. In addition to acquiring data on the four principal evaluation questions, this pilot would also help us evaluate three other important questions: (1) Is the training received by the LRAs adequate? (2) What is the optimal number of LRAs and mix of expertise and certification levels for a clinical department? (3) What is the best way to handle clinical trials— within a support unit with highly diversified portfolios or through a specialized, central clinical trials unit?

The new research administration model calls for all central services (e.g., contracts and grants, extramural funds accounting, certain regulatory activities, administration of gifts for research, relations with industry, legal support, conflicts of interest) to come together under a single umbrella to form the CRSU. Although this unit would retain some processing responsibilities (e.g., approving contracts with private sponsors), because the vast bulk of processing would eventually be decentralized to the academic units, the CRSU's major responsibilities will be to conduct training, disseminate information, maintain technology, provide expertise, solve problems, and interpret, develop, and promulgate policy. The CRSU itself might be divided into teams, each one responsible for providing support to a group of LRSUs if, indeed, this support would enhance CRSU service to LRSUs. Evaluation of the effectiveness with which the CRSU carries out its functions, and how well the team approach works, will allow us to optimize CRSU activities in support of the academic units.

## THE ROAD TO IMPLEMENTATION

Implementation of the new research administration model at UCSF will be difficult and complex, and almost certainly, at times, contentious. In an institution like UCSF, with a tradition of strong shared governance, the organizational changes required cannot simply be imposed from the top down as they might be in an industrial or military organization. Therefore, our fundamental strategy to ultimately achieve a change of the magnitude we propose is to start small, work with a handful of pioneers to demonstrate the superiority of the model in delivering high-quality service to selected academic units, and expand implementation as skeptics become believers.

### Managing Change

It is impossible to foresee all of the problems we might encounter. A few of the factors that can be predicted to create problems, and will have to be managed, are general resistance to change; organizational shifts—central vs. local responsibilities; shifts in the locus or balance of power, or both; changes in job duties; and fear of exercising authority.

## Providing Technological Support

Technologically, UCSF is not as fully developed as some other campuses; completing a network that serves all core facilities is a very high priority. In addition, UCSF has many smaller campuses scattered throughout San Francisco and beyond. Network issues notwithstanding, however, the complex, comprehensive software required to support the whole spectrum of research administration functions exists only in parts here and there. As a result, the technological challenges of this project abound. Among them are:

- Providing network access for all who require it.
- Providing research administration software that will support the entire spectrum of research administration needs.
- Offering training and support for users.
- Providing for data security and protection of confidentiality.

## Finding Financing

Implementing change of this magnitude is not cheap. There are one-time costs for conducting the RAP itself, and, of course, there will be ongoing operating costs of the model. Nevertheless, UCSF recognizes that the university cannot provide appropriate support to faculty in a time of intense competition for research funding with a decades-old, anachronistic system.

During the course of this project, the Work Group has never asserted that we would be able to deliver a research administration system that would save the campus money, at least in the long term. We believe that over both the short- and midterm, the model will cost somewhat more to operate than does the current system due to the need for more highly skilled (and therefore better paid) personnel, better and more extensive training, and advanced technological support. However, in the long term, after the model has been fully implemented, we believe it will pay handsome dividends through gains in the efficiency and effectiveness with which services will be delivered to the faculty and to sponsors. Therefore, we regard the RAP not merely as a short-term expense but as a long-term investment in UCSF's future.

We anticipate that the financial issues with which we will have to grapple will be fulfilling technological needs, financing personnel upgrades, financing the transition period (i.e., the costs of simultaneously operating the old and the new research administration systems), and sustaining the new system.

## Managing the Ripple Effects

Almost certainly, implementation of the new research administration model will have effects on other, nonresearch administration functions at UCSF. For example, the process of "defragmenting" personnel in order to generate full-time research administration staff will force administrative units to reorganize nonresearch administration staff. We believe it is probable that the new research administration model that delivers client-oriented services close to the site of need via better trained, technologically supported staff will quickly be seen as an attractive model adaptable to nonresearch administration.

## CONCLUSION

We have described here an ambitious endeavor to establish at UCSF a model for research administration that will be client oriented and technologically advanced and will create a wholly new cadre of research administrators dedicated to supporting the UCSF research enterprise. We believe it is essential to put such a system in place because our current transaction-based system is widely deemed by staff and faculty to be unsatisfactory and, in the emerging funding climate, may soon be unaffordable. We believe that a research administration model such as the one we describe will be an asset to UCSF faculty, supporting their competitiveness for research funding in what promises to be an intensively competitive environment in the 21st century.

# THE CLINICAL ENTERPRISE: CREATING NEW STRATEGIES AND STRUCTURES

*Robert J. Baker*

OR MANY YEARS, ACADEMIC HEALTH CENTERS occupied a privileged position. Standing above the fray, they were shielded from many of the competitive forces experienced in other portions of the health care economy. But the rules have changed. The contribution of academic health centers and their faculties to society at large is being questioned; as a result, the academic health center is being forced to achieve its longstanding tripartite mission of education, research, and service while using organizational structures that were not built to respond rapidly to market forces.

This report summarizes the market forces that threaten the clinical service portion of the three-way mission and adaptive strategies that will secure their futures. It should be viewed as a progress report as academic health centers must continue to experiment and to modify their strategies to keep pace with evolving markets. Today's academic health center leaders are more challenged than ever before. They entered the field when the clinical portion of the mission was, in many ways, a byproduct of its more sacred aspects: research and education. (For some centers, the clinical enterprise was, by definition, a laboratory in which research and education were performed.)

*Robert J. Baker is president and chief executive officer of the University HealthSystem Consortium.*

In a university with an academic health center, much of the academic health center's economic engine is often based in the medical school. If they are to serve as responsible stewards of their organizations, academic health center leaders must reinvent all three parts of the center's mission in response to the new, ever-changing health care economy.

## THE SUNSET OF A GOLDEN ERA

The academic health center responses to the major funding changes that occurred with the coming of Medicare and Medicaid are nearly perfect reflections of what society valued at the time. Medicare and Medicaid were launched in an era when universities were viewed as the sole source of the nation's innovation, freedoms of all types were being expanded, and, because society's problems were thought to be fixable through government intervention, money was pouring into the health care economy at an unprecedented rate. In such an environment, the opportunities for growth and development were so plentiful that medical school budgets and faculty practice plan and hospital earnings grew dramatically.

Thus, in the last quarter-century, four forces have shaped the nature of academic medicine:

• Government beneficence—Under Medicare and Medicaid, the promise of a single standard of care became a reality for much of America. Many of the nation's poor and elderly could be cared for by some of the nation's finest physicians in academic health center hospitals and clinics. Medicare and Medicaid programs also supported the training role of the academic health center through graduate medical education payments and disproportionate share funding.

• The promise of science and technology—The improvement in the public's health because of new technologies and drugs led to additional public and private support for research and the expansion of payments for specialty and subspecialty treatments and new procedures. Continuous growth in public support (especially at the National Institutes of Health) and in private support for biomedical research fueled growth in academic health center research programs.

• Growth of subspecialty medicine—Increased government funding supported the growth and development of the health care workforce and encouraged the training of additional physicians and nurses. Academic health centers were paid to increase the size of their residency programs and to develop the finest supply of health care professionals in the world. Growth in specialty residency programs and subspecialty fellowship training programs mirrored the growth of academic faculties.

• Enrichment of clinical departments and faculties—The growth of faculties, practice plans, and research revenue provided powerful, stable support for academic departments, equalizing compensation between academic physicians and their community counterparts and fostering a sense of entitlement among tenured faculty for a certain practice environment, lifestyle, and income.

## SOCIETY CHANGES ITS MIND

Each of these forces had a positive effect on academic health centers; the centers, in turn, met society's expectations. Today, however, society has changed its mind. The government is under fire for inefficiency and ineffectiveness. Former free-spending Democrats are espousing fiscal policy that is more conservative than that of Reagan-era Republicans. Health plans, politicians, and business leaders suspect that academic health centers may have wasted some of the money given to them. The scientific community has been criticized for being incapable of wiping out AIDS and cancer; focusing on pure or basic science while ignoring some of the systematic public health changes that could have saved many more lives; and spending public money unwisely. At the same time, the health care economy's rate of growth in expenditures is slowing as health plans and capitated groups learn to control costs. The frail and the ill are being forced into managed care systems designed to care for people who are essentially well, placing the frail and ill in a frustrating situation.

It was John Dewey, the educator and philosopher, who held that every perfect solution to a set of problems creates a new set of problems impossible to predict. Less-than-perfect solutions have an even worse effect. An extension of Dewey's logic to the recent changes in the health care economy implies that we should have expected problems and that rather than be frustrated by them, we should be stimulated by them. Academic health center leaders are being challenged to sustain the critical elements of their centers in an economy that has changed course. Indeed, the centers must stay ahead of the market, putting significant effort into trying to receive and interpret signals of the next revolution in health care so that they are not caught unprepared.

The most powerful segment of the health care industry today is the managed care industry. Health maintenance organizations (HMOs) are working as agents for large employers and the government in an effort to organize the health care system and control costs. Although the nation's health care spending in aggregate is not declining, premium costs have leveled off in many markets, as have enrollee premiums. This situation masks the underlying effects on providers overall and academic health centers in particular. A massive redistribution of the premium dollar is in motion. The big winners in this redistribution have been HMOs; these so-called arrangers-of-care have been richly rewarded by Wall Street (figure 1); the big losers have been hospitals and specialists.

## UHC MARKET CLASSIFICATION TOOL

The Market Classification Tool, developed by the University HealthSystem Consortium (UHC) in 1992 to track market development over time, provides a framework for examining underlying market structure, summary measurements of the relative role of payers and providers in creating change, and a shorthand to be employed in analyzing the relative impact of shifts in market structure.

---

Figure 1
**ESTIMATED HMO INDUSTRY EARNINGS BY TWO SURVEYS**

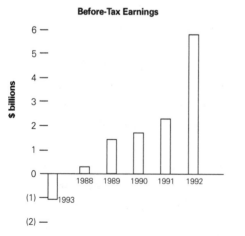
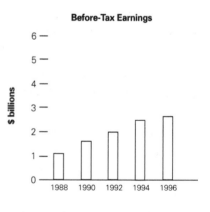

Source: Group Health Association of America. *Annual HMO Industry Survey*, 1995. Washington: GHHA.

Source: *The Warren Surveys Presents the HMO Salary Survey.* 1996. Rockford, IL: DeMarco Associates.

Dividing the health care market into four distinct stages of market competition—unstructured, loose framework, flux and consolidation, and hypercompetition—the UHC Market Classification Tool uses a number of variables, including HMO penetration, premium levels, and level of prepayment to physicians) to define the four stages. No one variable can accurately reflect the distinguishing characteristics of markets. For example, a standardized set of benefits in Boston (which has 44-percent HMO penetration) had an average monthly premium of $197 in 1995. In California's Orange County (which has 41-percent managed care penetration), the same level of benefits cost $123. It takes other variables to explain these differences.

*Stage 1, unstructured,* includes markets in which purchasing power is unfocused and providers are fragmented. Most reimbursement is through traditional fee-for-service, and reimbursement levels are relatively high. These markets offer health plans the opportunity to reduce payments to providers and share the savings with corporate payers.

In *stage 2, a loose framework* for financing and delivering services develops. Many health maintenance and preferred provider organizations pursue the market opportunity described in stage 1, enter these markets, and vie for growth and market position. Reimbursement quickly moves toward discounted charges and per diems, utilization begins to be managed, and excess capacity develops. Providers begin to affiliate.

A period of turmoil and rapid market development typifies *stage 3, flux and consolidation.* Dominant health plans emerge and look beyond price to utilization management to reduce costs. Big plans get bigger, acquisition occurs, and prices move to the lowest common denominator. Inpatient-use rates decline even further, and providers consolidate to remain clinically viable. Providers form virtual or vertically integrated networks to establish a stronger negotiating position with health plans and to share in the development of the infrastructure required to operate in a managed care environment. HMO enrollment is at 30 to 50 percent of the population. Specialist fees become heavily discounted, especially in markets where primary care physicians have organized. Risk-based reimbursement becomes more prevalent, and purchasers begin to measure their expectations in terms of cost per covered life and to profile physicians carefully so they can select those who contribute to reducing costs.

In *stage 4, hypercompetition,* a few large integrated provider systems, organized virtually or vertically, compete to provide comprehensive services to defined populations. The shape of the provider entities varies by market and can include independent practice associations (IPAs), proprietary physician networks, integrated delivery networks (IDNs), and proprietary hospital systems. Some markets, such as southern California, are dominated by large physician networks, others by aggressive payers. Payer alliances and large managed care organizations create a high degree of leverage, and payments to providers decline. As long as there is excess capacity in a market, endowments, funded

---

**Table 1**
**UHC MEMBER MARKET CLASSIFICATION, 1993**

| Stage 1– Unstructured | | Stage 2– Loose Framework | | Stage 3– Consolidation | | Stage 4– Managed Competition | |
|---|---|---|---|---|---|---|---|
| Nashville, TN | 1.5 | Chicago, IL | 2.3 | Los Angeles-Long Beach, CA | 3.2 | Minneapolis-St. Paul, MN-WI | 3.4 |
| Newark, NJ | 1.5 | Salt Lake City-Ogden, UT | 2.3 | Orange County, CA | 3.1 | | |
| New Orleans, LA | 1.5 | Tucson, AZ | 2.3 | San Diego, CA | 3.1 | | |
| Oklahoma City, OK | 1.5 | Cincinnati, OH-KY-IN | 2.2 | Portland-Vancouver, OR-WA | 3.0 | | |
| Toledo, OH | 1.5 | Dallas, TX | 2.2 | Sacramento, CA | 3.0 | | |
| Galveston-Texas City, TX | 1.4 | Houston, TX | 2.2 | Worcester, MA | 3.0 | | |
| Harrisburg-Lebanon-Carlisle, PA | 1.4 | Madison, WI | 2.2 | San Francisco, CA | 2.8 | | |
| Nassau-Suffolk, NY | 1.4 | Cleveland-Lorain-Elyria, OH | 2.1 | Denver, CO | 2.7 | | |
| Little Rock-North Little Rock, AR | 1.3 | Washington, DC | 2.1 | Seattle-Bellevue-Everett, WA | 2.4 | | |
| Pittsburgh, PA | 1.3 | Columbus, OH | 2.0 | | | | |
| Raleigh-Durham-Chapel Hill, NC | 1.3 | Philadelphia, PA-NJ | 2.0 | | | | |
| Augusta-Aiken, GA-SC | 1.2 | Albany-Schenectady-Troy, NY | 1.9 | | | | |
| Lexington, KY | 1.2 | Gainsville, FL | 1.9 | | | | |
| Omaha, NE-IA | 1.2 | St. Louis, MO-IL | 1.9 | | | | |
| Columbia, MO | 1.1 | Atlanta, GA | 1.8 | | | | |
| Charlottesville, VA | 1.0 | Richmond-Petersburg, VA | 1.8 | | | | |
| Morgantown, WV | 1.0 | Birmingham, AL | 1.7 | | | | |
| | | Hartford, CT | 1.7 | | | | |
| | | Indianapolis, IN | 1.7 | | | | |
| | | Middlesex-Somerset-Hunterdon, NJ | 1.6 | | | | |
| | | New York, NY | 1.6 | | | | |

Variables Included/Sources
• HMO penetration (double-weighted)/Interstudy Competitive Edge/Sachs Group
• HMOs with more than 100,000 enrollees/Interstudy Competitive Edge
• Percentage of total enrollees in the top three HMOs/Sachs Group
• Hospital occupancy/Interstudy Competitive Edge/Sachs Group
• Days/1,000/Interstudy Competititve Edge/Sachs Group
• Beds in systems (double-weighted)/Sachs Group
• Preferred Provider Organization consolidation/HMO/Preferred Provider Organization Directory
• State employees in HMOs/Seagal Co.
• Percentage of beds in systems that contract together/American Hospital Association
• Average pre-payment in groups with more than 15 physicians/ Interstudy Competitive Edge

depreciation, and retained earnings, providers seem to be willing to operate at a loss on their managed care business. Plans exploit the excess capacity to their advantage. Choice once again becomes important to consumers, who require providers to be low cost.

Contrary to widespread opinion, stage 4 should not be considered the end of the health care market evolution. Instead, it should be viewed as one stop on the way to a more substantive set of evolutionary changes that will change the process of care at least as much as the financing of care has done.

The classification tool is revised and updated periodically with the latest change occuring in 1996. Market stages are important when describing national differences and general market characteristics. Many markets have evolved to higher stages in the years from 1992 to 1996. The UHC Market Classification Tool provides a directional view of each market based on the best available nationally collected data (table 1). Strong local and regional variations within stages and markets require academic health centers to analyze their own markets rigorously, treating the classification of any specific market as a starting point and amending classification with the most reliable local data sources. Consideration must also be given to other factors ƒe.g., local culture, patient and customer attitudes, degree of physician integration, employer activism, and consumer sophistication ƒ that do not lend themselves to accurate quantification.

The reason to invest in continual market tracking is clear, namely, to be one of the organizations that has the advantage of advance knowledge. In 1996, UHC conducted extensive analysis and review of the major markets of UHC members (table 2). Three findings were clear.

1. Prices fall as markets move from stage 1 to stage 4.
2. Funds available to providers are now going to organizations that organize care and manage utilization.
3. Markets consolidate as evolution proceeds.

## MARKET IMPLICATIONS FOR THE TRIPARTITE MISSION

Changes in market structure affect each part of the academic health center mission (figure 2). The acceleration of provider consolidation and the growth of managed care (especially the channeling of increasing amounts of care paid

## Table 2
## UHC MEMBER MARKET CLASSIFICATION, 1996
**(Remaining original variables plus five new variables)**

| Stage 1– Unstructured | | Stage 2– Loose Framework | | Stage 3– Consolidation | | Stage 4– Hypercompetition | |
|---|---|---|---|---|---|---|---|
| Augusta-Aiken, GA | 1.5 | Gainesville, FL | 2.0 | Salt Lake City-Ogden, UT | 2.9 | Minneapolis-St. Paul, MN-WI | 3.5 |
| Charleston-North Charleston, SC | 1.5 | Harrisburg-Lebanon-Carlisle, PA | 2.0 | Milwaukee-Waukesha, WI | 2.8 | Sacramento, CA | 3.5 |
| Iowa City, IA | 1.5 | Lexington, KY | 2.0 | Denver, CO | 2.7 | Portland-Vancouver, OR-WA | 3.4 |
| Knoxville, TN | 1.5 | Pittsburg, PA | 2.0 | Baltimore, MD | 2.5 | Los Angeles-Long Beach, CA | 3.3 |
| Middlesex-Somerset-Hunterdon, NJ | 1.5 | Indianapolis, IN | 1.9 | Memphis, TN | 2.5 | San Diego, CA | 3.3 |
| Mobile, AL | 1.5 | Nashville, TN | 1.9 | Worcester, MA | 2.5 | San Jose, CA | 3.3 |
| Shreveport-Bossier City, LA | 1.5 | Hartford, CT | 1.8 | Cincinnati, OH-KY-IN | 2.4 | Orange County, CA | 3.2 |
| Charlottesville, VA | 1.4 | New Haven, CT | 1.8 | Seattle-Bellevue Everett, WA | 2.4 | San Francisco, CA | 3.2 |
| Little Rock-North Little Rock, AR | 1.4 | New York, NY | 1.8 | Albany-Schenectady-Troy, NY | 2.3 | Madison, WI | 3.0 |
| Morgantown, WV | 1.4 | Syracuse, NY | 1.8 | Boston, MA-NH | 2.3 | Tucson, AZ | 3.0 |
| Columbia, MO | 1.3 | Nassau-Suffolk, NY | 1.7 | Cleveland-Lorain-Elyria, OH | 2.3 | | |
| Greenville, NC | 1.2 | Newark, NJ | 1.7 | Kansas City, MO-KS | 2.3 | | |
| | | Birmingham, AL | 1.6 | Atlanta, GA | 2.2 | | |
| | | Galveston-Texas City, TX | 1.6 | Chicago, IL | 2.2 | | |
| | | Greensboro—Winston-Salem—High Point, NC | 1.6 | Columbus, OH | 2.2 | | |
| | | Omaha, NE-IA | 1.6 | Houston, TX | 2.2 | | |
| | | Raleigh-Durham-Chapel Hill, NC | 1.6 | Philadelphia, PA-NJ | 2.2 | | |
| | | | | Richmond-Petersburg, VA | 2.2 | | |
| | | | | St. Louis, MO-IL | 2.2 | | |
| | | | | Toledo, OH | 2.2 | | |
| | | | | Washington, DC | 2.2 | | |
| | | | | Ann Arbor, MI | 2.1 | | |
| | | | | Dallas, TX | 2.1 | | |
| | | | | Oklahoma City, OK | 2.1 | | |

Variables Included/Sources
- HMO penetration (double-weighted)/Interstudy Competitive Edge/Sachs Group
- HMOs with more than 100,000 enrollees/Interstudy Competitive Edge
- Percentage of total enrollees in the top three HMOs/ Sachs Group
- Hospital occupancy/Interstudy Competitive Edge/Sachs Group
- Days/1,000/Interstudy Competititve Edge/Sachs Group
- Beds in systems/Sachs Group
- Percentage of specialists capitated (new variable)/ Interstudy Competitive Edge
- Percentage of the Medicare population in HMOs (new variable)/Interstudy Competitive Edge
- Percentage of the Medicaid population in HMOs (new variable)/ Interstudy Competitive Edge
- Commercial HMO premium (double-weighted) (new variable)/Milliman & Robertson
- Medicare average annual per capita cost (area wage adjusted) (new variable)/Health Care Financing Administration

Figure 2
PERCENT CHANGE IN DAYS AND DISCHARGES OF UHC MEMBERS
BETWEEN 1993 AND 1996

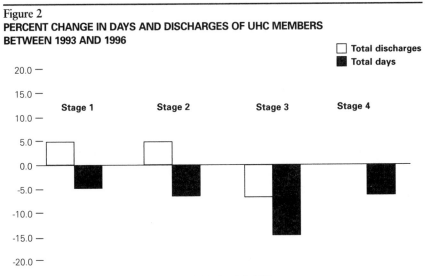

Source: University HealthSystem Consortium database. 1997. Oakbrook, IL: UHC

for by Medicare and Medicaid into managed care) are combining to threaten the ability of academic health centers to support their clinical, research, and education missions financially. As Medicare shifts to capitation, clinical revenue (especially hospital revenue) declines and, as of this writing, payments for teaching disappear. Grant funding remains concentrated. (Nearly half of all NIH dollars go to only twenty medical schools.) Faculty income continues to decline, causing a reduction in academic compensation. In short, academic health centers may no longer be able to carry out their mission.

Reduced reimbursement for clinical services inhibits clinical research, teaching, and training in two ways. One, referring physicians who are at risk for some or all of the cost of patient care may choose not to send patients to academic health center specialists who could cost more than other specialists because of subsidization, inclusion of patients in clinical research studies, or the additional costs incurred by involving trainees and students in the process of care. Two, academic health centers, which often receive contracted per diem or per case reimbursement, are aggressively examining their clinical, operational, and financial processes to determine if they can continue to provide indirect support for clinical research, teaching, or training from these fixed, limited reimbursements. As a result, traditional perquisites that support clinical research, teaching, and training will be identified, quantified, and subjected to investment criteria similar to those applied to other uses of funds.

Some academic health centers are also experiencing the explicit channeling of patients away from clinical trials and the refusal of managed care organizations to support any form of research that could eventually result in new, high-cost benefit requirements. Listen to what four health care providers from different parts of the country have to say:

> Stage Three cancer patients are counseled into hospice. We haven't been involved in any protocols since the mid-70s.— Capitated physician and group medical director in the West

> We might contract with an academic health center for tertiary care—but your physicians will want to put them [patients] into protocols. We can assure you that the minute you do that, you've blown the economics.— HMO CEO in the Midwest

> We offered to put the patient into the protocol at our own expense. We were confident it would work. We couldn't get an authorization. If it works, eventually they will have to pay for it.—Academic health center executive in the West

Most academic health center leaders are well acquainted with the need to develop integrated delivery systems, networks, and primary care capacity. As fig-

**Figure 3**
**CONTEXT FOR CONSOLIDATION IN HEALTH CARE**

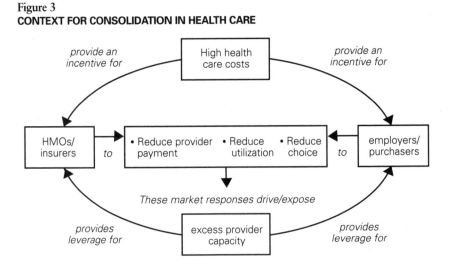

ure 3 shows, costs drive many of the changes in the market. High health care costs provide the incentive for HMOs, insurers, employers, and purchasers to find ways of reducing payments to providers, utilization of services by patients, and consumer choice of providers. Excess capacity gives insurers and purchasers leverage to insist on further cost reductions, which reduces the use of and need for inpatient care even more in maturing markets. Thus, collaborative linkages are becoming increasingly attractive to academic health centers.

The accelerated consolidation in the hospital industry directly affects support for the underfunded aspects of the academic health center's tripartite mission, as well as care for the poor. For-profit hospitals entering into ownership agreements with academic health center hospitals will be closely examining these kinds of support and will limit them. It is not clear, for example, whether formal support for research, contracted for as part of the sale, will completely replace the informal, unquantified support that existed for that purpose before the sale. New entities composed of university and community hospitals must also address these issues as these new organizations attempt to become cost-competitive. Many academic health center leaders believe that the underfunded costs of safety-net services, teaching, and research cannot be sustained in the new environment. Explicit levels of funding for each must be agreed to and managed.

Managed care affects physician revenue later than it affects hospital revenue. In the early stages of market evolution, specialist physicians are still being paid through a fee for service reimbursement system, although at a discount. Many patients still have direct access to academic physicians. In fact, revenue grew for most academic health center faculty group practices in early-stage markets. This trend reverses in later market stages as at-risk, primary-care referring physicians rechannel patients. Specialists, in turn, assume more risk through global fee arrangements or by accepting capitation themselves, either directly or as part of a physician group or clinical enterprise that contracts to provide care to a defined population.

The declining physician revenue directly affects the ability of academic health center faculty to engage in underfunded activities. A number of academic health centers are developing methods for clinical faculty to define their teaching, research, and patient-care activities more accurately. The funding support for each area is then explicitly identified. Standards of productivity for clinical faculty are also being developed, often using nonacademic production measures. Both developments will make it more difficult for academic health center faculty to devote time to academic activities unless the activities have a defined source of funding.

All these changes underscore the need for academic health centers to be closer to the center of the policy and operational decision-making process. Academic health centers are better off serving as masters of their own fate than remaining passive recipients of policies made by those who don't understand the full implications of market changes for patients, science, and health care in the United States.

## THE NEED FOR EFFECTIVE STRUCTURE
## AND LEADERSHIP

Responses to the current reimbursement changes and market requirements differ from, and also are more difficult than, those required in the past. Today, academic health centers are being asked to spend and do less, and the required changes are interdepartmental instead of departmental, and clinically driven instead of academically driven. They have led to the emergence of the clinical enterprise* as the organizing entity, rather than the university, medical school, or hospital taking this role. Fundamental changes in academic health center ownership, governance, and management structures—not simply different tactics—are required.

Some academic health center ownership structures set up barriers that impede the organization's ability to respond quickly to changes in the market. These barriers vary according to institution and can include civil service requirements, political interference, and financial considerations. In an environment that demands absolute flexibility, timely decision-making, risk-taking, and freedom to act, such structural impediments complicate the academic health center's ability to act aggressively and decisively. They place the center at risk for failing economically and for being unable to fulfill its missions.

When structural barriers to speedy decision-making and flexibility seem insurmountable, a change in the ownership of at least the clinical enterprise com-

---

* The clinical enterprise comprises the following components of an academic health center: hospital, group practice, and network partners.

ponent of the academic health center may be appropriate. Governing bodies that can focus specifically on the issues facing the clinical enterprise are more able to take decisive, risk-oriented action than those that are responsible for a broader entity. When current ownership structures are retained, academic health centers must focus on removing legal requirements and processes that hinder the ability to be competitive.

In sum, although no single organizational structure can guarantee success in the current health care market, all academic health centers need a structure that will enable them to make decisions quickly, take and manage risk, respond in a unified manner, collaborate with other providers and insurers, and demonstrate value in terms of cost, quality, and service.

The academic health center's governing board must be committed to achieving the center's three-part mission while supporting a bias for action. It must have sufficient authority to improve organizational performance and accountability, and the ability to enable or create the capacity for change within the organization. The board must also have the time and energy to focus on the needs of the market and the clinical enterprise if it is to fulfill its responsibilities. The clinical enterprise cannot afford to compete for the time and attention of the governing board.

The board should be close enough to the CEO and other leaders to understand and support strategic initiatives, yet be willing to provide considerable freedom to the organization's leaders so they can operate and make decisions quickly. They should be selected to ensure the mix of skills required to operate in the current health care environment and have sufficient stature to add value to the organization's external relationships. Board members must be committed, informed, accountable, and free of conflicts of interest. They should represent multiple constituencies, including the hospital, education, research, group practice, the community, and business.

The traditional academic health center culture is quite risk averse, but in today's health care environment, risk-taking has become essential. At all levels of the academic health center, quality of leadership is the critical variable determining how well the organization manages the changes required in a rapidly evolving environment. Within a supportive ownership and governance structure, leaders must be willing and able to take substantial risks in making changes that often conflict with the tradition and culture of the organization.

Academic health center leaders must focus clearly on developing and articulating the organization's mission and must overcome the divisive forces that seek to preserve traditional prerogatives. They must:

- Break down internal boundaries and barriers
- Alter the flow of funds throughout the organization
- Change control points
- Modify power structures
- Redefine values

Leaders must also clearly understand the market and environment in which the academic health center operates, define and communicate a common vision, reward risk-taking, build trust, develop external relationships, recruit excellent people, and be consistent, disciplined, focused, and politically savvy.

## STRATEGIC PORTFOLIO APPROACH

Academic health centers must also be equipped to consider new strategies and tactics. In this era of continuous change and chaos, the systematic pursuit of clearly defined, stable strategies is not an option, and, at many academic health centers, the change process has been significant and continuous. Leaders are devoting their efforts to a process of strategic management—putting processes and work groups in place to pursue the development, implementation, and continuous revision and fine-tuning of market-based strategies in a fluid and changing environment.

Successful center leaders compare the strategic management process in which they are engaged to portfolio management, which involves the simultaneous execution of multiple change processes each one addressing one element of the strategic change portfolio being pursued. The most common elements that make up the academic health center strategic change portfolio are channel management strategies, infrastructure development, lobbying and government relations, cost management and reduction (including the implementation of new economic systems), group practice formation, physician development, and the development of a full range of providers within the network. These elements should not be looked at as the total package but only as suggestive of the range of elements that might be included in an academic health center strategic portfolio.

Each year, different elements of the strategy may gain prominence in response to changes in the market. The process of strategic portfolio management is not fixed and is never complete. Midcourse corrections are necessary as the organization is buffeted by the changing market.

## Integrated Delivery Network

A core element of academic health center competitive strategy is the development of an integrated delivery network (IDN). A network organized around value creation can result in a vehicle that rebalances the competitive positions of payers and providers in local markets. The road to successful network development is developed over time, and often is littered with bad ideas, poor timing, unworkable structure, and muddy thinking. This discussion reflects what academic health centers have learned in network development so far. It is the best of what is known, not the answer.

Many of the arguments made in favor of IDN development are protectionist rather than market-oriented. A common assertion is that the network will create economies of scale. However, such economies are elusive, especially initially or when a virtual network is the preferred structure. A network might defray the costs of new infrastructure development, especially in network management and information systems. A network might also accommodate the movement of specialists into affiliated hospitals, which can increase the stability of specialty programs. Finally, a network might allow the academic health center to control or effectively intercept the patient channels established by payers or physician groups. Each of these arguments reflects benefits to the academic health center, not benefits to the market. In the experience of academic health center network builders, these arguments may have some appeal in selling the network internally but are better looked at as byproducts of the development of a market-responsive clinical entity with real staying power, not as products themselves.

The first premise of network development is that it needs to be market-driven. Extensive research with payers, including managed care organizations, business coalitions, and large employers indicates that the networks should have the following characteristics if they are to demonstrate distinctive and sustainable value in the marketplace.

- Costs that are at or near market levels, with a premium available only for services that are unique or especially desirable to the payer, patients, or physician groups.

- Accessible, well-located physicians and sites that are attractive to employers and patients.

- A stable and growing network with high service standards that has loyal patients, primary care physicians, and specialists.

- The ability to take and manage risk for all segments of the payer market, including global packages, subcapitation, full capitation, and discounted fee for service across all segments of the payer market.

- Innovative service design, especially as a result of the scientific inquiry that is at the heart of the academic health center.

- Selected service uniqueness and many of the most attractive providers in the market that allow the academic health center network to stand toe-to-toe with purchasers in negotiations.

- The ability to execute complex strategies to maintain differentiation. In many ways, every provider is trying to network to create market power. Academic health center IDNs need to be "differently better," that is, differentiated in a way that is difficult for others to replicate.

- The ability to shift strategy to respond to market changes. To sustain its edge in the market, the network needs to be a "learning organization."

The academic health center network must be built to serve the market so well that it surpasses other networks in competitiveness. The appeal of belonging to a network is often overplayed, for example, when it is viewed as a magic bullet that could protect the organization from the effects of the market. At a recent eastern urban academic health center planning retreat, one department chair said, "Once they (a community hospital and its management service organization [MSO]) are in our network, we can just make them use us for all specialty care." However, an important tenet of network development can be stated as follows: No network can indemnify a network participant from the effects of changes in the market for its services. The corollary is that the only network participants who will willingly participate in an activity not in their best interest on a sustained basis are merged participants who can see some other benefit for themselves within the organization.

Finally, a network cannot be organized around protectionism; if it expends its precious resources supporting dying programs, or overcompensating some network members at the expense of others, it will fail. Instead, a network should be viewed as a way to create new linkages with participants that can each benefit from the delivery of better care to patients under contract with payers. It provides the opportunity for additional exchanges among participants, is more closely linked to the community, and provides a more organized and responsive structure for systematic innovation in product and service design in response to market signals.

An academic health center can use one of four options in developing a role in an integrated delivery network: build, join, serve, or exit. Each approach has its pros and cons, and each has been successfully pursued by more than one academic health center. There is no one right answer for all academic health centers, only a number of observations and key lessons from those pursuing these strategies.

*1. Build.* The appeal of building an academic health center network or becoming a network integrator is strong. But the costs are very high. In the rush to be in control, the cost of the system, including acquisition payments for hospitals, physician groups, and other network development elements, is often underestimated. In addition, the competitive response of the market to the formation of a powerful new academic health center network could close off referrals and bring on formation of stronger competing networks. The potential moves of competitors should be considered in depth. To assess the effects of organizing a large portion of the market on those not included, academic health center leaders should play out the strategy of each competitor in response to each strategy under consideration.

For many providers not accustomed to working in a managed care environment, the potential downside of absorbing operating losses is often ignored. The shock of these losses, as well as their sheer scale, is one of the early moments of truth. Dividing dollars within the system across academic and nonacademic participants is another challenge for network builders. They must show supreme wisdom if they are to maintain balance within the network. Yet, University

## Table 3
### OPTIONS FOR BUILDING HOSPITAL NETWORKS

| Acquire | Merge | Create Operating Company | Share Managed Care Hub or Contracting Network | Divest Hospital |
|---|---|---|---|---|
| Initiator appoints other's board<br><br>Older owner generally distressed or very visionary<br><br>AHC as acquirer or seller | New, shared corporation<br><br>Both must be willing to cede control for common good | Quasi-merger— much easier for public institutions<br><br>Operating company leases facilities from individual boards<br><br>Operating company has total budget purchasing and capital authority | Hospitals stay independent<br><br>Strong strategy: jointly financed, formed, managed<br><br>Weak or start-up strategy: contract jointly/PPO<br><br>Market position but not operating control | Use capital from sale to build network or other academic components, retaining access to AHC facility or faculty |
| *Cleveland*<br>*UMass*<br>*NYH* | *BJC*<br>*Stanford/UCSF*<br>*Methodist/*<br>*Indiana* | *Cincinnati* | *Chicago*<br>*UMass*<br>*OHSU* | *Tulane*<br>*Minnesota* |

Hospitals of Cleveland Health System, University of Chicago Health System, Pennsylvania HealthCare System and Partners HealthCare System in Boston, as well as major systems in other states have all succeeded in this role (table 3). Strong leadership, financial acumen, market knowledge, and adequate capitalization are required to succeed in network building.

*2. Join.* Many academic health centers are choosing to join with other dominant nonacademic providers in a network that is not managed by the academic health center but is a partnership anticipated to be extremely successful in the local market. This strategy can be highly successful, but like the other options, poses significant risks. However, it may not require as dramatic a shift in role for the academic health center, and allows the academic health center leadership to remain somewhat partisan to the academic health center mission.

One risk of participating in a network built by others is that management might not appreciate the academic mission. In many ways this mission may become incidental to the network's clinical strategy. On the other hand, many enlightened, large community-based systems and provider-related health plans have embraced the need to move training to the community and HMO-practice setting. One of the most difficult issues in the negotiation of these relationships is assessing the relative commitment of the potential partner to the academic cause. The Health Alliance of Cincinnati, Penn State Geisinger Health System, and Clarion Health Care (Indiana University/Methodist) have each pledged financial and programmatic support to the academic mission. Thomas Jefferson University Hospital/Main Line Health System and Washington University/BJC Health Systems, Inc., in St. Louis are also successful examples of academic health center-community hospital mergers with promise.

3. *Serve.* A Swiss strategy—in which the academic health center remains nonaligned, in service to all with luck, and leverages its unique clinical programs—is possible where a unique market position can be achieved. The major risk here is that the large community hospitals populated by academic health center trainees will replicate many or all of the highly specialized treatments currently available at the academic health center. This situation can leave the academic health center with the costs of serving as a safety net, the costs of the underfunded parts of the academic health center missions, and the costs of the remaining highly specialized services that cannot yet be performed profitably in a community hospital setting.

The nonaligned strategy is the most common in children's hospitals, which have been successful in negotiating for higher reimbursement from health plans, and is also more common where only one academic health center is available regionally. The newly merged Stanford/University of California, San Francisco organization, the University of Utah, and the University of Washington are three organizations that are pursuing this strategy with some success.

4. *Exit.* The final strategic option is to exit by selling the hospital to another entity and then focusing the energies of academic health center leaders on research and education. Several academic health centers have followed this strategy, employing the proceeds of the sale and usually an ongoing payment from the acquirer as support for academic programs.

Decisions to exit are usually made by organizations that view the sale of the hospital as a way to achieve a market position and to overcome some insurmountable barriers to responding to the market as a stand-alone entity. In some cases, the hospital is losing money and is perceived to be a threat to the financial viability of the university. In other cases, the region has consolidated into a small number of health systems, and the academic hospital has found its network-building limited to the for-profit chain in the area. Some academic health centers are handicapped by an impossible governance structure that limits their ability to successfully respond to the market. To them, selling the hospital to an organization that is not so limited might be the only option. Often, the businesslike behavior of the partner, and its sheer discipline in management, have great appeal.

The risks involved in the sale of the hospital are relatively clear. First, good business people do not provide financial support to worthy, but money-losing programs. Second, the symbiosis between the hospital and faculty in the current academic health center environment can fade away. The experiences of academic health centers that have chosen this route lead to the conclusion that all supports and transactions need to be explicitly included in the contract at the time of sale; renegotiation is unlikely. In fact, all sellers should be aware that the team that made the deal, as well as the company, might be sold at any time. In one case, a highly visible transaction for the purchase of a large integrated health care system by a for-profit corporation was executed on a Friday. The purchasing corporation announced its sale to another for-profit the following Monday. And all but one of the executives who made the deal to acquire the system were gone from the new for-profit.

Another risk is created by the permanence of the deal. It is highly unlikely that the sale of the hospital to another entity can be reversed. Many academic health centers are in hypercompetitive markets and are still very profitable. In that case, the sale of a hospital that is unprofitable may be the wrong move. A better move might be to recruit new management that can return the center to profitability. The faculty should be made aware of the freedoms they could lose in the sale—from purchasing to maintaining an information system that supports their special research interests. Nevertheless, several academic health centers have made this move and believe they will be very successful. St. Joseph Hospital of Creighton University in Omaha was one of the first university hospitals sold to a for-profit. Tulane University, Medical University of South Carolina, the University of Oklahoma, and others have sold or are close to having the necessary approvals to sell. Creighton University and Tulane University have reported success in their respective relationships with Tenet Healthcare Corp. and Columbia HCA Healthcare Corp.

The role of the managed care contract within an integrated delivery network is often overstated by people with little experience in a managed care environment. Early in the development of managed care, faculty would say, "Why do we need to do anything different? All we need is the right contractor to get us a contract to bring us all the patients we need." Managed care contracts only rarely "herd" patients, like cattle, to the door of a provider. Instead, managed care creates new financial relationships and boundaries within which consumers can exercise choices. A managed care contract is like a fishing license. It allows a provider to dip a line in the pond, but it doesn't guarantee that the provider will catch its limit. Therefore, the network should be organized so that each of its elements consists of providers that compete effectively in their own segment of the market.

It is also worthwhile to reflect on the core product of the managed care plan. Managed care plans are extremely dependent on their contracted providers. Except for staff model and close group/network model HMOs such as HIP and Kaiser-Permanente that "sell" their own providers, a managed care plan sells its network of contracted providers, its price, and on occasion its hassle-free product design and administrative systems. In many markets, the price band within which plans sell is so narrow that all that can be sold are the network and the level of choice offered the enrollee.

If an academic health center has signed with a plan, the academic health center and the plan's network must both successfully call two "moments of truth" before the first patient visit can take place. The first is when the vice president of human resources or the benefits plan manager of a potential corporate buyer is in the process of selecting a plan. If the benefits director is assured that the right providers are in the network for the employee population and the price/product is right, there is a sale. The second moment of truth occurs when the enrollee reviews the health plan's directory of providers. If the enrollee's preferred provider is in the network, has an open practice, and the financial incentives are right, the plan is selected. Now the plan's physicians compete the old-fashioned way, that is, by being the preferred option for individuals when they seek medical care.

Physicians can no longer attract many patients directly. Instead, they must attract enrolled lives. If the academic health center does not offer physicians who can compete effectively, or have close ties with or own practices, it will be incapable of sustaining an adequate volume of patients to carry out its three-part mission. The scale of specialty and tertiary care required to teach subspecialty medicine, as well as the need to train clinicians in all aspects of patient care (including primary and ambulatory care), argues for a solid network strategy. Otherwise, clinical trials will not fill, and patient volumes will decline to a level that sends the faculty practice and the hospital into financial difficulty. A powerful network strategy can help academic health centers avoid this ending.

Network builders from some of the most successful academic health center networks in the nation have created a common set of network elements and core infrastructure requirements based on their experience (figure 4). According to them, the successful IDN has the following features:

• Primary care—Despite the advent of "open access" models, primary care physicians will form the first line of patient management and system access for the foreseeable future. Consumers, insurers, and employers demand neighborhood-based, physically attractive, easily accessible offices staffed by primary care and high-volume specialists. It is impossible to compete for enrolled lives without primary care physicians.

• Specialty care—The primary care network needs to be backed by a well-integrated group of excellent specialist clinicians willing to work as partners with primary care physicians and play by the financial and process rules of managed care medicine with energy and vigor. The effective interdisciplinary and longitudinal management of the chronically or seriously ill populations is essential to the success of any prepaid network and will be one of the most significant points of differentiation in the future.

• Hospital networks—Hospital networks are an essential element in network development in many markets. Often, hospital consolidation has preceded physician organization and consolidation. Typically, the only organizing force within the market is the hospital; physicians remain poorly organized and lack important infrastructure. Hospital networks have also been very successful in removing excess hospital capacity from overbedded markets and in stabilizing the delivery system while doing so.

## Figure 4
### ELEMENTS OF THE INTEGRATED DELIVERY NETWORK

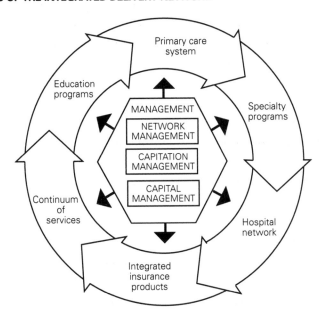

• Integrated insurance products—A number of academic health centers have sponsored the development of local health plans to attract enrolled lives for their networks and to develop the capacity to accept and manage partial and global risk. In some markets, the development of a competing health plan motivates other health plans to exclude the academic health center. The strategy is, again, market-specific. With or without a health plan, every academic health center must be able to accept capitation, bundled payments, or packages and share risk without political strife or financial losses.

• Continuum of care services—The reduction in hospital use is one of the greatest areas of savings in a managed care environment. Managing hospital-use ethically and responsibly demands close clinical and administrative relationships with a host of home care, step-down, subacute, and nursing home services. Many academic health centers are developing owned services. Others are developing them by extending their networks beyond community hospitals.

• Education programs—Three major reasons for education programs complete the continuum. First, the principal reason most academic health centers develop networks is to sustain their clinical base and to have access to additional teaching sites so they can continue to have outstanding training and educational programs. Second, many community networks are attracted to the academic health center because it provides the capacity to train new primary care physicians and assist in developing managed care physicians. Third, there will be a significant educational effort in retraining staff and physicians. The lack of a workforce that is knowledgeable about managed care is perhaps the greatest barrier to success.

Although each of the above network elements is important, the dual strategy of building primary care capacity and developing specialty services deserves a more detailed discussion.

The primary care physicians who form the "front door" for enrollees to join the network should share the objectives of the network and its customers; be responsive to network medical management, service, and administrative process requirements; and maintain open panels for network patients. Network integrators must assemble a large cadre of primary care practitioners who will fulfill these requirements. In many markets, this approach has required acquisition of practices or direct hiring of physicians. Alternatives include network funding of group practice and IPA formation, expanding clinical faculty, and creating service organizations aimed at managing independent community practices more efficiently and effectively (thus, in theory, allowing physicians to increase volume and decrease costs).

Primary care strategies have been among the most successful and important for many academic health centers. In many cases, building a primary care network is the only means of sustaining access to full-service managed care populations. However, this strategy requires new skills, new infrastructure, and often the recapitalization or buyout of the primary care practices themselves, and the market is requiring a premium for all these costs.

The sum of these costs—new information technology platforms, new staff and overhead, new organizational costs and start-up, and debt service on practice purchase—substantially burdens the primary care organization. These costs should be accounted for across the network. More often, they are added to the profits and losses of the primary care practices. What were essentially break-even cottage businesses now appear to be essentially uneconomical.

However, when the collateral revenues saved as a consequence of incremental managed care market share are factored into the equation, the value of the primary care network becomes clear. Moreover, information management, physician management, contracting, and coordination skills critical to a network's competitiveness are often most rapidly and effectively developed through the primary care physician management system.

Finally, without such networks, most network members would be suffering significant loss of market share. With them, despite persistent profitability problems in the practices and practice management organization itself, the network gains crucial advantages, for example:

- Essential skills that otherwise would need to be capitalized elsewhere.
- The ability to contract for and keep clinical control over fully covered lives.
- The skill base and credibility required to negotiate for risk and management-related portions of the premium dollar.

Specialty programs, long a strong fundamental distinction for all academic health centers, have become vulnerable. But specialty services are fundamental to academic health center strategy, and the centers do have significant opportunities to build strategic advantage and maintain margins. Academics can capitalize on unique clinical developments and excellent outcomes. They can coordinate resources to span and integrate services and sites of care. Opportunities exist to create multispecialty clinical teams to render comprehensive, well-managed care. Academic health centers can also redouble their efforts in a few "legacy" strategies that have worked for decades. Academic health centers that have launched effective networks have cautioned that developing specialty services is so attractive it might shift attention away from the other vital aspects of building an IDN.

However, no home run strategies exist in specialty care. Successful strategies rely on enrollee-referral volume from multiple contracts plus relationships to sustain patient access to specialty programs. Academic health centers should also begin to take chances and experiment. They must foster entrepreneurship among clinicians, creating an environment in which innovation, service orientation, and patient care are valued and compensated in accordance with their contribution to the ultimate survival of the organization.

Specialty strategies are idiosyncratic. No one strategy works across all markets. Academic health centers must develop strategies that take into account the characteristics of major diseases treated by clinical specialties. Disease characteristics affect how payers view contracting opportunities and determine the feasibility of financial terms and the extent of geographic coverage considered essential.

Legacy strategies continue to show significant return on investment in most markets. These strategies should not be abandoned as they continue to attract substantial patient volume by establishing strong referral relationships, delivering on the promise of service, and reaffirming the reputation of the academic health center for unparalleled technological innovation and expertise.

Marketing and contracting support will have to become much more sophisticated to support the development of specialty care products. Current academic health center investment in marketing and contracting is not adequate to support specialty product development. The centers must invest heavily in professional marketing and payer contracting capacity while expanding their information systems and medical service organization infrastructure to support specialty product development and the crucial reorganization of faculty practice plans. Service line management should be considered as a way of supporting the delivery of innovation to the market.

Finally, it must be realized that specialty networks complement, but do not replace, broad primary care initiatives. The most successful specialty physician organization will include physicians who are attractive to payers because of their clinical productivity, economic efficiency, accessibility, reputation, and sometimes outcomes. Academic health center breadth and depth can be turned into an advantage.

There is an immediate need for innovation, as well as stability, in the specialty market. Fragmented product design may overwhelm payers and block specialty product advances. Collaboration and market research can deliver a manageable portfolio of specialty services to the market. Academic health centers should be critically introspective, emphasizing programs that are truly exceptional, and should work to improve others before promising excellence to the market. By maintaining internal standards of differentiation, academic health centers can reinforce their credibility.

## Integrating the Clinical Enterprise

Many faculty, upon reading this paper, will say that their personal goals are inconsistent with the vision so far articulated and that even if they share the vision, they are not operating in an environment that will allow them to achieve it. However, a number of key internal organizational changes can help stream-line decision-making and extend participation in the change process beyond a select group.

A complex web of relationships demands that academic health center integration efforts be carefully considered. Driving the need for integration is an ever-widening circle of strategic desires that dictate more complex and inclusive developmental levels (figure 5). Most academic health center faculty today have

---

**Figure 5**
**DRIVER FOR CLINICAL SYSTEM INTEGRATION: ACADEMIC HEALTH CENTER STRATEGY IN THE MARKETPLACE**

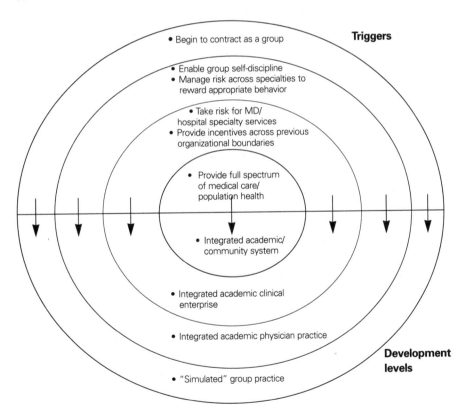

simulated a group practice so they can respond to contract opportunities with a single signature. However, more integration is necessary as the center's strategy in its marketplace becomes more expansive and includes managing risk, either as a physician group or an integrated physician-hospital organization, and perhaps also includes providing a full spectrum of medical care to a defined population.

As clinical integration at the academic health center progresses, the faculty group practice organization needs to exercise leadership and generate the maximum value from its resources by focusing on the functions that are most efficiently performed by the physician group. These functions are:

- Representing the interests of the clinical faculty as a group in clinical system governance.
- Coordinating faculty matters between the college of medicine and the clinical system.
- Providing medical staff functions, such as credentialing and quality improvement.
- Disciplining the members of the group when quality, service, or contractual deficiencies are identified.
- Coordinating recruitment of new clinicians so that appropriate clinician workforce sizing and mix is maintained and "turf issues" are resolved.
- Developing innovations that lead to superior quality and lower costs.

Academic faculty physician organizations face three key challenges. First, they need to maintain profit margins in the face of marketplace pressures. Second, they must learn to become "model partners" by overcoming traditionally weak governance, diffuse leadership, and an institutional history and culture that favors the status quo. Third, they need to create a state-of-the-art infrastructure supported through the ongoing infusion of capital. Furthermore, all of these initiatives must be achieved within the context of the academic mission.

Successful physician organizations have developed competency in ten key areas: mission and vision, governance, physician leadership, funds flow, capital, physician workforce, physician compensation, market initiatives, management systems, and clinical process improvement (see table 4 for definitions). Although all are important, the requirements for success for a particular faculty physician organization may not require excellence in all ten areas.

Academic health center faculty physician organizations are a powerful untapped resource and a vital component of the successful clinical enterprise. The academic health center's faculty physician organization is potentially the largest multispecialty group in nearly every market. Leveraging the size and scope of the physician faculty through effective integration (both horizontal and vertical) could establish new contracting opportunities and increase strength in the market.

The faculty physician organization is also the revenue engine of the academic health center and a potentially valuable source of capital. Through the wise integration of their economic, work, and human systems, faculty physician orga-

---

**Table 4**
**CRITICAL SUCCESS FACTORS FOR FACULTY PHYSICIAN ORGANIZATIONS**

*Mission and vision*
Develop a well-defined and collectively embraced mission and vision that are responsive to both market and academic imperatives.

*Physician workforce*
Determine and maintain the appropriate size and mix of physician faculty required to support the academic and clinical enterprise.

*Governance*
Establish a governing body and governance process that foster a shared strategic vision; promote rapid, coordinated decision-making; and build confidence.

*Physician compensation*
Implement a compensation program that is aligned with organizational goals, provides individual inceotives, and rewards clinical service at market-competitive rates

*Physician leadership*
Empower department chairs and other physicians to manage organizational goals to achieve both the academic and the clinical parts of the mission.

*Market initiatives*
Design desirable programs, products, and services that meet market demands and organizational goals and communicate such initiatives to customers.

*Funds flow*
Design a single integrated funds flow model that measures and manages revenues and expenses.

*Management systems*
Develop a single, clearly defined management structure and set of efficient, cost-effective, service-oriented business operations for the group practice.

*Capital*
Secure capital to support strategic investments required by the vision of the organization.

*Clinical process improvement*
Implement a clinical management program that promotes, supports, and rewards delivery of high-quality, cost-effective clinical care that is patient-oriented and comprehensive.

nizations can enhance their effectiveness and generate important competitive advantages for the center's clinical enterprise.

## Advantages

One key advantage of integrated systems is the ability to innovate. A study on vertical integration and organizational networks reported in the Spring 1996 issue of *Health Affairs* recognized that the delivery systems that maintain their advantage under managed care have the ability to innovate continually in evaluating their own performance, improving their own quality of care, and controlling their own costs.

Academic health centers have always been recognized as innovators. However, much of the innovation at centers has focused on scientific discovery and efficacy of individual drugs and technology. This type of innovation can be pursued independently by a single innovator or a small team and can be easily transferred to other organizations. Thus, sustainable competitive advantage is not possible.

Application science, in contrast, involves the implementation of multiple complementary innovations in a systems approach. These innovations cannot be easily transferred to other organizations or competitors and provide a sustainable advantage. The academic health center clinical enterprise provides the infrastructure and incentives for systemic innovation and improved application.

Another advantage of the integrated clinical enterprise is that it provides the structure for understanding funds flow across organizational components. This understanding can lead to structured and measured support of education and research while ensuring accountability for purchased services, investments, and research support. A detailed, systematic funds flow analysis and restructuring promote desirable behavior, partly by making interdependencies explicit. Because a funds flow analysis establishes a common financial language for the organization, it can create an open process that leads to group buy-in. Academic health centers have found that they cannot change the deals until the deals have been identified and their economic basis is understood. By explicitly defining the costs for activities that do not generate revenue, it is possible to measure the return on academic investment objectively and to allocate resources based on program imperatives and productivity. Finally, a commonly accepted approach to describing fund transfers can establish internal and external benchmarks for performance.

At the University of Alabama at Birmingham, one of the first UHC members to invest extensively in analyzing intrainstitutional funds transfers, a detailed funds flow analysis alleviated distrust among parties and helped them recognize their interdependencies. Balances that had not been viewed as accessible for investments now became a source of capital for program development because funds were now viewed as interchangeable. The initial reaction to attempts to identify all sources of revenue and expenditure had been that it was an attempt to control and centralize programs. Later, it was recognized that a funds flow model that was open, auditable, and used common financial language promoted decentralization of the organization and programmatic ownership.

Academic health center ownership and governance may dictate or preclude different forms of clinical enterprise integration. When full clinical enterprise integration is not possible, a virtually integrated entity may be desirable—one in which relationships and contracts allow coordination of efforts for a common purpose.

It is important to appreciate the subtle but important differences between a fully integrated clinical entity and one that is virtually integrated (table 5). Much has been written about the relative advantages of one against the other, especially in a dynamic marketplace. The measure of success for either form is the ability of the organization to effectively execute its selected strategy and to maximize the benefits of integration.

## Challenges

Integration of the center's clinical enterprise—whether faculty group prac-

**Table 5**
**DIFFERENCES BETWEEN VIRTUAL AND FULL INTEGRATION**

|  | Virtual Integration | Full Integration |
|---|---|---|
| Governance | Separate | Single |
| Leadership | Separate | Single |
| Mission and vision | Complementary | Single |
| Agendas | Shared | Single |
| Business processes | Separate or contracted | Single |
| Finances | Separate | Single |

tice development, hospital and physician integration, or community-hospital-physician integration—presents significant challenges. The desired operational efficiencies and smoothness that are so attractive are very difficult to achieve. Conflict inevitably arises over control and money. Large systems create complexities that are difficult to manage and can detract from execution. Most important, however, is the reliance of academic health center integration on successfully bringing together variable cultures—especially important for organizations with entrepreneurship and creativity, attributes that must be maintained.

## Developing and Honing Core Competencies

The strategic portfolio approach emphasizes the development of networks and the core competencies needed to support them. It allows academic health centers to respond quickly to market changes and to be a force in developing new products that redefine the market. A focus on core competencies has been credited with sustaining the competitive edge of companies such as 3M, Johnson & Johnson, and Canon Inc.

In fact, academic health centers led the development of specialty programs because of their core competencies in the science of discovery. Their discoveries of new chemical entities, surgical procedures, and other leading-edge technologies earned them a reputation as innovators when advances such as stem cell transplantation were heralded in the media as potential cures for cancer. But these innovations no longer provide academic health centers with a sustainable competitive advantage. Unlike the pharmaceutical industry, which has patent protection and licensing fees, many of the academic health center discoveries in transplantation, cardiology, infectious diseases, and oncology are quickly replicated in other settings, often by physicians trained by an academic health center.

Although the science of discovery may be critical to sustaining technological leadership in the long term, today's health care market is rewarding a new type of science—the science of application—with more systemic innovations that are difficult to transfer outside the "incubator" organization (figure 6).

Specialty care strategies need to address the three ways in which academic health centers can compete: end products or services, core products, and core competencies. Using the metaphor of a tree, we can describe the core competencies as the root system. The end products are the leaves of the tree. The core

Figure 6
**ABILITY TO ENGAGE IN APPLICATION OF INNOVATIONS
ACCORDING TO TYPE OF PRACTICE**

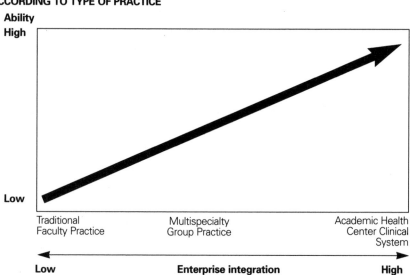

products are the trunk of the tree.

In the manufacturing world, 3M's Post-its represent a well-known end product. The company's ability to integrate its experience in combining its core products of substrates, coatings, and adhesives represents a core competency.

In academic health centers, a bypass or transplant procedure was a commonly known end product supported by core competencies in surgical techniques, patient care, and immunology research. In the new market for specialty care, however, the new end products may be a coronary artery bypass or heart transplant procedure package that adds an element of financial risk to the range of clinical services. The new end products require the application of core clinical competencies and the development of new market-focused ones.

Based on the attributes of a core competency, four market-focused competencies have been identified for specialty programs. Described below, they comprise cost management, medical management, channel management, and service management (table 6).

In this era of increased competition and decreased revenues, academic health centers must manage their costs better. Funds flow analysis can accom-

## Table 6
### CORE COMPETENCIES THAT SPECIALTY PROGRAMS NEED

| Competency | Expands Market Access | Creates Perceived Benefit | Not Easily Reproduced |
|---|---|---|---|
| Cost | It is easier to be competitive if costs are in line. | Good cost management can be transformed into value. | Sustainable focus on cost management requires a culture that is difficult to achieve. |
| Medical Care | Medicine is both art and science. The market is requiring both evidence-based norms and good communication skills. | Being the one who sets the standards creates a "halo" effect. Consumers use the *US News and World Report* rankings. | Leadership in medical management requires core competencies at the heart of AHCs—the science of what works best and the art of professional consensus. |
| Channel Management | Consolidated market requires new approaches to contracting and marketing and the systems to support channels. | Good channel management creates partners that share in the productivity gains. | People and systems working together between organizations is difficult to achieve. |
| Service | Focus on meeting customer needs builds long-term relationships and loyalty. | Good service creates a feel-good value. | Organization of complex functions into a seamless operation requires a healthy culture. |

plish the following:

- Reveal the anatomy of deals that have been made for decades; many are at odds with present priorities and provide the wrong motives.
- Make interdependencies explicit, thus allowing the alignment of financial incentives.
- Create open process that leads to group buy-in.
- Facilitate the allocation of resources based on program imperatives and productivity.
- Define explicitly the costs of subsidies for activity that does not generate revenue.
- Measure return on academic investment objectively.
- Clarify and establish common financial language.
- Establish internal and external benchmarks for performance.

With regard to the last item, funds flow analysis can lead to calculations of performance measures such as productivity ratios, efficiency ratios, and dependency ratios. These ratios can motivate improved performance by comparing the organization's performance to that of similar academic health centers and a performance ideal. Physician compensation and proper incentive structures can also motivate improved performance. An appropriate compensation program reinforces the organization's mission, vision, and culture. It promotes organizational performance while enhancing individual performance by linking incentives to organization, team, and individual goals. Finally, the ideal compensation program fosters effective recruitment and retention of high-caliber physicians and rewards clinical service activities at market-competitive rates.

Academic health centers must be able to deliver clinical care in the most cost-effective manner. Clinical resource management is a means of planning, directing, and controlling health care services cost-effectively while maintaining high-quality patient care. In 1993, UHC conducted a survey that identified four key recommendations for implementing a successful clinical resource management effort:

- Articulate the importance of clinical resource management to the entire institution.
- Seek physician ownership of projects.
- Establish clear and measurable objectives.
- Build central support.

From the analysis of both the survey and site visit results, UHC found that clinical evaluation is in its infancy both in academic health centers and in many teaching hospitals. One-third of the centers surveyed had no formal clinical evaluation program. Twenty-two respondents reported having a clinical evaluation unit. Fourteen of these units were established in the last two years, and six were less than one year old.

Education and teaching are crucial to a successful evaluation effort. Clinical evaluation unit managers must educate other clinicians about the importance of these efforts through meetings, presentations, and department conferences. They must also work to fully integrate clinical resource management into traditional medical education activities.

These units must demonstrate improvement in the process of care in ways that will ultimately save money and improve medical outcomes. Medical culture often emphasizes doing the right things for patients; clinical evaluation emphasizes doing the things the right way. Benchmarking, establishing clinical pathways, and conducting clinical research are all ways that an academic health center can manage its clinical resource.

In 1996, UHC took the concept of clinical resource management a step further and introduced Targeted Patient Management (TPM) to its membership. TPM is the coordinated clinical management of patient populations with a specific disease across all providers and sites of service to prevent or slow disease progression while reducing costs. TPM will support the management of high-cost disorders, attracting capitation dollars to specialty providers. To succeed at TPM, academic health centers must begin to act in an entrepreneurial fashion; marry clinical, administrative, and data collection functions to achieve and document results; and sell the results to purchasers through sophisticated marketing and contracting efforts.

Academic health centers should be aware, however, that TPM is not applicable to all academic health center specialty strategies. It is suitable for management of complicated, high-frequency, high-cost disorders such as cancer, renal disease, and diabetes. Furthermore, TPM is not a "home run" strategy. It supports risk contracting by generating incremental returns from many programs over extended periods (similar to scoring runs with singles and doubles rather than with home runs).

How the physician practice is organized, its relationship with the hospital, and its ability to accept risk influence an institution's capacity to provide cost-effective, high-quality clinical care. Several UHC studies have warned that the traditional academic model is inadequate for competing in the emerging managed care environment. The rotating attending system doesn't work. Physicians who spend little time in the clinical setting typically underproduce, and the demands of payers for continuity and service go unmet. The center's three-part mission cannot be sustained. It does not appear possible to maintain existing levels of research and clinical service at the same time. Research dollars increasingly go to full-time researchers, and clinical service requires constant attention and a strong time commitment. Efforts to "simulate" group practice won't suffice. In general, fragmented, department-governed faculty practices have proven unable to support the service, efficiency, and capital investment requirements of the new clinical market.

Having accepted the proposition that historic faculty practice organizations are unable to meet market demands, clinical faculty groups are evolving on several levels and in many different ways. Many are attempting to form multi-specialty groups. Some are attempting to establish community physician networks. No single structure or form is the key to success; how effectively the structure functions is what determines success or failure.

UHC research has identified a number of key functions of the physician organization in a mature academic health center clinical system. The physician organization must represent the interests of the clinical faculty as a group in clinical system governance. It coordinates faculty matters between the college of medicine and the clinical system and provides medical staff organizational functions, such as credentialing. It is responsible for group discipline, group "birth control," and innovation for superior quality and cost.

Academic health centers must realize a fact already well-known in other industries, namely, that customer satisfaction can make or break a relationship. When customer service fails at an academic health center, patient volume falls. Networks divert cases, providers with deficient customer service lose market share, and contract renewal is in jeopardy.

To compete, academic health centers must begin focusing on how to best serve their customers: patients, referring physicians, employers, and health plans. Each group has its own perceptions about how an academic health center should improve service levels to meet its needs. Therefore, academic health centers must consider and treat each group individually. Customers are powerful. Over the years, these customer groups have redefined the academic health center product. They have forced academic health centers to include referral management, travel planning, family assistance, financial counseling, and other services as part of the core product.

Academic health centers must be able to manage the channels through which patients enter the health care delivery system. This task involves managing relationships with affiliated providers, health plans, payers, and networks. Previously, academic health centers had associated themselves loosely with referral networks and anticipated that the physicians would refer patients to the centers because of the centers' superior quality. Today, academic health centers must sign contracts that explicitly specify referral relationships so they can ensure referral volumes. Successful channel management embodies patient (or enrollee) acquisition, plan/referrer management, and retention.

Many academic health centers are pursuing channel management through network development at both the hospital and primary care levels. Hospitals are forming networks in a variety of ways, and mergers and acquisitions are common. Primary care is being placed in a variety of locations within the academic health center, including departments, the faculty group practice plan, the medical school, the hospital, and the integrated delivery network. Academic health centers vary greatly as to where their primary care groups are anchored, and some have them in multiple locations. Capital investments required to develop these networks can be significant, but so can returns.

Specialty contracting is important when managing patient channels. Academic health centers have reported that their top contracting priorities focus on providing specialty care and building risk-management capacity. Unfortunately, there is no "home run" strategy when it comes to contracting. Successful contractors have patched together hundreds of agreements to sustain patient access to specialty programs.

## CONCLUSION

In summary, academic health centers need to accept the fact that the market continues to change and to understand that, to remain competitive, academic health centers must begin to develop such strategic responses to market changes as capitation, hospital consolidation, and managed care.

One successful strategy has been development of an integrated delivery network. UHC has identified six elements critical to IDN development: building primary care capacity, restructuring specialty programs, creating a hospital network, developing or participating in integrated insurance products, providing subacute care, and maintaining the education and research portions of the academic health center mission.

A second successful strategy is building an integrated clinical enterprise. Although not an easy task, it can create an organizational climate in which academic health centers respond quickly to market demands, capitalize on innovations originating in the education and research enterprise, and regulate funds flow, thereby generating capital.

An essential strategic approach involves the successful management of excellence in four critical areas—cost, medical care, service, and patient channels. Excellence in these areas will also support other strategies adopted by the academic health center.

Finally, academic health centers must adopt certain characteristics correlated with success. The most important is a leadership that is willing to accept risk for the benefit of the center.

We hope that this paper stimulates discourse and action to secure the important missions and progress of academic health centers.

# HEALTH CARE DELIVERY: A MARKETPLACE IN EVOLUTION

*Alan L. Hillman, MD, MBA*

ANY EXPERTS HOLD THAT THERE ARE four stages to change in a marketplace. The situation in health care is no exception. In this paper, we look at the changes taking place in the health care marketplace, with a case study of the situation in Philadelphia serving as a reflection of the first four stages. We also postulate the coming of a fifth stage and suggest ways to become an active participant in the marketplace evolution.

## THE TRADITIONAL STAGES OF CHANGE

The first stage of change in the health care marketplace is simply the great old past, a time when physicians and hospitals operated independently and indemnity fee-for-service prevailed; it is a place to which many doctors would like to see us return.

In the second stage of the health care marketplace, we see a loose framework of health maintenance organizations (HMOs), preferred provider organizations (PPOs), (other) provider networks, and what I call "grouping up," that is, purchasers and providers group-up to garner economies of scale and efficien-

*Dr. Hillman is director, Center for Health Policy, Leonard Davis Institute of Health Policy, and associate dean, School of Medicine, University of Pennsylvania. This paper is excerpted from his remarks at the Annual Meeting of the Association of Academic Health Centers, Indian Wells, California, September 26, 1997.*

cies so that they can negotiate with each other and focus on discounts. Hospitals remain profitable during this period despite excess capacity. And we start to have efficiencies and economies of scale.

The third stage is a period of more rapid consolidation and integration, with the developments of stage two continuing. Competition among the large buyers and sellers of health care leads to reduced choices and best buys for certain employers. Lots of deals are taking place. For the first time, there is a shift in risk-taking, or financial risk-sharing, to the providers. Risk-sharing in a financial sense becomes a major difficulty, especially for academic health centers.

Price pressure is mainly responsible for this wave of consolidation and integration. Seen another way, the consolidation is a response to inefficient fragmentation, with providers looking to create efficiencies and economies of scale. Also, referrals to academic health centers based on prestige alone start to fall. In economic theory, we call this situation "the patient leverage theory," that is, academic health centers have a competitive advantage because people generally believe that academic health centers have the best and the brightest and the latest equipment. (This theory may explain why academic health centers could wait so long to take action after the marketplace started to change and still be in the running.)

In the fourth stage, the mature phase, the market is completely driven by managed care and mature purchasing coalitions consisting of labor unions, employers, business coalitions, etc. These are integrated systems—large buyers and sellers of care who are managing large populations. With full integration of all services, the hospital is no longer playing a central role on the health care scene.

This fourth stage, however, cannot really be considered mature; it is still evolving and its future shape is still uncertain. Every marketplace that I have visited, regardless of whether it is in health care or another field, or if it is stage one, two, three, or especially four, is continuing to change. Thus, as part of the effort to find the right organizational structure for academic health centers in the future, I suggest that we investigate the probability of a stage five.

## A CASE STUDY: THE PHILADELPHIA
## MARKET STAGES 1-4

We must look more closely at the way health care provision is actually developing in the market to discover new models of care. A relevant case study of the four stages of change is the City of Philadelphia, which *The New York Times* has said "is dominated by the health care industry more than any other city per capita. It has the highest costs, the highest cost per patient, the longest length of stay."

In stage one, Philadelphia has six medical schools, a half a million people in managed care, five million hospital days, eighty teaching and community hospitals, and—very important—significant cost shifting.

In later stages, a reduction in the number of medical schools occurs, the first time ever since the Flexner Report in 1910, as a result of the merger of Hahnemann University and the Medical College of Pennsylvania. Managed care grows to cover 2.5 million people, a five-fold increase in just ten years. There is a 20 percent reduction in hospital days, from 5.2 million to 4.6 million. Most important is the emergence of an uninsured population, partially as a result of the loss of the city's public health hospital and because the system no longer allows cost shifting. Employers got tired of paying more than their fair share and absorbing more than their fair share of costs, and the 80,000 doctors and all of the hospitals merged into four major health care systems with four different strategies for providing care; the situation is actually a reflection of a four-stage systematic approach to changes taking place in the health care market.

## The Allegheny Health and Education
## Research Foundation

The Allegheny Health and Education Research Foundation has two academic hospitals, eleven community hospitals, and an emphasis on the purchase of physician practices. The foundation came to Philadelphia because its strategic plan called for an academic health center as the central part of its program; the University of Pittsburgh apparently didn't want to be a part of its system. This situation supports the patient-leverage theory.

## Jefferson University/Main Line

Jefferson University/Main Line has fifteen community hospitals, emphasizes collaboration instead of purchasing, and is pursuing a more decentralized strategy.

## Temple University

Temple University has four community hospitals and an emphasis on primary care practices. This system was bailed out by the state; indeed, it will always be bailed out by the state and thus has an advantage over the other systems.

## The University of Pennsylvania Health System

The University of Pennsylvania Health System has three core teaching hospitals and five community hospitals. With an emphasis on the purchase of physician practices and full-risk contracts, it has a more centralized view of how an academic health care system should be organized.

## STAGE 5

But the four-part systematic change model represented by Philadelphia cannot possibly capture the future. It is, therefore, important to speculate on the future, both in general and with respect to academic health centers, by considering a fifth stage.

I believe this fifth stage will be marked by new forms of integration and consolidation and new kinds of organizations. There is going to be a rethinking of the managed care approach that is considered mature in stage four. Ten years ago, we knew exactly what an HMO, a PPO, and a point-of-service system meant. But now it is impossible to take one system and put it in a given basket because there is a spectrum of managed care.

In stage 5, we are continuing to test new organizational strategies. Because there are so many specialists, they will have to be "retooled" to deliver primary care. Centers of Excellence will emerge. Not every provider in a marketplace will have to do everything, and thus there will be no need for three or four academic centers, each with helicopters and trauma units. The unique competencies of each program will take hold, and there will be an understanding within the marketplace that certain places should do some things and other places should do others. (Clearly, some in-patient facilities will close, as has already happened in Philadelphia in terms of floors or wards or even hospitals themselves—an experience mirrored throughout the country in the closure of excess facilities.)

## The Role of Technology

Information systems are going to be absolutely paramount for health care in the future. True integration of information systems is going to lead to new efficiencies that prolong our ability to keep the system under control. Although we have currently reached a quasi-equilibrium in the cost of care (i.e., the fat has been cut out of the system), I think that new fat will be found and new efficiencies will be needed. The latter will become possible as information systems become integrated and can report all resource-use and all information about a given patient.

New efficiencies will come from the integration of information and the testing of outcomes research in a timely fashion and will lead to feedback about what works and what does not work. If the interventions work, we can defend them statistically and reliably. If they do not work, we can retool and change them. Such tests proofs demand a comprehensive information system that precludes the need to search for information in several different areas, departments of an academic health center, or other type of health center. Once we obtain the results of disease management research, we want to be able to use them in the most efficient way possible. We will be able to look, for example, at four diseases with four possible interventions and consider the possible cost of each intervention and the likely outcome in terms of life years.

Thus, if a health care organization has $100,000 to spend on new initiatives next year, what are the different ways they could use the money? One option would be to buy A and B and get 350 quality-adjusted life years as an outcome measure from the disease management protocol that was applied to people with disease A and disease B (one protocol for each). Or, it could reduce spending on disease D and the disease management protocol in place for disease D and, with the resulting savings, put A, B, and C in place, increasing the overall production of quality-adjusted life years from 350 to 360. But to make these decisions and to make them in a moral fashion, the organization must know if cutting back on the disease D protocol or intervention, which has not been shown to work, is ethical. If A, B, and C have been shown to work in a statistically reliable way and the organization is just guessing about D, then D should not take precedence.

Although many people in health care believe that disease management makes sense and is the right thing to do, any protocols that are written must then be tested scientifically before the protocol can be put into practice.

In my opinion, major problems will arise as new technologies drive up prices for care and thus further limit the availability of insurance. I think that the current equilibrium in the cost of care will be lost as the products of genetic engineering, monoclonal antibody research, and other new devices and technologies coming out of the pharmaceutical and device pipeline and going through the Food and Drug Administration. These developments will lead to magnificent new changes and advances in patient care. But as with all health care technologies, they will entail additional costs. I do not think the current system can absorb these costs. The changes will require a entity like the Securities and Exchange Commission (SEC) to emerge, where the government and marketplace come together to establish an unbiased board of people to deal with allocating resources and determining levels of coverage.

I also think there will be a basic level of insurance and, I hope, a moral imperative to bring the uninsured into the system. However, what does seem likely is that there will be a basic level, basic-plus, and full-coverage insurance, which an SEC-like entity will put together, and that we will eventually have overt rationing in this country rather than rationing by default or ability to pay.

## The Role of the Government

The question remains: Who is going to take charge of the changing health care providers of the future. Eventually, the government will realize that legislative micromanagement does not work and that the financial incentives, protocols, guidelines, and so forth that managed care uses are actually the heart of managed care. You cannot manage care if you cannot influence the people who prescribe that care. At some point, Congress will recognize this fact and stop producing legislation in response to each individual clinical situation, such as the drive-through delivery and the gag-rule problems. These kinds of actions on behalf of the entire country result in as many problems as solutions.

## CONCLUSION

Clearly, academic health centers are always going to be more expensive than other health care providers. But there will always be a premium for teaching and research. I think it is important, however, to call attention to some things that do need change or correction in our system.

The furor over whether or not Medicare is going to continue to support academic health centers has to end; an institution cannot plan strategically for the next ten years when it does not know if it will have a source of income for those years. It would seem that government must eventually realize what a mistake it would be to undermine our nation's extremely powerful academic health centers system by stripping away the support it receives through Medicare. Unfortunately, there is no legal requirement for any of these subsidies or for any government entity to support academic health center training of doctors and fellows.

(There is some hopeful news. For example, the Health Care Financing Administration is paying New York State $1.25 billion over the next five years to reduce the number of residents and fellows and to create a new organizational entity that will allow academic health centers to exist and to deliver good quality care in stage five. It is to be hoped there will be more New York State-like initiatives in the future.)

In general, there will be two basic choices to make regarding the organization of the academic health centers in the future. One is to integrate the academic health center into every new form of care and put teaching and research into every acquisition. Alternatively, academic health centers could maintain a separate facility for teaching and research, and a separate facility, maybe even a for-profit entity, to bring in revenues to support the teaching and research mission.

Of course, Medicare and Medicaid will continue to add to the pressure on the system, and academic health centers will have to begin doing something that they don't like to do—namely, real marketing. They will have to develop a strong brand loyalty for their product and convey this message to the public consistently and repeatedly. They must become, like it or not, the Kellogg's Cornflakes of health care. They will have to adjust to the fact that marketing is necessary to sustain the Centers of Excellence concept. There is plenty of room to maneuver.

Hospitals could learn from the pharmaceuticals industry's marketing efforts and take a look at the percent of their revenues that goes toward marketing.

In addition, academic centers will have to become comfortable with full-risk contracts. They may even develop academic health center insurance products that offer one-stop shopping for the buyer or the employer. This approach will be a necessary part of the effort to seek efficiencies, economies of scale, and more control for academic health centers so they can accomplish their triple, traditional mission of teaching, research, and service. Some help toward this mission has been forthcoming, including funding from major organizations on projects that encourage greater collaboration between academic health centers and managed care organizations.

In 1899, Charles Duel, the director of the U.S. Patent Office, advised the President of the United States to close the office, saying, "Everything that can possibly be invented has already been invented." Duel reminds me of many people in academic medicine who are defending the status quo at all costs. The alternative is to become more realistic and fruitful, namely, to recognize that the best way to cope with change is to help create and organize that change, rather than simply react to it.

# LESSONS FROM CORPORATE AMERICA AND THE INTERNATIONAL SCENE

THE CHANGING SHAPE OF
AMERICAN COMPANIES:
IMPLICATIONS FOR ACADEMIC
HEALTH CENTERS

THE GLOBALIZATION OF
HEALTH CARE

# THE CHANGING SHAPE OF AMERICAN COMPANIES: IMPLICATIONS FOR ACADEMIC HEALTH CENTERS

*Charles C. Snow, PhD*

S PART OF THE PROCESS OF REASSESSING THEIR missions for the next century, academic health centers are turning to corporate America for useful ideas. American companies have been concerned about their missions, too, particularly since the troubled times of the late 1980s and early 1990s. This paper, therefore, traces the changing shape of American companies and identifies those features most likely to be relevant to academic health centers.

## HISTORY OF ORGANIZATION FORMS

The development of the large American corporation can be traced to the period immediately following the U.S. Industrial Revolution in the 1860s. Over the next century and a half, five major forms of large-scale organizing were developed (Miles and Snow 1994). When a new organizational form appeared, it typically solved the main problems associated with the previous form, and it added to the capabilities available to all companies wishing to adopt the new

*Dr. Snow is Mellon Bank Professor of Business Administration, The Smeal College of Business Administration, The Pennsylvania State University.*

form. The five major organizational forms and the periods during which they thrived appear in figure 1.

## Traditional Organizations

The oldest corporate structure is the functional organization. It was invented primarily by the railroads in the latter part of the nineteenth century and was based on previous organizational models such as the Catholic Church and the military. The functional organization made two major contributions to the capabilities held by companies of the time; the contributions are still influential today.

One achievement was specialization. By focusing on narrow product or service lines, companies were able to improve on their limited offerings continuously. The second contribution, developed around the turn of the century as the functional structure was adopted by steel and other manufacturing companies, was the practice of scientific management. This approach, championed by people such as Frederick Taylor (1911), focused on cost reductions, improved work methods, and other efficiencies that could be obtained throughout a company's operations.

Eventually, every company of any significant size was functionally organized. However, the price that companies paid for the twin benefits of specialization and efficiency was a lack of responsiveness; the rigidity of the functional

Figure 1
EVOLUTION OF MAJOR ORGANIZATIONAL FORMS, 1850–2050

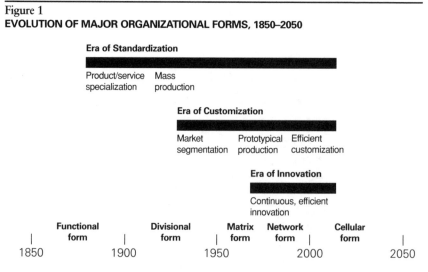

structure made it difficult for firms to do new and different things.

Nevertheless, the functional organization dominated American industry until the end of World War I. When the war was over, companies that wanted to take advantage of growing national markets felt constrained by the functional structure. The time was ripe, therefore, for the invention of a new way of organizing. The primary inventor of the new form was General Motors, with significant help from Sears, Roebuck, the first company to adopt the new form—divisional organization—in retailing (Chandler 1962).

Although General Motors developed the main features of the new form in 1921–25, the Depression and World War II delayed the widespread use of divisional organization until the late 1940s and 1950s. Compared to the functional form, the divisional structure was much more flexible. By forming a series of product groups (divisions), and targeting each one toward a particular segment of the market, divisionalized companies began to offer their customers products that were customized to customer needs and tastes. However, the ability to customize came at a price; this price was inefficiency. The divisional organization required high overhead, was subject to resource duplication, and frequently suffered from suboptimal economies of scale.

The movement from standardization to customization continued into the late 1960s and 1970s as firms adopted mixed organizational forms, such as the matrix, that allowed a dual focus on both stable and emerging market segments and clients (Davis and Lawrence 1997). For example, by employing a matrix organization, an aerospace firm such as TRW could produce standard products for the civilian and military markets in one or more divisions, and also simultaneously transfer some resources from those units into project groups that designed and built prototypical products for space exploration.

The matrix organization provided companies with a more finely grained mechanism for exploiting their know-how across a wider range of both standardized and customized products and services. However, the powerful capability of simultaneous specialization and customization was accompanied by a tremendous amount of administrative complexity.

All three traditional organization structures (functional, divisional, and matrix) were hierarchically based. They relied heavily on rules and procedures to accomplish work objectives, and they used extensive control systems to make

**Table 1.**
**STRENGTHS AND LIMITATIONS OF FIVE MAJOR ORGANIZATION FORMS**

| Organization Forms | Strengths | Limitations |
| --- | --- | --- |
| Functional | Specialization, efficiency | Rigidity |
| Divisional | Segmentation, customization | Inefficiency |
| Matrix | Dual focus on specialization and customization | Complexity |
| Network | Collective assets, speed | Overdependence of suppliers on lead firms |
| Cellular | Continuous learning and adaptability | Scarcity of personnel with range of required skills |

sure work was performed efficiently. The main strengths of each organizational form, as well as its key limitations, are summarized in table 1.

## Today's Popular Organizational Form: The Network

The 1970s was a period of major upheaval for the hierarchical organizations that had developed over the previous one hundred years. The scene in which companies functioned now included greater global competition, widespread national economic reform (including deregulation and privatization), and the development of new communications and computer technologies. Such changes both forced and facilitated the development of new ways of organizing, and a new organizational form—the network—ultimately emerged.

Network organizations came about in two main ways. One common route was downsizing, de-layering, and disaggregating formerly hierarchical organizations (*Business Week* 1993a). No longer did the big American firms try to do everything; many became smaller, leaner, and more focused. The other route, usually chosen by newer companies, was to eschew hierarchy from the outset by forming key partnerships and by outsourcing noncore functions to suppliers.

In either case, the end result was that a firm focused on perfecting and leveraging its core competencies. In addition, companies became much more sensitive to their customers' needs and requests, and began to respond to customer demands with uncommon speed. If a company was able to select partners whose core competencies complemented its own, then the resulting multifirm network could act like an all-star team, entering new markets at exactly the right scale, reconfiguring itself as appropriate, and efficiently customizing activities at each stage of the industry value chain.

A well-known example of a multifirm network organization is NIKE. Actually, the "Just Do It" company does not do everything. For example, it is not a manufacturing company. All of NIKE's products are manufactured by the firm's production partners located in Asia and elsewhere. Nor is NIKE a retailing company. Although NIKE has some retail operations (e.g., Niketowns and sports apparel shops), most of its products are sold in stores operated by The Foot Locker and other retail partners. NIKE focuses primarily on its core competencies: R&D and marketing; it is also very good at managing relationships with its network partners (variously called "horizontal," "relationship," or "supply chain" management). Thus, NIKE's "organization" includes not only its own assets and capabilities but those of its partners as well.

Another networked company is the Dell Computer Corporation. Dell has taken relationship management to new heights by working with its various partners and suppliers to do the right things at incredible speed and at the lowest possible cost. Even when Dell makes a mistake (such as its poorly received laptop computer in the early 1990s), it has the flexibility and know-how to recast key relationships quickly and effectively and to fix its mistakes (such as reentering the market with a much-improved laptop computer within a year). Today, Dell is a model of just-in-time manufacturing, inventory management, customer service, and electronic commerce.

NIKE, Dell, and other network companies of the 1980s and 1990s are built on horizontal rather than vertical organizational principles (*Business Week* 1993b). Rather than do everything themselves through the traditional command-and-control model, network firms rely on a business model that includes (1) the collective assets of their partners; (2) close relationships with their partners, suppliers, and customers; and (3) internal managerial mechanisms that are market-based rather than rules-based.

Counteracting these benefits of networking, however, is the possibility that suppliers can become stale if they grow too dependent on the "core" or "lead" firm. Alternatively, a lead firm may be tempted to manage some of the internal operations of its network partners and suppliers. If such managerial incursions expand, the network may be transformed into something resembling an old-style vertically integrated firm (Miles and Snow 1992).

## Anticipating Tomorrow's Organization: The Cellular Form

What will be tomorrow's competitive environment? What type of managerial mind-set will emerge? What type of organizational structure will be required to serve the business interests of companies in the twenty-first century? In tomorrow's business world, some markets will still be supplied with standard products and services, while other markets will demand large amounts of customization. However, the continued pull of market forces and the push of ever-increasing know-how honed through network partnering is already moving some industries and companies toward what amounts to a continuous process of innovation. Beyond the customization of existing designs, product and service invention is becoming the centerpiece of value-adding activity in an increasing number of companies. So-called knowledge businesses—such as design and engineering services, advanced electronics and biotechnology, computer software design, health care, and consulting—not only feed the process of innovation but feed upon it in a continuous cycle that creates more—and more complex—markets and environments.

The managerial mind-set appropriate for this vision of the future might include the belief that a company should be able to do "anything, anytime, anywhere." To do so would require an ambidextrous organization, that is, one that could compete and cooperate simultaneously. And, quite obviously, such an organization would be severely constrained by traditional features such as hierarchies, rules, and extensive control systems. Thus, the organization of the future is more likely to be self-managing.

Recently, we have begun to refer to this type of organization as the cellular form (Miles et al. 1997). The cellular metaphor suggests a living, adaptive organization. Cells in living organisms possess fundamental functions of life and can act alone to meet a particular need. However, by acting in concert, cells can perform more complex functions. If shared across all cells, evolving characteristics, or learning, can create a higher order organism. And, like cells in living organisms, a cellular business organization is made up of cells (self-managing teams, autonomous business units, firms, etc.) that can operate alone but can also interact with other cells to produce a more potent and competent business mechanism. It is this combination of independence and interdependence that allows the cellular organizational form to generate and share the know-how that produces continuous innovation.

In the future, complete cellular business organizations will achieve a level of know-how well beyond that of earlier organizational forms by combining entrepreneurship, self-organization, and member-ownership in mutually reinforcing ways. Each cell will have an entrepreneurial responsibility to the larger organization. The customers of a particular cell can be outside clients or other cells in the organization. In either case, the purpose is to spread an entrepreneurial mind-set throughout the organization so that every cell is concerned about improvement and growth. Indeed, giving each cell entrepreneurial responsibility is essential to the full utilization of the firm's constantly growing know-how. (Of course, each cell must also have the entrepreneurial skills required to generate business for itself and the overall organization.)

Each cell must be able to reorganize continually in order to make its expected contribution to the overall organization. Of particular value here are the technical skills needed to perform its function, the collaborative skills necessary to make appropriate linkages with other organizational units and external partner firms, and the governance skills required to manage one's own activities. Application of this cellular principle may require the company to strip away most of the bureaucracy that is currently in place and replace it with jointly defined protocols that guide internal and external collaboration.

For this organization to function well, each cell must be rewarded for acting entrepreneurially and operating in a business-like manner. If the cellular units are teams or strategic business units instead of complete firms, psychological ownership can be achieved by organizing cells as profit centers, allowing them to participate in company stock-purchase plans, and so on. However, the ultimate cellular solution is the actual member ownership of the cell assets and resources that they have created and that they voluntarily invest with the firm in expectation of a joint return.

Technical Computing and Graphics (TCG), a privately held information technology company based in Sydney, Australia, is perhaps the best example of the cellular approach to organizing. TCG develops a wide variety of products and services, including portable and hand-held data terminals and loggers, computer graphics systems, bar-coding systems, and electronic data interchange systems.

The thirteen individual small firms at TCG are the focus of the organization's "cellularity." Like a cell in a large organism, each firm has its own purpose and ability to function independently, but it shares common features and purpose with all of its sister firms. Some TCG member firms specialize in one or more product categories, while others specialize in hardware or software.

Each of the TCG member firms came into the group with existing high levels of technical and business competence. However, the operating protocol at TCG assures that systemwide competence will continue to grow. The process is called triangulation, and it is the means by which TCG continually develops new products and services (Mathews 1993). Triangulation is a three-entity partnership between (1) one or more TCG firms, (2) an external joint-venture partner (e.g., Hitachi, Ltd.) that also provides equity capital to the venture, and (3) a principal customer (e.g., Telstra Corporation, Ltd, an Australian telephone company) whose large advance order wins it contractual rights as well as providing additional cash to the venture. Each TCG firm is expected to search continually for new product and service opportunities. When a particular venture shows concrete promise, the initiating firm acts as project leader for the entire venture.

The first step in the triangulation process is to identify and collaborate with a joint-venture partner, a firm with expertise in the proposed technology. TCG receives partial funding for the project from the joint-venture partner, and it also gains access to technical ideas and distribution channels. Next, the project leader firm identifies an initial large customer for the new product. TCG also collaborates with the customer in the sense that it agrees to custom-design a product for that client. By working together with the joint-venture partner and the principal customer, TCG is able to efficiently develop a state-of-the-art product that is tailor-made to the principal customer's specifications.

According to TCG's governance principles, the project leader firm is also expected to search among the other TCG companies for additional partners, not only because the firms are needed for their technical contribution, but also because the collaboration itself is expected to enhance overall organizational know-how. The process of internal triangulation thus serves a dual purpose. It produces direct input to the project, and it helps to diffuse competence in areas such as business development, partnering, and project management.

The three principles of cellularity are tightly interconnected at TCG, mutually reinforcing each other and producing a strong overall organization. First, acceptance of entrepreneurial responsibility is required for admission to the group and is increasingly enhanced by the triangulation process. Second, self-organization gives the individual firm both the ability and the freedom to reach deeply into its own know-how to create responses to a continuously evolving set of customer and partner needs. Third, each firm's profit responsibility, as well as its opportunity to own stock in other TCG firms, provides an ongoing stimulus for the growth and utilization of know-how.

A close examination of cellularly structured companies such as TCG indicates that these companies also share some of the features of earlier organizational forms. Just as in the past, each new form incorporates the major value-adding characteristics of the previous forms and adds new capabilities to them. Thus, the cellular form includes the dispersed entrepreneurship of the divisional form, customer responsiveness of the matrix form, and the self-organizing knowledge and asset-sharing of the network form.

The cellular organizational form, however, offers the potential to add value even beyond asset and know-how sharing. In its fully developed state, the cellular organization adds value through its unique ability to create and utilize knowledge. For example, knowledge-sharing occurs in networks as a by-product of asset sharing rather than as a specific focus of such activity. Similarly, matrix and divisionalized firms recognize the value that may be added when knowledge is shared across projects or divisions, but they must create special-purpose mechanisms (e.g., task forces) to generate and share new knowledge. By contrast, as illustrated at TCG, the cellular form lends itself to sharing not only the explicit know-how that cells have accumulated and articulated, but also the tacit know-how that emerges when cells combine to design unique new customer solutions (Nonaka and Takeuchi 1995). Such learning focuses not on the output of the innovation process, but on the innovation process itself: It is know-how that can be achieved and shared only by doing.

Beyond knowledge-creation and -sharing, the cellular form has the potential to add value through its related ability to keep the firm's total knowledge assets more fully invested than do the other organizational forms. Because each cell has entrepreneurial responsibility and is empowered to draw on any of the firm's assets for each new business opportunity, high levels of knowledge utilization across cells can be anticipated. Network organizations aspire to high utilization of know-how and assets, but upstream firms are ultimately dependent on downstream partners to find new product or service uses. In the cellular firm, the product-service innovation process is continuous and fully shared.

The tradeoffs one must make to obtain the benefits of a cellular organization are not yet clearly evident. However, two potential drawbacks of the cellular form can be postulated. The first involves high-caliber human resources needed to staff a cellular organization. In most cases, finding people who possess a combination of technical, entrepreneurial, leadership, and self-governing skills will be difficult. Second, the approach required to manage such people has not been clearly defined. If cells (teams, small firms, etc.) are expected to be essentially self-directing, then "management" becomes a service provided on request. What form managerial services should take, and how they should be provided, are not clear.

## MISSION: THE PURPOSE OF ORGANIZING

All of the organizational forms discussed above have been developed to serve an economic purpose. A particular company's purpose is (or should be) embodied in its statement of mission. Mission statements are valuable managerial tools; they communicate a company's purpose to a variety of stakeholders including investors, customers, managers and employees, governmental authorities, and local communities. But a mission statement needs to be clearly defined before an organizational form is chosen to support it.

In general terms, a mission statement describes who we are (company identity), what we do (domain), and where we're headed (direction). A mission statement should be agreed upon and written so that it is neither too general nor too narrow. A general or bland mission statement that could be applied to almost any firm does not define a company's identity or domain for its stakeholders clearly. On the other hand, a narrow mission statement, even if it is specifically stated, can feel restrictive to organization members who have grander, more ambitions about the company's direction and growth. And, ideally, a mission statement should generate enthusiasm and support among stakeholders. It is this behavioral aspect of a mission statement that is most important for company success.

The mission statements of three well-known companies—NIKE, Inc., Ben & Jerry's Homemade, Inc., and Starbucks Corporation (coffee)—each have a particular feature worth noting.

NIKE's mission statement, for example, has generated widespread agreement, passion, and commitment among its employees. In contrast to many companies, NIKE's managers and employees understand the company's mission and strongly support it. On a day-to-day basis, employees make decisions and take actions that are consistent with the company's mission, which, in turn, serves to perpetuate the mission. The managerial lesson to be learned from NIKE is that it is important to state a company mission in appealing terms, communicate it widely, and abide by it consistently.

**Mission Statement**

**NIKE, Inc.**

**Our mission is to enhance people's lives through sports and fitness. We do so by designing, developing, and globally marketing high-quality sports footwear, apparel, and accessories.**

Ben & Jerry's, the ice cream company, has a somewhat controversial mission statement, particularly when viewed from an investor's perspective. A traditional investor simply searching for an investment that offers a good financial return is likely to see a tension, if not a contradiction, between Ben & Jerry's economic mission and its social mission. Traditional investors want to support their own social causes, and not have a company do it for them. On the other hand, one can argue that investors can learn from the mission statement that Ben & Jerry's is committed to social activism and can then avoid investing in the company if they believe that its social mission is hurting profitability. Here, the managerial lesson to be learned is that the company's mission must be stated

**Mission Statement**

**Ben & Jerry's Homemade, Inc.**

Ben & Jerry's is dedicated to the creation and demonstration of a new corporate concept of linked prosperity. Our mission consists of three interrelated parts:

Product mission: To make, distribute, and sell the finest-quality, all-natural ice cream and related products in a wide variety of innovative flavors made from Vermont dairy products.

Social mission: To operate the company in a way that actively recognizes the central role that business plays in the structure of society by innovative ways to improve the quality of life of a broad community: local, national, and international.

Economic mission: To operate the company on a sound financial basis of profitable growth, increasing value for our shareholders, and creating career opportunities and financial rewards for our employees.

Underlying the mission of Ben & Jerry's is the determination to seek new and creative ways of addressing all three parts, while holding a deep respect for individuals, inside and outside the company, and for the communities of which they are a part.

unambiguously, and its various pieces must have a collective as well as an individual rationale.

The mission statement of Starbucks is notable for the balance between its business domain and its guiding principles. By reading this informative statement, we understand what the company wants to be ("the premier purveyor of the finest coffee in the world") and how it intends to accomplish its vision (via six guiding principles). More than most companies, Starbucks is forthcoming about its identity, domain, and direction. By divulging its corporate personality, Starbucks allows stakeholders (whether customers, employees, or investors) to make informed decisions about the company.

## IMPLICATIONS FOR ACADEMIC HEALTH CENTERS

In setting out their missions and in developing the organizational structures and processes necessary to pursue them, American companies have learned a great deal that is of relevance to academic health centers. I, therefore, offer three broad recommendations to academic health center policymakers and administrators who are responsible for charting the course of their organizations.

## 1. Review, redefine, and communicate the mission of the academic health center.

Because of the ever-changing health care environment, every academic health center needs to review its mission periodically. Can the academic health center continue to support all of its current research activities? Should it offer more services to the local community? What should be its relationship to the rest of the university? A thorough mission review requires input from all key constituencies. Once consensus has been reached on the nature of the mission, the statement itself must be carefully written following the guidelines and examples discussed above. Finally, the academic health center must communicate its mission both internally and externally, in a manner that generates wide support.

**Mission Statement**

**Starbucks Corporation**

**Our mission is to establish Starbucks as the premier purveyor of the finest coffee in the world while maintaining our uncompromising principles as we grow. The following six guiding principles will help us measure the appropriateness of our decisions:**

**Provide a great work environment and treat each other with respect and dignity.**

**Embrace diversity as essential to the way we do business.**

**Apply the highest standards of excellence to the purchasing, roasting, and fresh delivery of our coffee.**

**Develop enthusiastically satisfied customers all of the time.**

**Contribute positively to our communities and our environment.**

**Recognize that profitability is essential to our future success.**

## 2. Bring organization structure and management processes into alignment with the mission.

Most academic health centers use some type of matrix organization to pursue their missions. It is a traditional structure that allows a focus on both specialties and programs, and has served many organizations well for many years. In the future, however, some academic health centers may want to explore a network structure that allows more collaboration with external partners of various sorts. Companies migrate to network structures as they abandon the do-it-yourself mind-set and replace it with a cooperative approach in which the collective resources of multiple organizations are used to pursue company missions. A few academic health centers may even wish to explore the cellular organization structure in order to generate maximum amounts of entrepreneurship and innovation.

## 3. Reengineer the academic health center as appropriate.

The reengineering wave has not hit academic organizations with the same force as it hit companies, particularly in the 1980s. Nevertheless, both the philosophy and process of reengineering have continuing relevance for academic health centers. It is essentially an approach that removes unnecessary activities, streamlines those that remain, and instills a belief in continuous improvement (Hammer and Champy 1993). Although reengineering usually requires difficult and unpleasant decisions, it is a key accompaniment to mission and organizational change.

### CONCLUSION

An organization's mission is something that needs to be managed. In the constantly evolving health care environment, the mission of every academic health center must be regularly reviewed and evaluated. Moreover, as the mission changes, so too must the organization's structure and management systems. Managers of academic health centers can find worthwhile ideas and approaches in corporate America, which, in its approach to viability during changing economic times, has been at the leading edge of organizational change for a century and a half.

## WORK CITED

*Business Week*, 1993a. What big companies can learn. Special Issue on Enterprise, 190–257.

*Business Week*, 1993b. The horizontal corporation. December 20, 76-81.

Davis, S.M., and P.R. Lawrence. 1997. *Matrix*. Reading, MA: Addison-Wesley.

Hammer, M., and J. Champy. 1993. *Reengineering the Corporation: A Manifesto for Business Revolution*. New York: HarperBusiness.

Mathews, J.A. 1993. TCG R&D Networks: The triangulation strategy, *Journal of Industry Studies* 1:65–74.

Miles, R.E., and C.C. Snow. 1992. Causes of failure in network organizations, *California Management Review* 34:53-72.

———. 1994. *Fit, Failure, and the Hall of Fame: How Companies Succeed or Fail*. New York: Free Press.

Miles, R.E., C.C. Snow, J.A. Mathews, G. Miles, and H.J. Coleman, Jr. 1997. Organizing in the knowledge age: Anticipating the cellular form, Academy of Management Executive 11, 7–20.

Nonaka, I., and H. Takeuchi. 1995. *The Knowledge-Creating Company: How Japanese Companies Create the Dynamics of Innovation*. New York: Oxford.

Taylor, F.W. 1911. *The Principles of Scientific Management*. New York: Harper.

# THE GLOBALIZATION
# OF HEALTH CARE

*John Wyn Owen, CB*

GRADUAL EXPANSION OF HEALTH CARE HAS
taken place from the 1960s to the present time. I believe
that the first decade of the new century should and will
focus on its global aspects. Indeed, a recent study by Moran
and Wood (1996) on international political economy states that "if we discover
that internationalization is indeed taking place in health care, a policy sphere
which hitherto has been parochial, then we have a striking demonstration that
the trend toward internationalization is significant." The authors define internationalization as a process through which the authority and autonomy of the
nation state is challenged or supplanted by structures, processes, or policy development that cut across national boundaries.

If the health care scene is being penetrated by a global approach, something fundamental must be afoot. In this paper I sketch out the main features of
recent pronouncements by important United States and United Kingdom organizations on involvement of their nations in current health concerns and discuss
trends in international health. I then go on to provide an analytical framework
for examining globalization; put an American perspective on globalization; and
consider some of the specific implications of these international developments for
academic health centers. Finally, some personal concerns and issues that need to
be explored further and with some urgency are addressed.

---

*John Wyn Owen is secretary of The Nuffield Trust, London.*

## LOOKING TO THE FUTURE

### Why America Must Act

The 1997 Institute of Medicine report, in its discussion on advancing the U.S. international interest, states that "the United States has unique strengths to improve global health yet the potential has not been fulfilled." The board concludes that, to remain in a position of leadership in global health, the United States must increase investment in biomedical research on major global health problems through expanded partnerships and cost-sharing with other governments and international donors. There must be an investment in the education and training of physicians and researchers from around the world for health leadership.

The United States must also pay its dues to the United Nations; for example, $145 million is owed to the World Health Organization (WHO). This sum must be repaid if the United States is to regain the influence that it so urgently needs to reform the system. The board also advocated a form of global partnership with governments, private sectors, and other interested parties.

### International Partnerships

Although America's participation in global health is vital, it cannot do the job alone. Global problems are most likely to be solved by global action. The theme of partnership in health also pervades the recent U.K. Technology Foresight Project. The policy initiative embraces the dual themes of partnership and wealth creation, bringing together industrialists and scientists to identify opportunities in markets and technologies likely to emerge during the next ten to twenty years and the investment actions needed to exploit them. The foresight panels, such as the panel on Health and Life Sciences (1997), have generated visions of the future that will lead to more informed decision making in health in both the public and private sectors. Similar initiatives have occurred in other countries, including Australia and the United States.

The U.K. experience provides a useful picture of across-the-board advances in basic knowledge made over the last two decades that are now being translated into new treatments for illness, new products, and new industries. The pace of discovery is accelerating, innovative opportunities are widening, and important new areas of demand, such as those of an aging population, are emerging. Mark Ferguson, the chairman of the Health and Life Sciences Panel, has said that "a biological science revolution is underway, the impact of which will be greater than the industrial or the atomic revolutions."

## THE WORLD HEALTH SCENE
### An Aging Population
The best documented trend in health needs is the aging of the population. In the United Kingdom in 1961, 11.7 percent of the population was more than 65 years old; this figure will rise to 17.5 percent by the year 2015. This situation will increase the prevalence of illness and disability, particularly degenerative conditions such as cataracts, osteoarthritis, neoplasms, and cardiovascular and neurodegenerative diseases.

The future is far from clear; medical need may be affected by further increases in life expectancy or changing health and lifestyles among those currently middle-aged. The impact of this situation on service and products may be magnified by attitudes to elderly people, the increasing political power of the elderly, attitudes to care by caregivers, and the increased affluence of some elderly subgroups, as well as technical opportunity.

### Economic and Cultural Change
Long-term changes in economy and social structure, although more difficult to foresee, may have an even greater impact. In the most stable, affluent societies, lifestyle, working environment, family, wealth, and social disparity still have clear effects on health. The effects of unemployment, poverty, overcrowding, drug and alcohol abuse, and violence will become much more marked if current prosperity, social equality, cohesiveness, and human environments cannot be sustained over coming decades.

Cultural change is another variable. Public understanding of science and medicine, and attitudes to individual responsibility, determine to a large extent the effectiveness of preventive medicine. We already have more literate, more aware health consumers with high expectations. If this trend continues, it may have a positive effect on the quality and effectiveness of care and communications and the transparency of decision making.

In developed countries, a high proportion of hospital admissions, premature deaths, and disability is due to accidents and trauma. Better treatment is important and feasible to ensure the return to a healthy, productive life, but the most obvious need is for more effective preventive and deterrent measures. Cultural, political, and economic forces, however, make accurate predictions impossible.

Worldwide population growth will be concentrated in Africa, Asia, and South America, and the proportion of people living outside the current developed world will reach 83 percent by the year 2020. The health needs of the poorest countries will probably be dictated by congestion, poor nutrition and sanitation, and environmental degradation. Infections will remain a major killer, and the main needs will be for basic preventive measures, such as clean water, health education, and vaccinations. Among the more prosperous developing countries (e.g., Southeast Asia), the median age at death will increase, and diseases of affluence and age will mix with the problems specific to culture, climate, and infrastructure. Markets for high-cost, high-benefit treatments will certainly broaden.

Some needs cannot be predicted or extrapolated from current trends. In the last four decades, we have had to respond to major new or reemergent infections and environmental and iatrogenic diseases during a period marked by greater population diversity and mobility, environmental degradation, and antibiotic resistance. We must assume that new threats will continue to emerge.

Western lifestyles are also invading the developing world, bringing with them an epidemic of chronic disease. Cancer cases are expected to double in developing countries over the next twenty-five years, and there is a similar growth in diabetes. "We are truly messengers of death worldwide," Dr. Paul Kleehouse, a WHO director said when presenting the annual global health report of WHO (1997). "There is a dramatic trend for the globalization of Western lifestyle and a parallel globalization of the associated diseases. We had expected this, but we are nevertheless surprised at the pace at which this is happening. Cancer rates are soaring in countries which hardly knew the disease a few years ago."

Changes in diet and the rise of smoking in Asia and Africa appear to be mostly to blame. "The smoking habit is one of the greatest importance for cancer and the pace this is spreading round the world is remarkable," said

Kleehouse. He blamed Britain, Germany, and the Netherlands for blocking all attempts within the European Union to protect minors from smoking. While the habit has been cut to 25 percent of the population in the United States and 40 percent in Western Europe, the Eastern European and Asian figures have risen to 70 percent.

Dietary changes to typical Western fare–heavy in fats–are changing the kinds of cancer people have. Whereas there was a prevalence of stomach cancers in the developing world, there is now also a surge in breast, prostate, and lower bowel cancers. Heart disease and obesity, also closely linked to diet, are increasing rapidly in developing countries as their populations adopt unhealthy eating habits. Diabetes, also associated with Western-style diets, is showing a rapid increase.

## Service Trends

It is not always easy to understand why policy makers feel pressure to restrict spending on health care in the face of continued demand by patients for the provision of such services. One explanation is that the mind-set of policy makers is determined by the values and assumptions that they have about health care expenditure levels. The result is that any general pressure to cut costs is bound to involve health. Since the long boom, all capitalist systems have been under that sort of pressure. National economies have increasingly become enmeshed in this problem.

A number of trends common to developed countries throughout the world are likely to dominate the health care scene over the next decade or two. "Cost containment strategies worldwide are placing increasing emphasis on evaluation of procedures and technologies, improved resource allocation, health promotion, and the prevention and early detection of disease" (Feedbaum and Hughesman 1997).

Improved measures of cost benefits will create some new markets while eroding old ones. Strategies involving shared costs or copayments for patients' insurers and those based on encouraging competition will change the way demand for technologies will evolve and the way it is met. Australia now requires that drugs on the public benefit reimbursement scheme must meet cost-benefit criteria as well as efficacy and safety (Maynard and Bloor 1997).

A narrowing of the role of the hospital, with shorter-stay surgery, more specialist consultation outside the hospital environment, and greater use of separate centers for convalescent, geriatric, and terminally ill patients all demonstrate the increasing proportion of services now being provided off-site. Such decentralization has acutely increased the need for effective communication and information transfer systems.

People have a desire for care close to home together with greater emphasis on prevention and shorter hospital stays. There is also a recognition of the importance of primary care and the demand for technologies and communication systems that enhance the capability (in advanced diagnostics and telemedicine) of primary care organizations.

The distribution of expertise and information systems seems to be gradually changing with less dependence on medically qualified individuals and greater emphasis on teamwork and expanding roles for different professional groups. Moves toward protocol—based care will contribute to redefining the role of the medical profession.

The key uncertainties with regard to services are the speed of progression and the interaction of current trends with political and sociocultural change nationally and internationally–especially the degree to which society and individuals value health care relative to other areas of public or private expenditure.

## Business Trends

The pharmaceutical industry has begun to plan for partnerships at various levels of operation. The last few years have seen several of the largest companies take over or ally with pharmaceutical benefit management firms or other health management business. Particularly in the United States, the trend may produce new types of health care companies with portfolios encompassing insurance, care, health education and prevention, diagnosis, treatment, and rehabilitation. Prescription drugs are now only a part of the product line. Inte-gration not only provides a means to advance sales but also ensures that, within the overall cost of disease management, drug price is not subject to undue pressure. A further benefit is access to high-quality information and disease management, treatment, and outcomes to inform development strategies and evaluation.

Pharmaceutical R&D portfolios are becoming tightly focused, partly to contain costs and partly because success increasingly depends on innovation rather than general developmental work. At the same time, larger businesses are looking at alliances with small biotechnology companies or groups of academics to complement in-house R&D and to improve the rate of innovation, particularly at a time of accelerating advances in biological knowledge and the development of new techniques and new technologies.

## Technological Trends

On a broader scale, we expect that the advances made over the last three decades in the science of molecular genetics and information technology will have the greatest effect on the technologies and methods of health care and other life science-based industries over the coming decade.

Developments in information technology will create opportunities for more advanced medical information systems as well as for systems to inform users of services. Key areas are telemedicine, which includes remote monitoring, remote consultation (doctor-to-doctor and patient-to-doctor), remote intervention, and virtual reality. The necessary communications infrastructure is being put into place, although there are legitimate concerns about security and confidentiality.

Some simple applications are already practical and may soon enter use in some specialist areas. Systems with more local intelligence than those currently available will be needed before widespread use is possible. Issues of integration with other health care information systems and with other forms of service provision and training are becoming significant. We can see information technology affecting image and interpretations, supporting clinical decision making, and providing information analysis or options to assist in investigations, diagnoses, therapy, and treatment plans.

There is a close link here with evidence-based medicine. The role of a decision-support system is to provide the clinician and other health care staff with information on history, methods of investigation, diagnosis, and prognosis (including genetic considerations), and trials, studies, and treatment options relevant to a particular patient. Such systems will thus represent an essential complement to other forms of medical information technology.

Meeting this demand will involve long-term research into computational methods and both organizational and behavioral issues. There is also the potential of information systems and technology to enhance interventions, including developments in robot-assisted surgery and image-guided surgery. Mechanical and conventional electronic issues are important, but advanced information technology will enable systems to adapt to individual anatomy and pathology.

The science of molecular genetics has accelerated enormously in its acquisition of human knowledge of animal and plant biology, not the least through genome analysis, and it now forms the basis of much of the biotechnology industry and current trail-blazing work on gene therapy, early detection of cancer pathogens characterization, and prenatal diagnosis of defects. It is also revealing new therapeutic targets and approaches for novel drug creation. In the longer term, understanding the inherited factors that predispose people to common illnesses, such as heart disease, and interaction of these factors with lifestyle and environment, may revolutionize medicine, allowing individual measures of tailored plans, risk, and better-informed choice of treatments.

## The International Health Care Industry

The magnitude of world spending on health is huge (World Bank 1993). Public and private health care expenditures in 1990 amounted to $1,700 billion, 8 percent of the world's product; 41 percent of this amount was consumed in the United States, amounting to 12 percent of its GNP, or about $1,500 per person. Developing countries spent 4 percent of their GNP on health, or about $41 per person.

Furthermore, spending has risen rapidly over twenty years. The United Kingdom, the United States, and France have doubled their expenditure in real terms as a result of changing needs and expectations of aging, affluent populations; the uptake of new technology; and inefficiency in current systems. Policies have been dominated by cost-containment using methods of shifting cost closer to the user, increasing competition, limiting activity or spending, or improving utilizations of resources.

Closely related to health care are the pharmaceutical and medical device and diagnostic industries with global sales of $208 billion and $75.2 billion, respectively. Despite cost-containment measures, worldwide markets show steady growth.

The pharmaceutical industry is fragmented, with no company accounting for more than 4 percent of the world market. Fourteen of the top thirty companies are European or part-European; the others are based in the United States and Japan. Business success is primarily determined by the ability to innovate and supply new products.

The medical devices and diagnostic industries are less fragmented: a few large manufacturers account for a large percentage of the market, particularly for the most advanced instruments and devices, although there are large numbers of very small businesses in the diagnostic sector and at the low-tech end of the medical devices market. Here, the United States is particularly strong and accounts for two-thirds of the world production.

The biotechnology sector comprises a diverse set of innovative enterprises. Some are medically oriented, developing novel therapeutics and diagnostics based on advances in genetic modification and molecular and cell biology.

Taken together, there are over 1,500 biotech companies worldwide, of which 265 are publicly quoted. More than 70 percent are based in the United States. Of the 25 percent in Europe, the largest percentage is in the United Kingdom. The majority of enterprises are in medical biotechnology: therapeutics, 42 percent; and diagnostics, 26 percent. Most of the companies were set up in the 1980s and are small, with about 100 employees. In many cases, a larger partner is essential to support the commercialization of products and to maintain capital flow. The larger established companies formulate partnerships with small biotechnology companies.

## The International Political Environment

Philip Cerny (1996) writes that, in the modern world, international and crossnational economic relations have formed a dense web of power constraining activities and shaping the activities of people and governments. As we approach the next century, security is dependent less on military power and more on economics. Economies are more global, and the politics of states are caught up increasingly in autonomous patterns of trade, international capital flows, global markets, and transnational institutions, both public and private.

Skidelsky (1989) writes that the decade of the 1980s was a watershed. It marked the demise of what, in 1905, Dicey in his book, *Introduction to the*

*Study of the Law of the Constitution*, called the Age of Collectivism. Collectivism is the doctrine that the state knows best. Dicey described it color-fully as "government for the good of the people by experts and officials," the antithesis of classical liberalism according to which governments exist for the sole purpose of protecting the life, liberty, and property of its people.

We now live in a postcollectivist age, and the most dramatic evidence of this is the collapse of communism. All over the world, governments, in response to public opinion or mounting complications, have given up shaping the future. Furthermore, we have seen the revival of economic liberty within nations and between them. We now live in a global economy where national frontiers have become increasingly unimportant in determining the flow of money, goods, and services.

There do exist, however, regulators of activities that are no less powerful for being less visible than the national governments and parliaments. We see institutions of transnational governance—the World Trade Organization is an example—and regional groupings, of which the European Union is the most advanced. Private insurance can well take over many of the security functions hitherto provided by welfare states.

## A FRAMEWORK FOR EXAMINING GLOBALIZATION IN HEALTH CARE

What is the extent of globalization in health care and how should we look at it? Moran and Wood provide a useful analytical framework. It is based, first, on the structure of policy making; second, on implementation or application of policy on product markets in health; and finally, on an understanding of inter-nationalization in the context of policy making.

### Structure of International Policy Making

There are two striking examples of the internationalization of the policy-making process. The first is the network of health policy experts working with each other in professional and other circuits across national boundaries. For example, the American Alain Enthoven (1985), a key figure in health reform in Europe, popularized the idea of internal markets in a number of European states, particularly the United Kingdom, the Netherlands, and Sweden. This sharing of policy expertise has been further helped by activities of international organizations concerned with the analysis of health care policy such as the Organization for Economic Cooperation and Development (OECD), which has compared inputs and outputs of OECD nations and sponsored a series of comparative policy studies.

As global health needs and opportunities change, the international agencies (in particular, those of the United Nations) are being forced to review their roles to identify how they can best respond within their resource constraints. Because global health policy is likely to be strongly influenced by the shape these organizations take in the future, all countries have a direct interest in their development.

The international health institutions include the UN agencies, programs, funds, development banks, and multilateral development agencies. The lead UN agency in health is WHO, created in 1948 with the objective of guaranteeing the attainment by all people of the highest possible level of health. Another important group is represented by the development assistance agencies of developed countries. Among the more notable nonprofit organizations participating in the world health systems are international foundations, professional bodies, health and medical assistance groups, and consulting agencies. The private sector is also a key player.

The international health agencies have developed a unique set of human resources, organizational abilities, and knowledge that has enabled them to achieve such ambitious goals as the eradication of smallpox and the near-eradication of polio. Over the years, the world's health system has grown in capacity, in the number of participants in the field of international health, and in the complexity of programs. In particular, the World Bank has taken an increasingly influential role.

The bank has encouraged governments to pursue an economic growth policy that will benefit the poor including, where necessary, adjustments to policies that preserve cost-effective health expenditures; expand investment in schooling, particularly for girls; and promote the rights and status of women through political and economic empowerment and legal protection against abuse.

A second change in policy advocated by the World Bank is to improve government spending on health. The challenge for most governments is to concentrate resources on compensating for market failure and efficiently financing services that will particularly benefit the more deprived. There are several policy directions for this, namely the reduction of government expenditure on tertiary facilities, specialist training, and interventions.

A third World Bank policy is that of encouraging diversity and competition. Government finance of public health and of nationally defined packages of essential clinical services would leave the remaining clinical services to be financed privately or by social insurers within the context of a policy framework established by government. Governments can promote diversity and competition in provision of health services and insurance by encouraging social or private insurance and encouraging suppliers to compete both to deliver clinical services and to provide inputs such as drugs. Domestic suppliers should not be protected from international competition. Information on provider performance, essential equipment and drugs, the cost and effectiveness of interventions, and accreditation status of institutions should be generated and disseminated to the public.

In addition to the networks and the enforcement of agencies such as WHO, OECD, and the World Bank, another feature affecting policy-making networks is the rise of the European Union. The new Treaty of Union, Maastricht, has significantly expanded the European Union's potential jurisdiction, particularly in public health. And for the first time, a ministerial council for the European community has been established and now meets regularly. In this way, the structure of policy making has the potential of becoming internationalized. The rise of the modern state as a significant actor in health care policy has largely taken place inside national boundaries. The expansion of the state's role in health care has been closely connected to the wider development of the welfare state, and the welfare states have in turn been closely connected with the creation of entitlements based on national citizenship.

The internationalization of these hitherto distinct national policy-making systems in health care occurs in two ways. International networks can develop between policy actors in different systems, leading to the diffusion of policy innovation from one national environment to another. And international or supernational actors can penetrate the policy-making systems of individual nations. It is not surprising, therefore, that the various reforms in different countries resemble each other.

## Internationalization of Health Care Services and Products

Independently of how policy is made, internationalization can take place in the delivery of health care services via the movement of deliverers across national boundaries in search of work or the movement of patients in search of care. Patient travel across the world to the Mayo Clinic is a well-known phenomenon, as has been travel to London. Again there is nothing new here: Spa towns in Europe were favored visiting places. Outside the world of the rich, however, the flow of patients in search of medical treatment is very limited. Transferring citizen entitlements across national boundaries is not easy.

The mobility of providers is different. There is an established history of mobility in the medical professions, particularly in research and education. Furthermore, the European Union directives now require member states to recognize qualifications obtained in other member states. In theory, a single market exists in Europe. In practice, a striking feature of the market for medical professions is the extent to which national or even subnational factors have remained determining forces. Patients rarely cross national boundaries to seek care. When doctors move across boundaries, their movements are shaped by national priorities and national institutions and considerations of language. Thus, whereas the world markets are opening up generally in some sectors, such as medical practitioners, national states still continue to regulate movement strongly and attempt to restrict entry.

## Internationalization of Health Products Market

Health care systems involve more than the delivery of personal services and the development of personal service markets. They also involve the product markets in health care. The *British Medical Journal* (1996) not too long ago carried an editorial about American companies looking for international markets. A month before, leaders of the U.S. managed health care plans had met in Mexico to look at doing business internationally. Here, workshops looked at market opportunities in Israel, Korea, Venezuela, Canada, Mexico, Russia, France, Singapore, Brazil, New Zealand, Puerto Rico, Australia, South Africa, and Argentina.

Tom Friedman, of the *New York Times* recently said that countries were going to be forced increasingly to open their economies to global competition. The businessmen who run for-profit managed care plans in the United States see no reason why they should not follow the paths of their colleagues in other businesses and compete globally. Indeed they may have to—Wall Street expects them to keep growing which means signing more people to their plans. As one chief executive put it, "We are soon going to run out of people in the United States." Managed health care plans already cover 100 million people. The *BMJ* questioned whether the world needs what these managed care plans have to offer. The World Bank clearly thinks that the world does and that the opportunities are greatest in the developing countries.

In the past ten to fifteen years, development has come to be seen as a matter for the private sector rather than for governments, and health services are a key part of development. The economies of most developing countries are growing faster than those of developed countries primarily because of private investment. In most developing countries the private sector is proportionately much larger than in developed countries and in many of these countries, for example Malaysia, Indonesia, and Bangladesh, the private sector is expanding. The old reason was said to be equity, but in most public health systems inequity remains a problem. Particularly because health spending has been concentrated in city hospitals, the rural poor have been subsidizing the urban wealthy.

The World Bank is now concentrating on public and primary health care for the poor. It believes in increased private health care for the wealthy in order to release public money for the poor and to raise the efficiency and quality in the private sector: "Managed care holds the biggest hope for developing health services in the developing world." Health care systems are even more than the delivery of personal services, however organized. They also involve the creation, marketing, and consumption of a wide range of products. These products include hospitals, medical equipment (from syringes through to the complex scanners) and the pharmaceutical products that can amount to one-sixth of the total spend of any health care system. The internationalization of markets in health care products can in turn mean one of two things: the organization of production and supply on a scale that transcends the boundaries of individual nation states or the regulation of those markets and products by institutions other than the nation state.

## THE CONTEXT FOR
## INTERNATIONALIZATION OF POLICY

Another way of thinking about internationalization focuses on the health care system itself, that is, the context in which health policy making takes place. The issue of cost-containment has dominated health care debates in recent years. Moran and Wood (1996) maintain that the desire to contain costs continues to be the most important driver of policy innovation, with respect both to system organization and delivery and to innovations designed to restrict entitlements to care and oblige patients to contribute more.

Success or failure in the international market depends on maintaining competitive advantage. Policy is driven not by what happens in health care institutions but by the wider context of economic policy; no national economy can insulate itself from wider economic global forces. In the United States, there is a growing conviction among the economic elite that American noncompetitiveness lies in the high cost of health care and the way much of that cost is shouldered by large enterprises. Research suggests that this assumption is debatable.

## AMERICAN CONTRIBUTIONS
## TO GLOBAL HEALTH

All nations, whether rich or poor, are struggling to contain spiraling health care costs as people live longer and demand for medical care rises. All countries need strong international health organizations to provide leadership and set standards. Yet the bodies currently engaged in international health (e.g., those in the UN system) are widely seen to be inadequate to the new challenges they face.

Without the active engagement of the United States, the global health gains of the twentieth century threaten to falter and Americans' own health, wealth, and security will suffer. But American investment in international health has been falling. By 1995, only 0.1 percent of the nation's GNP was being spent on global health assistance.

According to the 1997 Institute of Medicine report, the United States should increase its involvement in global health for a number of reasons.

1. *To protect the American people.* Preventing illness saves money as well as lives. American investment in the eradication of smallpox, for example, has saved an estimated $1 billion annually in vaccination costs. The IOM board con-

cluded that the United States should work with its partners to build an effective surveillance network for monitoring infectious disease and to guard against bioterrorism. Also, since certain diseases such as AIDS are much more prevalent outside the United States, drugs and vaccines against these diseases may be tested and developed only in collaboration with other countries. United States citizens have much to gain from such collaboration.

2. *To enhance the American economy.* Healthy populations abroad make healthy, growing markets for U.S. business. For example, if the United States invests in improving the health of other populations by studying and developing treatments for their major illnesses, its economic returns will be enhanced. The IOM board concluded, in particular, that the American pharmaceutical, vaccine, and medical product manufacturers could contribute more to global health than they are doing now.

Currently some two billion people worldwide have no access to essential drugs. To help U.S. industry meet global needs without suffering losses, the government should act to reduce regulatory barriers to product development, allow multitiered pricing, safeguard intellectual property rights, increase incentives for development (e.g., by extending certain patents and, where necessary, forge private-public sector partnerships to ensure the development of certain essential products).

U.S. responsibility for health concerns rests with a large number of Federal agencies, including the Department of Health and Human Services, the Department of Agriculture, and the Agency for International Development. Fragmentation and lack of coordination are keeping each agency from contributing to its full potential. The IOM board recommends that an interagency task force on global health within the U.S. government be established to anticipate and address global health needs and to take advantage of opportunities in a coordinated and strategic fashion.

## IMPLICATIONS OF GLOBAL TRENDS FOR
## ACADEMIC HEALTH CENTERS

The first priority for academic health centers must be to adopt the recommendations of the Institute of Medicine. They must also maintain an overview of what is happening internationally, particularly because biology is the science for the new century. The centers should be encouraging a collaborative approach to research and to new knowledge, such as research integrating molecular biology and genetics with cell and tissue biology and whole-organism studies to accelerate progress in basic research.

Second, academic health centers should sponsor research in neuroscience and the cognitive sciences, particularly research into progressive degenerative diseases and nonspecific, age-related cognitive decline. They should further encourage an assessment of genetics in risk evaluation and patient management. They should be enhancing drug creation and delivery based on biological, molecular, and chemical science that support new classes of therapeutic agents; supporting recombinant technology, research into key metabolic pathways, metabolic engineering, and sciences relevant to biological manufacture and industrial products; diagnostic applications of molecular biology by applying research into disease at genetic, molecular, and cellular levels to develop new generations of diagnostics; immune manipulations including research into the control of the immune system and applications in specific interventions in inflammatory and immune disease, vaccines, transplant, and other areas.

Another important consideration for the academic health centers is supporting basic research into aging and disabling degenerative diseases, coupled with technologies for sustaining a reasonable quality of life for the elderly infirm.

Academic health centers should also be assessing the health service and care opportunities offered by human animal and plant genome projects and other advances in molecular genetics and informing the public in the United States and internationally. They should contribute to the development of relevant and informed health care policies and health service organizations. They should seek to achieve local patterns of vertical and horizontal integration in health-related industries. Considerable opportunities lie in recognizing the importance of information technology and communications in medicine and the life sciences, particularly telemedicine, which extends services beyond the institution and internationally.

Academic health centers must also be responsive to and support industries that typically congregate around them. They should promote cooperative programs. They should link to technology incubators. They should ensure the maintenance of investment in physical infrastructure of life science research. They should maintain a strong clinical research base that underpins the development and evaluation of new products and methods and support for basic research. In particular, the academic health centers must appreciate community needs and how they can best help meet these needs.

The centers must also appreciate the way in which business organizations are readjusting themselves to cope with global markets. One of the key themes in documents issued on international health has been the importance of collaboration and partnerships. Academic health centers in the United States have a key part to play in fostering collaboration that will erase or, at least, greatly reduce the global divide in health research and also help provide answers relevant to both developing and developed countries. These countries are often viewed separately in terms of their health problems and health services research. Thus, although more than 90 percent of the lost years of potential life belong to the developing world, only 5 percent of global research funds are devoted to world health problems.

Chronic diseases—cancer, heart disease, and mental illness—are problems of equal significance to the developing world. Morbidity and mortality from communicable disease are now problems of the developing world and, with the exception of AIDS, the solutions are all the same for many health care problems. But developing countries have two further constraints: 1) the task of introducing the interventions within existing health services and 2) cultural sensitivity.

Further high-quality collaborative research performed in developing countries can provide evidence of relevance and value to the developed world. U.S. academic health centers may, therefore, see many advantages to conducting research in developing countries. The advantages include the availability of significant cases, the existence of well-trained investigators, lower costs, and benefit to health systems and health institutions from financial involvement. Many of the trials of international relevance could be carried out in developing countries; indeed, the number of international publications on health services research from developing countries has increased steadily over the last few years (PAHO 1992).

Multinational collaboration is the surest way to answer questions of global relevance. Medical opinion in the United Kingdom also suggests that academic health centers might consider franchising their operational activities in other countries. For example, St. Thomas's Hospital in London now provides medical services for the armed services in Germany. There is no reason why academic health centers should not be competing in this type of market.

Then there are the prospects of twinning, a concept promoted by the Commonwealth Secretariat in 1992. At the beginning of the decade, the Commonwealth Health Development Programme saw human resource development as a key strategy to be pursued in strengthening health services. Human resource development could be assisted by the twinning, or linking, of institutions in developing countries with similar but more mature organizations in other parts of the world. The arrangement should be used to promote specific objectives. It should represent the desire of the institutions to share research, learning, and teaching experiences, enhance management and organizational capability, exchange ideas, and collaborate in the solution of common problems.

## ISSUES FOR FURTHER DEBATE

I believe that mining the many international opportunities in the field of health and health care must be based on relevance, cultural appropriateness, and ethical considerations. In the United Kingdom, our foreign policy now has a strong ethical dimension, particularly in the area of defense sales.

In the early 1980s, during my private-sector days at the British Association for the Advancement of Science, I spoke on the theme, "Are we selling the right things to the right people?" I emphasized then, as I do now, the importance of appropriate technology, that is, technology that is relevant to the given techno-socio-economic framework at a given point in time. This was very much the policy advocated by WHO when it recommended that, in meeting health needs, technology must be geared both to the problems to be solved and to the local conditions; that it should be significantly sound and acceptable to those who apply it and to those for whom it is used; and that it should be affordable to the nation. The IOM endorses this stance by stating that scientific advances from the United States must be relevant to the country.

With the benefit of hindsight and recent experience, I would add a further requirement, namely, the key messages of the World Bank to which I have already referred and the recent Ljubljana (Yugoslavia) Charter that says that the European health care system should be:

   i. driven by values of human dignity, equity, solidarity and professional ethics,

   ii.  targeted to protect and promote health,

   iii.  centered on people, allowing citizens to influence health services and take responsibility for their own health,

   iv.  focused on quality, including cost-effectiveness, and

   v.  based on sustainable finances to allow universal coverage and equitable access oriented towards primary care.

The charter also identifies principles for managing change, namely the development of health policy. Health care reforms should be a coherent part of overall policy for health for all that is consistent with the socioeconomic conditions of each country. Major policy and managerial and technical decisions on development should be based on evidence; governments must raise value-related issues for public debate and ensure equitable distribution of resources and access of the entire population to health services. The governments should also take facilitating legislative and regulatory initiatives and, whenever market mechanisms are appropriate, they should favor competition to ensure quality and use of scarce resources.

   The charter advocates listening to the citizen's voices and choices; governments reshaping the health care system based on self-care, family care, and informal care; and working with a variety of social institutions. It also advocates well-designed strategies to shift working capacity from hospital care to primary health care, community care, day care, and home care; regional health service networks; a policy of continuous quality development, reorientation of relevant human resources for health care, strengthened managerial capability, and the importance of learning from experience. There is a need to promote the national and international exchange of experience with the implementation of health care reforms and support of reform agendas. The support must be founded on a well-validated knowledge base with regard to health care reforms and proper understanding of cultural differences in health care, and must be appropriately valued.

## CONCLUSION

In their discussion of global health, Moran and Wood conclude their analysis of internationalization as a case "not proven," although there are plainly powerful international forces at work: We can see the policy advocate networks, powerful supply and national actors in the field of health care policy, significant movement of health professionals in search of work, all taking place across national boundaries. The pharmaceutical and medical goods industries are organized on a global scale. Above all, the sheer size of health care systems means that in the advanced capitalist nations, world health care policy is shaped by national policy makers and their belief about the wider needs of national economic competitiveness—needs that in turn are the result of forces created by independent global economies.

Changes in health services and patterns of health care across the world seem both inevitable and desirable to meet the changing needs of the twenty-first century. Among the strongest influences in this context is the international development of genomics, which will lead within the next few years to the ability to produce a genetic blueprint of each human life. This will enable earlier and more accurate diagnosis or prediction of major diseases and new opportunities for prevention and treatment.

In countries at all levels of development, practitioners will have access to global information on diagnosis, treatment, and outcomes as well as information about disease outbreaks. Taken together within the global system of communication created by the World Wide Web, the implications for patterns of clinical care and the expectations and demands of patients and medical ethics around the world will be enormous.

## WORK CITED

British Medical Journal. 1996. Global competition in health care—American managed care companies begin to look for international markets. (Editorial). Vol. 13 (September).

Cerny, P.G. 1996. International finance and the erosion of state policy capacity. In Globalization and Public Policy, Phillip Gummett, ed. Cheltenham, U.K. and Brookfield, U.S.: Edward Elger.

Enthoven, A.C. 1985. Reflections on the Management of the National Health Service. London: Nuffield Provincial Hospital Trust.

Feedbaum, E., and M. Hughesman. 1997. Health care systems: Cost containment versus quality. Financial Times. London.

Health and Life Sciences Panel, Technology Foresight Project. 1997. Progress Through Partnership. Her Majesty's Stationery Office: London.

IOM (Institute of Medicine). 1997. America's Vital Interest in Global Health: Protecting Our People, Enhancing Our Economy and Advancing Our International Interests.

Washington: National Academy of Sciences.

Maynard, A. and K. Bloor. 1997. Regulating the pharmaceutical industry. *British Medical Journal*. 315: 26 July.

Moran, M., and B. Wood. 1996. In *The Globalization of Health Care*, Phillip Gummett, ed. Cheltenham, U.K., and Brookfield, U.S.: Edward Elger.

PAHO (Pan American Health Organization). 1992. *La investigacion en America Latina. Estudio de paises seleccionades.* Washington: World Health Organization.

Skidelsky, R. 1989. *The Social Market Economy.* London: Social Market Foundation.

WHO (World Health Organization). 1997. *Conquering Suffering, Enriching Humanity.* WHO: Geneva.

World Bank. 1993. *Investing in Health: World Development Indicators.* Washington: World Bank.